Drugs & Drug Abuse

THIRD EDITION

Canadian Cataloguing in Publication Data
Main entry under title:

Drugs and drug abuse. — 3rd ed.

Second edition published under title: Addiction Research Foundation's drugs and drug abuse.
Includes index.

ISBN: 978-0-88868-252-9 (PRINT)
ISBN: 978-0-88868-937-5 (PDF)
ISBN: 978-0-88868-938-2 (HTML)
ISBN: 978-0-88868-939-9 (ePUB)

1. Drug abuse. 2. Drugs. I. Brands, Bruna. II. Sproule, Beth. III. Marshman, Joan A.
IV. Ontario. Centre for Addiction and Mental Health.

RC564D78 1998   616.86   C98-930536-8

P5530
Printed in Canada

This publication may be available in other formats. For information about alternative formats
or other CAMH publications, or to place an order, please contact Sales and Distribution:
Toll-free: 1 800 661-1111
Toronto: 416 595-6059
E-mail: publications@camh.ca
Online store: http://store.camh.ca

Website: www.camh.ca

This book was produced by CAMH's Knowledge and Innovation Support Unit.
2064 / 06-2013 / P5530

A REFERENCE TEXT

Drugs & Drug Abuse

THIRD EDITION

EDITORS:

Bruna Brands, PhD
Beth Sproule, PharmD
Joan Marshman, PhD

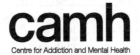

camh

Centre for Addiction and Mental Health

A Pan American Health Organization /
World Health Organization Collaborating Centre

TABLE OF CONTENTS

Section 1 — Understanding Drugs, Drug Effects and Drug Use

Section 2 — Major Drug Classes

Section 3 — Some Key Drugs

Section 4 — Other Drugs in Brief

Section 5 — Additional Drug Notes

Section 6 — Glossaries

Preface

If the experience of recent years tells us one thing, it is that the reality of substance use is continually evolving. Every year, new drugs and new ways of using them emerge, each bringing potential new benefits and new risks for users and for society as a whole. Simultaneously, each new generation develops and refines its own unique perspective on substance use in the context of its evolving world. Today, with the explosion of information technology, the flow of information — and misinformation — about drugs, drug use and drug abuse is virtually unlimited in both scope and audience.

These developments present challenges for individuals, families, institutions, communities, provinces, states and nations, all of whom make decisions (explicitly or implicitly) about the use, prevention and control of alcohol, tobacco and other drugs. Such developments are equally challenging for physicians who prescribe drugs for their therapeutic benefits, and professionals and others who strive to help substance abusers and their families resolve their substance use problems.

Recent years have seen breakthroughs in our understanding of drug receptors and the mechanisms of action of psychoactive drugs, as well as new drug-delivery technologies. These advances have led to the discovery and development of many new drugs and dosage forms in the pharmaceutical industry. Many of these new products — for example, the family of antidepressants known as selective serotonin reuptake inhibitors (SSRIs) — are more specific in their action than earlier generations of therapeutic agents and, used appropriately, achieve their desired effects with fewer disruptive side effects. However, illicit manufacturers have also been active, continuing to produce older drugs such as LSD, while adding newer "designer" drugs such as "ecstasy" (MDMA) to their major product lines.

While the development of new drugs is one dimension of drug use and abuse that is reflected in the third edition of this book, the experience of a new generation of users is another. It appears that in drug use and abuse, as in many facets of life, the more things change, the more they stay the same. LSD, for example, seems to be rediscovered by every generation of adolescents, and many LSD myths of the 1970s have re-emerged in the 1990s. Meanwhile, exotic drugs such as harmaline are a source of fascination for some young North American drug users today, just as they were for their parents' generation in the late '60s and early '70s, despite the fact that the availability of these drugs remains limited. The net result seems to be a generational cycle of increases and declines in the popularity of various drugs, especially hallucinogens, as each generation deals with drug use in the context of its own world — its music, its forms of entertainment and its value system.

Each generation also selects and develops its own information sources concerning drugs and their use and abuse. But never has a generation had the diversity of information sources that are available and readily accessible to today's youth. Unfortunately, with the explosion of information technology has come the globalization of misinformation as well as information. As a result, experimenters can readily identify new drugs to use, and new ways to prepare and use older drugs. Each new drug, whether crack cocaine, "ecstasy" or a new opioid analgesic, gives rise to both a knowledge base and a mythology, including distortions, exaggerations and simple mistakes of fact — all of which are transmitted to an audience of unprecedented breadth at an unprecedented speed. Such myths reflect, in part, society's need to understand how and why some of us use drugs. However, to separate fact from fiction and deal constructively with alcohol and other drug problems, drug users, parents, counsellors, professionals and the public at large need reliable information, presented in a clear, concise, and accessible manner.

This third edition of *Drugs and Drug Abuse* has been prepared to help meet that need. It is not intended to be encyclopedic in scope. Rather, it is designed to provide reliable, basic information in a readily accessible form. *Drugs and Drug Abuse* aims primarily to address the needs of three groups of readers: members of the general public, including students, who want information about psychoactive drug classes or specific drugs; addiction workers who require a basic understanding of the pharmacology and therapeutics of the psychoactive drugs used by their clients; and professionals in various types of general practice — as diverse as social work, education, nursing, pharmacy, medicine, journalism, the criminal justice system and corrections — who may encounter drugs and/or drug problems as part of their work. To meet the needs of this diverse readership every effort has been made to present information concisely and with a minimum of technical jargon.

The basic concept for *Drugs and Drug Abuse* was conceived by Eugene LeBlanc and Terry Cox. In 1975 they prepared *A Handbook on Drugs and Drug Abuse* for judges and lawyers, a group that needed an authoritative source of factual information not only about psychoactive drugs as commodities, but also about the dynamic interaction of those substances with the body, and the associated benefits and risks. As this resource became more widely used to meet increasingly diverse information needs, the Addiction Research Foundation decided to further develop the concept to address the needs of a broader readership. Thus in 1983 the first edition of *Drugs and Drug Abuse* was prepared by the original authors, Terry Cox and Eugene LeBlanc, together with Joan Marshman and the late Michael Jacobs.

Reader feedback strongly endorsed the book's concept, and led to the preparation of a second edition of *Drugs and Drug Abuse* in 1987 by Michael Jacobs and Kevin Fehr. This edition provided not only an update on rapidly changing information, but also coverage of additional topics suggested by a range of readers, from parents and teachers to addiction counsellors and law enforcement personnel.

New scientific advances and social developments since 1987, together with continuing demand for *Drugs and Drug Abuse*, dictated that a third edition be prepared. It is less the role of this new edition to profile those developments than to reflect their consequences — the wider range of psychoactive drugs in common use, our better understanding of their actions and effects, and the changes in the way people use drugs. These changes are evident throughout this volume, from the addition of new substances to the expanded and updated glossaries of drug trade names and street drug language.

This volume is an extensive update of the previous edition rather than a major re-structuring, and the general format of the previous edition that readers have found so easy to use has been retained. We have included information on some newer psychoactive drugs, including alfentanil, crack cocaine, and "ecstasy," as well as new formulations of older drugs, such as fentanyl transdermal patches, that have come into common use since the last edition. However, we have retained information about some drugs that are not currently widely available — STP and glutethimide, for example — but have a place in the history of drug abuse in North America.

One significant change is the inclusion of a chapter on psychiatric medications (in Section 2) as well as chapters on the individual therapeutic groups and substances within this family (in Section 4). This new material reflects recent developments in this field as well as the use of some of these drugs in treating intoxication or withdrawal symptoms. It also reflects the needs of staff in substance abuse treatment programs who recognize the coexistence of mental health disorders in many of their clients and need a basic understanding of the drug therapies prescribed for these clients. Another change is the expansion of the chapter on anabolic steroids because of the increased use of this class of drugs by young people involved in bodybuilding. Chapters have also been added describing newer drugs used in treating opioid dependence, such as buprenorphine, naltrexone and LAAM, while the nicotine chapter has been expanded to include new evidence on the health risks of tobacco use and information on nicotine transdermal patches as an aid in quitting smoking. In addition, greater attention has been given in many chapters to drug effects in pregnancy.

In making these and other changes the editors have made every effort to ensure that this edition is as easy to use as its predecessors. Readers familiar with earlier editions will find this volume retains their clear language and convenient layout, and they will welcome this edition's more detailed footnotes and suggested background readings.

Like previous editions of *Drugs and Drug Abuse*, this volume reflects the expertise, creativity and dedication of a great many contributors. There are few organizations as well staffed and as able as the Addiction Research Foundation to mobilize the scientific and professional expertise needed to produce this kind of reference text. Fewer still have the community programs base to provide an understanding of the types of information wanted and needed by a diverse readership. In making this updated information on alcohol, tobacco and other drugs so readily accessible to those who need it, *Drugs and Drug Abuse* typifies ARF's goal — using research-based knowledge to help users, families, professionals and communities deal appropriately with alcohol and other drug problems and reduce substance-related harm.

Bruna Brands, PhD
Beth Sproule, PharmD
Joan Marshman, PhD

Acknowledgments

The preparation of a volume as extensive and detailed as this edition of *Drugs and Drug Abuse* would not be possible without the expert knowledge, skills and commitment of a large number of individuals. The editors wish to thank the many present and former staff members of the Addiction Research Foundation* who made contributions to the preparation of this book.

In particular, the editors would like to thank Richard Frecker, MD, PhD, Pearl Isaac, BSc Phm, Meldon Kahan, MD, Harold Kalant, MD, PhD, and Anne Kalvik, BSc Phm, for their advice and their significant contributions to the writing, revising and reviewing of several chapters of the new edition.

We would also like to thank Usanda Busto, PharmD, William Corrigall, PhD, Douglas Gourlay, MD, Jina Hahn, BSc Phm, Eva Janacek, BSc Phm, Bhushan Kapur, DPhil, Kevin MacDonald, BSc Phm, David Marsh, MD, and James Tomarken, MD, for their contributions to and comments on material included in this edition.

We owe a debt of appreciation also to members of the Addiction and Mental Health Services Corporation's Marketing and Communications Department, including Myles Magner for copy editing and editorial co-ordination, and Nancy Leung for graphic design, and to freelance editors Dianne Broad for copy editing and indexing, and Sharon Kirsch for proofreading.

Thanks are due to Christine Cotie for her assistance with early revisions of the manuscript, to Michelle Furler for compiling the Glossary of Medical and Scientific Terms and the Glossary of Street Drug Language, and to Elizabeth Marshman for her diligent work preparing the final manuscript.

Finally, we would like to recognize the contributions of the dozens of people whose work on the first two editions of *Drugs and Drug Abuse* ensured the book's success, including, in particular, those of Terence Cox, MA, Kevin Fehr, PhD, Michael Jacobs, PhD, Eugene LeBlanc, PhD, and Joan Marshman, PhD.

---

* The Addiction Research Foundation is a Division of the Addiction and Mental Health Services Corporation.

The Editors

Bruna Brands is a scientist in the Addiction Research Foundation's Clinical, Social and Evaluation Research Department. She received her PhD in pharmacology from the University of Western Ontario, in London, Ontario.

Beth Sproule is a research scientist with the University of Toronto's Psychopharmacology Research Program at Sunnybrook Health Science Centre and an assistant professor in the Faculty of Pharmacy at U of T. She received her PharmD from Wayne State University, in Detroit, Michigan.

Joan Marshman is a professor in the Faculty of Pharmacy at the University of Toronto and is a past president of the Addiction Research Foundation. She received her PhD in pharmacy and completed post-doctoral studies in pharmacology at the University of Toronto.

An Important Note

Pharmacology and medicine are evolving sciences. As new research and clinical experience broaden our knowledge, changes in treatment and drug therapy are required. In revising this reference text, the editors and publishers have referred to sources that are believed to be reliable. The contents of this book are based upon information available as of 1996-1997. However, in view of the possibility of human error or changes in medical science, none of the authors, editors or publishers nor any other party who has been involved in the preparation or publication of this text warrants that the information herein is in every respect accurate or complete, and they are not responsible for any errors or omissions or for the results obtained from the use of such information.

Drugs and Drug Abuse is intended as a reference text for general and professional readers. It is not intended as a clinical manual or as a primary source of information on the clinical administration of drugs or on the diagnosis or treatment of medical or drug-related problems. Readers are encouraged to confirm the information contained herein with other sources.

Readers are particularly advised to check the product information sheet included in the package of any drug product they plan to administer or consume to be certain that the information obtained from this text or any other reference material is accurate and that changes have not been made in the recommended dose or in the contraindications for administration. This is of particular importance in connection with new or infrequently used drugs.

Understanding Drugs, Drug Effects and Drug Use

INTRODUCTION

Drugs have always been part of human life. For thousands of years plants have been used to benefit the body, mind and soul: opium has long been valued for relief of pain, diarrhea and coughs, as well as changing mood; beer has been brewed from plant materials for nearly 6,000 years; and the mescal cactus has long been used in religious ceremonies. But the words used to describe drugs have varied over time.

The ancient Greek word for drug, *pharmakon*, meant both medicine and poison. Similarly, *pharmakeuein* was either the practice of witchcraft or the use of medicine, depending on the context. These simplistic concepts, reflecting a certain ambivalence, represented an attempt by the Greeks to come to terms with the powerful effects of drugs on the mind and body of the individual.

Even in more recent times, society has had great difficulty in defining the word "drug." For many people, a drug is simply whatever a physician prescribes to treat their disease or discomfort. For others, the term "drug" has a much broader meaning, including any chemical agent[1] that affects living processes. This broader meaning is most useful in considering drugs in relation to drug abuse.

---

[1]   It is important to recognize that the term "chemical substance" includes substances that are produced naturally in plants and animals as well as those produced in laboratories.

Psychoactive drugs, which form the focus of this book, are those substances that can change sensation, mood, consciousness, or other psychological or behavioral functions. Thus, coffee and tea, alcohol, tobacco, anti-anxiety medications, cocaine, cannabis, LSD (lysergic acid diethylamide), heroin and solvents are all psychoactive drugs. Each is used to change the user's existing state: to speed us up, slow us down, or change how we perceive and react to ourselves and the world around us.

People use psychoactive (sometimes called mood-altering) drugs for many purposes:
- to treat medical problems
- to relax, especially in social situations
- to lower inhibitions
- to cope with or forget problems
- to attain a sense of "belonging" to a certain group
- for religious or ceremonial purposes
- for pleasurable sensations
- to satisfy curiosity about a drug's effect, and to experiment.

Psychoactive drugs fall into four main groups: depressants, stimulants, hallucinogens and psychiatric medications.
- The first group — depressants — includes alcohol, anxiolytics, sleeping pills and opioid drugs such as heroin, morphine and methadone. These drugs make people more relaxed and less conscious of their surroundings.
- The second group — stimulants — speeds up mental processes, making people feel more alert and energetic. Cocaine, amphetamines and even caffeine fall into this group.
- The third group — hallucinogens — alters our perceptions, and our sense of time and place. These drugs, including LSD, mescaline, and even marijuana and hashish, can produce hallucinations — making people see or hear things that aren't really there, or see or hear things differently than they would without the drug's influence.
- The fourth group — psychiatric medications — includes drugs used to treat chronic and temporary mental or emotional disorders. This group includes antipsychotic medications, antidepressants and mood stabilizers.

Depending on the drug and how it is used, we tend to think of a particular drug as either a valuable medicine, an important element of social, ceremonial or religious observances, or a source of problems. However, few drugs fit conveniently into just one of these groups. Generally we should recognize that any drug has the potential for both benefits and problems. Just as there are many types of drugs, there are also many types of drug problems. Typically, the user experiences the benefits of a drug, although, in some cases, the benefits may also extend to the user's family, friends and even the community. Some problems also affect primarily the drug user, but others affect people who live or work with the user and some affect the community as a whole. In some cases, the benefits may clearly outweigh the risks, while in others the risks seem to outweigh the benefits.

Users experience medical problems when a drug causes direct physical or mental harm. Heavy drinking, for example, can damage the liver, brain, stomach and other organs. Heavy smoking damages the lungs and heart. Many drugs, such as heroin, alcohol and cocaine, can be fatal when taken in high doses. Drug use may cause mental and emotional problems, or intensify problems that aren't evident without the drug. Feelings of persecution, for example, are common among heavy users of cocaine or amphetamines, and depression often follows such heavy drug use.

Drug use also poses the risk of dependence. Dependence refers to the users' compelling need to use a drug for physical or psychological reasons. Perhaps they have developed tolerance to a drug, meaning they now need to use more of the drug to get the same effects they once got from smaller amounts. Without the drug, they may feel desperate or lost, and they may also suffer physical symptoms known as withdrawal. Although each drug differs in this regard, dependence always means the user is in trouble, and may need professional help.

Some medical problems are linked to the way drugs are used, as much as the drugs themselves. Anyone sharing a needle to inject heroin, cocaine or any other drug, runs a risk of becoming infected with HIV (human immunodeficiency virus), the virus that causes AIDS (acquired immune deficiency syndrome). Hepatitis and other serious infections are also spread this way.

People who use illicit drugs or combine different drugs (including alcohol) rarely know their risk of encountering problems. People who use illegal drugs often don't know exactly what they are taking, so they cannot accurately predict the drug's effects. While prescription drugs are made and marketed in Canada under strict federal government standards, illegal drugs are often produced with little regard for purity and consistency, and they may be diluted, or "cut," with harmful substances. Furthermore, some users take alcohol with other drugs, or mix drugs, without realizing that this may increase their risk of problems. Combining alcohol and sleeping pills, for example, can be lethal.

Although medical problems are often considered to be the primary consequence of inappropriate drug use, use may generate a range of problems for users, their families, co-workers and the community. Drug use may result in family dysfunction and poor job performance. Drug use is linked to injuries and death through impaired driving, criminal activity, assaults, suicides and other high-risk behavior: some people who would never consider committing murder will nonetheless drive after they've been drinking — even though the consequences of their actions can be just as serious. All of these problems impose a heavy burden on the community — including costs of family and social, health care and police services.

This book examines drug use primarily from a human pharmacological viewpoint — the impact of drugs on the human physiological system. It is designed to increase the reader's knowledge as one component of the effort to reduce the harm linked to drug use. Section 1 discusses some general aspects of drugs, the ways in which they affect the body and are, in turn, affected by the body, and some concepts relating to drug use. Section 2 provides an overview of each of the major groups of psychoactive drugs and their use. Section 3 presents a brief outline of each of the major drugs in each group. Section 4 provides brief information on some psychoactive substances that are less commonly used. Finally, Section 5 includes short notes on additional drugs that may be of occasional interest. Glossaries of medical and scientific terms and of street drug language and a list of selected drug trade names and the non-proprietary equivalents are provided at the end of the book to assist the reader who is less familiar with such terminology.

Understanding Drugs

Sources of Psychoactive Drugs

Psychoactive drugs can be divided into three major types, according to source: naturally occurring, semi-synthetic and synthetic.

Naturally Occurring Psychoactive Drugs

Certain plants and animal tissues contain psychoactive drugs; the crude material is used as the drug preparation or it is extracted and purified. Both primitive and modern societies have relied heavily on naturally occurring drugs for both medical and non-medical purposes. In China, for example, the central nervous system (CNS) stimulant ephedrine has been extracted from a local plant, *ma huang* (*Ephedra equisetina*), and used in traditional medicine for thousands of years. Ephedrine has also been widely used in western medicine since its introduction in the early 1900s. Initially the drug was isolated from plant material, but today it is synthesized from chemicals. The stimulant cocaine, contained in the leaves of the *Erythroxylum coca* shrub, has been in both medical and non-medical use in Peru for hundreds of years. It is both a local anesthetic and a stimulant. The active alkaloid, cocaine, is easily extracted from the plant by chewing or pressing the leaves. Opium and its chief alkaloid, morphine, have long been used as painkillers and euphoriants in medical and non-medical circles. Opium is the dried form of the milky material that flows from slits made in the seed pods of the opium poppy, *Papaver somniferum*, and morphine is extracted from opium.

Most of the commonly used naturally occurring drugs have been used for centuries: folk medicine discovered and took advantage of the drug effects of plants (and occasionally animals) without understanding which constituents produced the desired effects, much less understanding their chemical nature.

Semi-Synthetic Psychoactive Drugs

Semi-synthetic drugs are prepared by chemically modifying substances prepared from natural sources. For example, heroin (diacetylmorphine) is produced in the laboratory by reacting the natural product, morphine, with acetic anhydride or acetyl chloride. Similarly, LSD is derived from certain ergot alkaloids — substances that occur naturally in certain *Claviceps* fungi that grow on grains. Both heroin and LSD are examples of semi-synthetic drugs with different types of effects than the substances from which they are derived.

Synthetic Psychoactive Drugs

Synthetic drugs are produced entirely by chemical reactions in a laboratory and do not depend on plant or animal substances as a starting material. While a synthetic drug produced by laboratory processes may be chemically identical to a naturally occurring or semi-synthetic drug, many of the drugs prepared synthetically have been designed to have some particular pharmacological property or properties that cannot be obtained in naturally occurring drugs. Methadone, for example, is a synthetic compound that was developed in Germany during World War II, when the opium poppy resin needed to produce morphine was difficult to obtain. Dextromethorphan is an example of an entirely synthetic cough suppressant. While structurally related to the opium alkaloids, it is designed to combat cough effectively without the risk of creating dependence — a disadvantage of most cough suppressants derived from opium.

Any pharmacological drug class may include examples of naturally occurring, semi-synthetic and synthetic drugs. For example, opium and morphine are naturally occurring analgesic (pain-relieving) drugs. Heroin, a semi-synthetic drug derived from morphine, is effective in relieving pain, but is also particularly attractive to people who abuse drugs because of its euphoric effects. Methadone and meperidine, which also have pain-relieving properties, are totally synthetic.

Legal and Illegal Manufacture of Psychoactive Drugs

In Canada, the legal manufacture of prescription drugs takes place in production facilities that must comply with government standards. Manufacturing functions include preparing the raw material; producing individual dosage units (such as tablets, capsules and suppositories); maintaining quality control processes; packaging and distribution to drug wholesalers, hospitals, pharmacies, and medical, dental and veterinary practitioners. The drugs are formulated into stable preparations of known strength and purity so that both prescribers and users can rely on dosages. Packaging is designed to protect the product from deterioration during storage, and labelling includes advice concerning storage, expiry dates and instructions for appropriate use. Many drugs may be obtained legally only with a prescription. However, drug products approved for over-the-counter sale are prepared under similar strict controls and are intended for safe self-medication. Finally, federal government regulations control advertising and promotion of medications, as well as alcohol and tobacco.

In contrast, the illegal manufacture of psychoactive drugs takes place typically in clandestine laboratories that lack safeguards for purity, safety and reliability. In some cases the production methods are crude and outdated and the producer's skills are quite limited. Indeed, anyone with a rudimentary knowledge of chemistry can manufacture some types of drugs, provided the clients' standards of acceptability are not very high. However, in certain large and well-organized illicit enterprises, both the equipment and the chemists' skills are very sophisticated. In general, though, buyers of the products of illicit laboratories are uncertain what drug they are getting, in what strength, or with what contaminants or adulterants. Illegal manufacturers direct their production, often through a distribution chain, toward dealers who sell the drugs illegally on the street.

It is important to note that not all drugs available on the street are manufactured illicitly. Some legitimate pharmaceutical products are diverted to the illicit market by theft, prescription forgery, or duping of physicians to obtain unnecessary medication.

Identifying and Analysing Drugs

Visual Identification of Drug Preparations

In general, legally produced drugs can be identified much more easily than illegal drugs. Original packaging and prescription containers for legal drugs provide label information and many dosage units of legal drugs bear unique identifying markings. Occasionally, however, illicit producers attempt to identify their products for the street market. For example, it has been possible to identify particular producers' LSD dosage units on blotting paper by the drawing on the paper, such as "Superman" and "Frog." Illicit producers may also counterfeit the size, color, shape and markings of a particular legal product. In general, however, it is impossible to identify visually with any certainty a drug that is encountered outside of legitimate channels.

The Problem of Reliability in Illegal Drugs

On the illegal drug market, drug quality poses a serious problem for the buyer, because neither the buyer nor dealer can be certain of the identity, purity or strength of the drug being sold.

Street-drug analysis in Canada and the United States has shown that a substantial proportion of samples do not contain the drug they were represented to be. For example, drugs submitted as mescaline to Canadian laboratories are often LSD, PCP (phencyclidine) or a combination of the two. LSD and certain amphetamine-like substances have been substituted for MDA (methylenedioxyamphetamine), which is another hallucinogen. The consequences of using improperly identified drugs range from unexpected drug effects to death. In the 1970s, for example, a number of users died after taking PMA (paramethoxyamphetamine), a highly toxic amphetamine analogue, possibly in the belief that they were taking MDA.

Purity is most likely to be a serious problem when the drug is in liquid form intended for injection. Unsanitary material and insoluble diluents are a major source of drug-related infections and tissue damage among injection drug users. Even drugs that are taken orally can cause illness from impurities. Impurities in a purchased drug product may result from sloppy purification of the crude drug made in the laboratory. They may also result from chemical degradation that occurs between production and sale, since illegal drugs are not stored under controlled conditions. In some cases, other drug substances are added to a drug to increase its effect, or to mislead the potential buyer who uses crude methods of "testing," such as tasting. In these cases, the buyer actually receives a drug mixture, rather than the single drug expected, and will experience the effects of both drugs.

In addition, even when the drug sold to the user is accurately identified and without impurities, the question of strength or concentration, often referred to on the street as potency, remains. For example, when a drug that is a white powder is mixed with some other white powder, such as sugar or talcum, to make it easier to weigh, the buyer cannot tell accurately, short of obtaining a laboratory analysis, how much of the actual drug is present. This means that the buyer may be "ripped off" by receiving a very low concentration considering the price paid, or may be at risk of medical problems or death from overdose as a result of an extraordinarily high concentration.

Users' ignorance about the identity, purity and strength or concentration of street drugs leads to greater and more frequent health-related problems than can be attributed to the pharmacological actions and effects of the drugs themselves. Overdose, life-threatening drug interactions, infections and tissue damage are everyday results of the unreliability of street drugs and the ways they are used. Typically, overdose and accidents occur when the concentration or strength of the drug is changed suddenly on the street or when the user is inexperienced with street drugs.

Laboratory Identification and Analysis of Drugs and Drug Products in the Body

Although visual inspection of a drug product sold illicitly is not a reliable means of identifying what it contains, law enforcement monitoring of illicit drug distribution has resulted in the development of the science of "pillistics." The punch-and-die sets used to produce tablets leave characteristic marks on the tablets that can be used to identify their production source in much the same way that rifling marks on bullets can be used to identify weapons. However, these markings provide no evidence concerning the actual drug contained in the dosage form, since the same punch-and-die sets could be used to manufacture dosage forms of several different drugs.

Therefore, the only way to learn with absolute certainty what drugs a particular product contains is through detailed analysis in a modern laboratory. This approach is useful in the following cases:

- when medical or law enforcement professionals or others concerned with drug abusers or drug abuse situations need to know what drug substances are being used by their clients or in their community
- when emergency medical personnel need to know what drug is involved in a case of drug intoxication or poisoning in order to treat the case
- when a pathologist or the coroner needs to know what substances were in a victim's body at time of death in order to assess the role that these substances may have played in the death itself
- when law enforcement agencies must identify a drug product so that they can monitor its distribution and criminal use.

Qualitative analysis involves identification of the drug substances present in the dosage form or body fluid presented for analysis and, in some cases, identification of the nature of contaminants. The identification process often begins with establishing the class of drugs to which the sample belongs (e.g., opioids), and only then focuses on the specific drug (e.g., heroin, as opposed to codeine or morphine). The process of qualitative analysis becomes more difficult if one has no idea of the nature of the substance to be analysed. In a worst-case situation, the physician will engage in symptomatic treatment (maintaining breathing, monitoring body temperature and so on) until the patient begins to recover or further information is available. Some testing procedures may be too time-consuming to be helpful in medical emergencies.

For a few of the drugs for which an effective antidote is available, such as acetaminophen, methanol and ASA (acetylsalicylic acid), identification of the patient's drug intake is important. For most other drugs, treatment is typically symptomatic. The physician may be able to obtain some useful information about the identity of the drug ingested by questioning the patient or friends of the patient who have brought him or her into the hospital, although the information obtained from these sources may be inaccurate and even misleading. Similarly, examining the drug material found in the patient's possession may be helpful, but there is no certainty that what is in the patient's possession is the same as what he or she actually used.

Qualitative analysis is further complicated by the fact that many drug preparations contain more than one drug. In such cases the component drugs of the sample must usually be separated before they can be identified. Yet another complication relates to the greater potency of some of the newer synthetic and semi-synthetic compounds. As potency increases, the amount of drug present per unit dose decreases. Thus only a minute amount of material may be available for analysis.

While qualitative data establish only the identity of the drug or drugs present in the sample (and in some cases impurities and/or additives), quantitative analysis establishes how much of the various drug components is present. Thus quantitative analysis is often as important a tool as qualitative analysis. It permits assessment of the quantity of the drug present in the drug product or in the patient's blood (or more commonly, the plasma part of the blood) at a specific time. This latter information may shed some light on the role of the drug in the problem under investigation. In medical emergencies, knowing the concentration of drug in blood plasma, and the usual rate at which the body metabolizes that drug, allows the physician to estimate the time it will take for the drug to be cleared from the patient's body.

A wide range of technologies are used in drug analysis. Qualitative methods range from classical color and crystal tests (which tend to be of low specificity and sensitivity); through paper, thin-layer (TLC), and gas-liquid chromatographic (GC or GLC) methods, high-performance liquid chromatography (HPLC), spectrofluorometry, and infrared (IR) and ultraviolet (UV) spectrophotometry; to X-ray diffraction and mass spectrometry (MS) (the last often coupled to a gas-chromatograph/computer system, i.e., GC/MS), and immunoassays. Quantitative analysis may involve use of some of these same technologies, notably ultraviolet spectrophotometry, GLC, GC/MS and HPLC.

Classifying Drugs

As more drugs were developed and we learned more about their actions and effects, it became useful to classify drugs in various ways. Classification emphasized the relationships between and among individual drugs and made it easier to refer to groups of drugs with similar attributes.

There are six basic methods of classifying drugs: by their origin, therapeutic use, site of action, chemical structure, mechanism of action or street name. Each approach is useful for certain purposes. For example, people interested in plants may find classification by origin helpful in understanding the relationships among drug substances found together in the same plant, or in closely related plants. However, a physician treating a drug-intoxicated patient may be more interested in knowing whether a new drug has the same or different mechanism of action as a more familiar drug.

Classification by Origin

Drugs derived from natural sources such as plants are often classified by source or origin. For many years the term "opiate"[2] was used to designate the group of morphine-like drugs obtained from the opium poppy, *Papaver somniferum*. Despite their common source, and their structural similarities, the different properties of the individual opiate drugs led to different uses. Thus morphine is a very potent analgesic used to relieve

---

2   It is important to note that, although different drugs within the class share a common profile of types of effect, they differ from one another in their intensity of effects and side effects, onset and duration of action, usefulness in treatment and risks.

severe pain, while codeine is a much weaker analgesic that also reduces coughing (i.e., has cough-suppressant or antitussive properties) and so is used in products for both pain relief and cough relief.

Classification by Therapeutic Use

Although classification of a drug by its therapeutic use is convenient for medical personnel, it often does not reflect accurately the basis for the drug's non-medical use and abuse. For example, morphine is commonly classified as an analgesic (painkiller), yet its considerable abuse arises mainly from its euphoriant property. Moreover, many drugs have more than one therapeutic use and should properly be included in several therapeutic classes; for example, codeine, which is used for both pain relief and cough suppression, is properly found in both therapeutic classes.

Classification by Site of Action

Classification by site of action is of limited usefulness, for any one drug may act on several areas in the body. Cocaine, for example, has both stimulant effects on the central nervous system and local anesthetic effects on the skin and mucous membranes. Therefore, to classify it as a CNS stimulant tells only one part of the story. Further, drugs that are chemically different and have markedly differing mechanisms of action and/or net effects may affect the same target organ or system. For example, the "CNS stimulants" include such widely different drugs as cocaine, amphetamine and strychnine, which are very different in their chemical structure, therapeutic use and risks.

Classification by Chemical Structure

Many purely synthetic compounds with no alternative natural source are classified by the chemical structure of the parent synthetic compound. The benzodiazepines are a good example of this type of classification: all drugs belonging to this group share a common core structure. However, pharmacological activity may vary both quantitatively and qualitatively within such a group. For example, there are great differences among the benzodiazepines in how rapidly and how long their effects are felt. As a result, while a short-acting one might be used for anesthesia, a longer-acting one might be used to treat anxiety.

Classification by Mechanism of Action

This classification is based on an understanding of how a drug produces its effects. Unfortunately, we do not yet understand the mechanism of action of many drugs, although this is an area of continuing pharmacological research. The drug tranylcypromine (Parnate®), for example, is usually classified by mechanism of action. It is commonly described as an antidepressant of the monoamine oxidase inhibitor (MAOI) type; that is, a drug that can reduce depression by preventing the enzyme monoamine oxidase (MAO) from working in its usual way.

Classifying drugs by their mechanism of action is useful because it emphasizes the fact that drugs in the same class are likely to have not only common desirable effects, but also common risks or undesirable effects based on their mechanism of action.[3] For example, tranylcypromine may relieve depression through its MAO-inhibiting effect, but, like other inhibitors of MAO, it impairs the body's capacity to destroy blood pressure-elevating amines present in some foods and beverages (such as old cheeses and red wine). As a result, the patient treated with MAO inhibitors must avoid dietary sources of such amines in order to avoid their excess buildup and a resulting surge in blood pressure.

Classification by Street Name

Non-medical use of drugs has also given us a form of classification that emerges from the drug-using community and especially from the street drug market. The slang names coined in these environments reflect a variety of associations, as in the numerous names for marijuana — pot, weed and so on. In some cases, these street names indicate pharmacological effects. "Speed," for example, is a reasonable description of the effect on the central nervous system of the stimulant methamphetamine. Conversely, sedative/hypnotic drugs are referred to as "downers." However, street names change with time and can be specific to geographical locations. Further, as in the case of "downers," drugs with the same street name may vary considerably in their potency. Therefore, street names must be interpreted with caution.

---

[3]   It is important to note that, although different drugs within the class share a common profile of types of effect, they differ from one another in their intensity of effects and side effects, onset and duration of action, usefulness in treatment and risks.

Naming Drugs

Considerable confusion and misunderstanding exists as a result of different approaches to naming drugs, and therefore the use of different names for a particular drug. Understanding how drug names are derived helps to reduce these problems.

Six types of names are often applied to a drug: the chemical name, manufacturer's laboratory designation, chemical group name, non-proprietary/generic name, proprietary name and common-use name.

The *chemical name* defines systematically, in numbers, syllables and word roots, the full chemical structure of a single drug molecule. It contains enough information to allow a trained chemist, regardless of the language spoken, to identify the drug unequivocally. For example, the chemical name of the drug diazepam is 7-chloro-1, 3-dihydro-1-methyl-5-phenyl-2H-1,4-benzodiazepin-2-one. However, this naming system cannot be applied when the drug's complete chemical structure is not yet known (such as in the case of some hormones and enzymes prepared from plant or animal sources). Further, most chemical names are too long, complex and unwieldy for common use.

The *manufacturer's laboratory designation* is usually a code name or a number given during the early stages of laboratory development and investigation — for example, RD 5-6901 for the sedative/hypnotic drug flurazepam (Dalmane®). When a compound appears to be highly promising, its code name is discarded and a non-proprietary name is adopted.

The *chemical group name* may be applied to a group of drugs with similar chemical structure. Generally, drugs belonging to the same chemical group produce a spectrum of similar effects. "Benzodiazepines" is an example of a chemical group name.

The *non-proprietary/generic name* is an official short name for a drug substance, used in the public domain in place of the more awkward chemical name. It cannot be trademarked and is not written with a capital letter. It can be used to refer to products marketed by different manufacturers. Such names typically reveal no useful information about the drug's nature or effects. Diazepam is the non-proprietary/generic name of the drug that is widely marketed under the brand names Valium® and Vivol®. Most of the drugs described in this book are referred to by their non-proprietary names.

The *proprietary (brand) name* is the name given by a particular manufacturer to its product. When several manufacturers market a product containing the same drug substance, each manufacturer will do so under its own proprietary name. For example, the drug diphenhydramine is marketed by different manufacturers under different trade names, including Benadryl® and Nytol®. Proprietary names are trademark names and are always capitalized.

The *common-use name* may be identical to the non-proprietary or proprietary name, or it may represent a rough classification according to type of use. In some cases a well-advertised proprietary name is used loosely by the public to refer to similar products marketed by different manufacturers. For example, laypersons use the name Aspirin®, which is a brand name in Canada, when referring to all brands of acetylsalicylic acid (ASA) tablets.

In Table 1, three examples are listed under their various drug names and classifications.

Table 1. Names and Classifications of Three Example Drugs

	Dextroamphetamine	Diazepam	Lysergic Acid Diethylamide
Chemical name	*d*-2- amino-1-phenyl-propane	7-chloro-1,3-dihydro-1-methyl-5-phenyl- 2H-1,4-benzodiazepin-2-one	N,N-diethyl-*d*-lysergamide
Manufacturer's laboratory designation	no longer in use	no longer in use	LSD-25
Chemical group name	amphetamine	benzodiazepine	indolealkylamine
Non-proprietary/generic name	dextroamphetamine	diazepam	d-lysergic acid diethylamide
Examples of proprietary names	Dexedrine®	Valium®, Vivol®	Delysid® (obsolete)
Common-use names	upper, amphetamine, "ice"	trank, tranquillizer, downer	acid, LSD

Different Chemical Forms in Which Drugs Exist

One of the complications of naming and classifying drugs arises from the fact that some drugs exist in more than one chemical form. For example, pentobarbital, a typical barbiturate-type sedative/hypnotic drug, has the chemical characteristics of a weak acid, and like other weak acids it is capable of reacting with bases to form salts. Thus, pentobarbital can be changed to pentobarbital sodium, its salt form, by placing it in a basic solution containing sodium ion. Both the "acid form" of the drug (pentobarbital) and the "salt form" (pentobarbital sodium) have the same pharmacological properties, although they differ in their physical properties (such as solubility in water, alcohol or other organic solvents; melting point; and pH of aqueous solution). Therefore, in cases where it is useful to have the drug dissolve rapidly in a water-based solution (including gastric juice), the more water-soluble form (pentobarbital sodium) will be preferred. However, because the two forms share the same pharmacological properties, many people refer to both as pentobarbital.

In contrast, most psychoactive drugs have the chemical characteristics of bases. That is, they are capable of reacting with acids to form salts. Like the salt of pentobarbital, these salts are more water soluble than the corresponding base form of the drug. Thus morphine, in its base form, will form a salt, morphine sulphate, in the presence of sulphuric acid. Similarly, amphetamine base will react with sulphuric acid to form the salt amphetamine sulphate. Many other psychoactive drugs are commonly available in the form of their salts produced by reaction of their base form with hydrochloric acid. These salts are commonly called "hydrochlorides," such as cocaine hydrochloride. Some drugs are available in the form of salts prepared by reaction with other acids (e.g., hydrobromides, produced by reaction of bases with hydrobromic acid, and citrates, produced by reaction with citric acid).

Drugs in their base form are commonly oily materials that tend to be less stable chemically, more easily vaporized when exposed to heat, and somewhat difficult to crystallize. In contrast, their salts are typically easier to crystallize, and thus easier to purify and weigh more accurately for preparing dosage forms. Therefore, most drugs are marketed in the form of a crystalline salt. The particular salt of a drug (hydrochloride, sulphate, citrate and so on) used in preparing dosage forms is typically determined by the relative costs of production, chemical stability, physical characteristics and so on. Just as the term "pentobarbital" is commonly used for both the acid and salt forms of the drug, so "amphetamine" is commonly used to refer to both amphetamine in its base form and amphetamine sulphate, the salt form. However, pharmacists and chemists are typically quite precise in their use of drug terms.

There are two contexts in which specification of the precise chemical form of drug is required — in expressions of drug dose and expressions of drug concentration in solutions or biological fluids. The actual amount of active drug available in a dosage unit (or present in a solution or fluid) depends on the number of drug molecules present. Since a molecule of the base or acid form of the drug differs in weight from that of the salt form, the number of molecules of drug present is known accurately only if the precise name of the drug used in the dosage form is specified along with the weight of drug used.

UNDERSTANDING DRUG EFFECTS

The intensity of a drug's effects is determined by many factors relating to the concentration of drug at the site of action (sometimes called the tissue site), and the drug's interactions with receptors at the site.[4]

The Concentration of Drug at the Site of Action

The concentration of drug at the site of action, at any particular time after drug administration, depends on the characteristics of the drug administered, the route by which it was administered, its distribution and metabolism in the body and its excretion.

Characteristics of the Drug

Although the amount of drug administered determines how much of the drug is potentially available, the dosage form used (e.g., tablet, powder, solution), and the (physico) chemical properties of the drug, together with the size and nature of the user's body, affect how much of the potentially available drug will actually reach its intended site(s) of action (and how much will reach other parts of the body), how fast this will occur, what the maximum concentration will be and how long it will stay. Usually we think about the way a drug acts on and changes the body, but we must also recognize that the body acts on and changes the drug, through the processes known as absorption, distribution, metabolism (or biotransformation) and excretion. When we describe a drug in relation to these processes, we refer to the drug's pharmacokinetic properties.

---

[4]   Although most attention is given to the concentration of drug at the site of action where the drug's desirable effects are achieved, it is important to remember that (with limited exceptions) drugs are distributed throughout the body and therefore are present in various tissues at varying concentrations. In some cases the interaction of drug with these other tissue sites is the basis for the drug's side effects.

An important drug property that affects virtually all of these drug-body processes is solubility in fat (i.e., lipid solubility) relative to its solubility in water. Most psychoactive drugs are highly lipid-soluble. In fact, their lipid solubility allows them to cross cell membranes to reach the brain where they exert their effect. However, if the drugs are administered in the form of a tablet or capsule, they must also be water-soluble enough to dissolve in the stomach or intestine, because only the dissolved drug molecules are able to pass into the blood in order to reach the brain.

In contrast to most other psychoactive drugs, ethyl alcohol (ethanol, beverage alcohol) is a very small and water-soluble molecule, which is poorly soluble in fat. Alcohol mixes freely with the water and, like water, flows readily through cell membranes. Therefore alcohol is both readily absorbed from the stomach and intestine and distributed quickly to all parts of the body, including the brain.

Routes of Administration and Drug Absorption

There are four principal methods of drug administration: swallowing (oral), direct application to mucous membranes and to skin (transdermal), inhalation and injection (parenteral).[5] Each method has advantages and drawbacks depending on the user's situation and the properties of the specific drug. The choice is usually based on convenience, desired speed of onset and duration of action, availability of sterile preparations, and the drug's water- and fat-solubility. The following brief descriptions outline the different routes of drug administration with some of their attendant risks, benefits and problems.

Swallowing (Oral): The oral route is the most common method of taking drugs provided as capsules, tablets, liquids and powders. Drugs taken orally are generally absorbed primarily in the small intestine rather than in the stomach. Absorption from the stomach and intestine is sometimes affected by the presence of food in the digestive tract. Food can delay stomach emptying or it can dilute the concentration of a drug, thus slowing its absorption and reducing the peak drug level in blood.

---

[5]   New drug delivery technologies include implantable dosage forms. These include small pellets containing medication that can be implanted surgically under the skin to release drugs on a continuing basis over weeks or months without the need for repeated injections. Such technologies are potentially useful in the treatment of chronic disorders when the drug cannot be taken orally or when patients have problems remembering to administer the drug on the required schedule.

Furthermore, food can occasionally cause the drug to pass out of the body in the feces without being absorbed.

An important feature of the oral route is the slow speed at which most drugs are absorbed into the bloodstream. As a result, drug users who are looking for an immediate or intense effect or "rush" avoid taking drugs orally.

The oral route is ineffective for certain drugs because the stomach destroys them or makes them less effective. Heroin, for example, is changed into morphine in the stomach, and once the morphine has been absorbed into the bloodstream, it passes through the liver on its way to the brain. During this initial pass through the liver, so much of the morphine is destroyed that only a small fraction of it ever reaches the brain. Therefore, swallowing heroin does not result in the rapid, intense euphoric effect sought by most users.

Absorption Across Mucous Membranes and Skin (Transdermal): Mucous membranes form the moist surfaces that line the mouth, nose, eye sockets, throat, rectum, vagina and so on. Compared with the epidermis (skin), mucous membranes are thinner and have a greater blood supply, allowing drugs to travel a shorter distance to reach the blood, from which they are distributed to other sites in the body. In addition, the cells of the mucous membranes lack keratin, a structural protein that reduces drugs' rate of travel through skin. For these reasons, fat-soluble drugs are absorbed rapidly across mucous membranes.

Certain drugs placed sublingually (under the tongue) are rapidly and effectively absorbed into the bloodstream. For example, drugs such as nitroglycerin are taken sublingually for the treatment of angina pectoris (heart pains due to poor circulation of blood to the heart). Similarly, nicotine from chewing tobacco and nicotine "gum" (e.g., Nicorette®) is absorbed through the mucous membranes of the mouth. However, the unpleasant taste of many drugs often makes sublingual administration problematic.

Sniffing or "snorting" (not to be confused with inhalation) allows a drug to be absorbed across the mucous membranes of the nose and sinus cavities. Examples of substances taken by sniffing are cocaine, amyl nitrite and tobacco snuff. In the case of the first two, sniffing is the most effective way of getting the drug into the bloodstream. (Glue "sniffing" is actually an incorrect description. Technically, glue and solvent vapors are inhaled and absorbed through the lining of the lung.) Most drugs cannot be effectively absorbed by sniffing, but for those that can, this route is very rapid and effective.[6] Irritating drug substances and those that interfere with blood flow may cause localized damage of the mucosal surfaces. For instance, when cocaine is sniffed, it restricts the flow of blood in the surfaces of the nose to such an extent that in heavy users it may perforate or entirely destroy their nasal septum and the lining of their nose.

Some drugs can be absorbed by the mucous membrane of the rectum. Rectal administration is sometimes chosen when oral administration would induce nausea and vomiting or when the patient is unconscious, is a small child or is otherwise unable to take the drug through more efficient routes. The drugs are usually inserted in the form of suppositories. Cafergot®, a medication used to treat migraine headaches, is an example of a drug that may be administered rectally. However, many drugs are not absorbed efficiently by rectal membranes.

Traditionally drugs were applied to skin (e.g., in ointments) when the skin was the intended site of the drug effects (e.g., antihistamines and local anesthetics). However, as new technologies have been developed (e.g., transdermal patches), application to skin has been increasingly used as a way of delivering low doses of drugs (such as nicotine) into the blood continuously over a period of hours or days.

Inhalation: In the case of inhalation, the drug is absorbed into the bloodstream across the lining of the lung (the alveolar membrane). Since the surface of the lung is large and the diffusion distance is short, this is a very effective way to achieve rapid absorption of certain drugs. For a drug to be inhaled, it must be in gas form (e.g., the vapors of solvents), in fine liquid drops or in fine particles of solid suspended in a gas (e.g., aerosols or the smoke from tobacco or cannabis). For many drugs, inhalation is the most rapid method of administration. Its major drawback is that only relatively small amounts of the drug can be absorbed at a single administration.

Injection (Parenteral): The term "parenteral" refers to the pathways through which drugs are injected directly into the body with a needle and syringe. Substances that would not be efficiently absorbed through other routes because of low fat solubility

---

6   Only those drugs that are very fat soluble are effectively absorbed by sniffing.

may be very effective upon parenteral administration. For other drugs, the rate of onset or duration of action may be altered with the appropriate choice of parenteral route and the appropriate type of drug product.

Since normal barriers that protect the body from micro-organisms (such as the skin and mucous membranes) are bypassed by the parenteral routes, systemic infections may result when non-sterile needles and/or solution are used. Street drug users who share needles and/or syringes are at increased risk of infection from, and contribute to, the transmission of hepatitis, HIV and other infectious diseases.

There are three main parenteral routes of injection: subcutaneous, intramuscular and intravenous. Subcutaneous injection — commonly called "skin popping" by street users — involves injecting the drug under the skin. Of the three needle routes, it requires the least technical skill and is commonly used by beginners. The rate of absorption from the site of injection is slower than from intravenous injection but faster than from the oral route. Various drugs including heroin can be administered subcutaneously. If the drug and needle are not sterile, infections may result at the site of infection (locally) or throughout the body (systemically). Furthermore, insoluble diluents used in drug preparations tend to stay at the site of injection rather than enter the bloodstream. Both problems may lead to marks (tattooing) or lesions of the skin. When several such marks appear in rows, typically along the arm of an injection drug user, they are referred to as "needle tracks" or simply "tracks."

Compared with subcutaneous injection, intramuscular injection involves deeper penetration of the drug into the body tissue. The drug is injected directly into the muscle mass, where it is slowly absorbed into the bloodstream. Drugs may be injected in the form of a solution or in suspension (i.e., very small solid or liquid particles suspended in a liquid, usually designed to slow the release of the drug). This route is often used by athletes administering anabolic steroids. Localized pain is a major drawback of intramuscular injection. Some drug abusers use this method because placement of the needle is not as critical as in intravenous injection, so that the injection can be made through the clothing. The risks of infection and of localized tissue damage are quite high.

Intravenous injection — popularly known as "mainlining" — involves injecting the drug directly into the veins. It is one of the fastest ways of getting a drug into the bloodstream and allows relatively large amounts of a drug to be administered at one time. Suspended particles may cause blood clots to form, which may block blood vessels. In a localized area, clots may lead to tissue damage; in a vital area, such as the brain or heart, they may lead to death. Intravenous injection takes the drug into the superficial veins of the body. Some skill is needed to use this route effectively. For example, in order to find a good injection site, it is sometimes necessary to make the veins more visible by using a pressure cuff on the heart or "upstream" side of the site. The forearms and elbow-joint area are common sites for intravenous injection, although some users may avoid them in order to hide their drug use. Since injection of high concentrations of drugs irritates veins, eventually a frequently used vein may become blocked and collapse, and another site must be found. A wide variety of sites on the body may be used, including the ankles, scrotum and underside of the tongue. Needle marks on the body of the drug user often indicate the duration and severity of the drug problem.

The Distribution of Drugs in the Body

Once a drug is absorbed into the bloodstream, it is distributed throughout the body.[7] Most drugs are not distributed uniformly to all parts of the body. Some drugs, for example, bind more strongly to blood elements such as plasma protein and therefore a larger part of the dose tends to remain longer in the blood, while others tend to accumulate fairly rapidly in tissue that is rich in fat. With limited exceptions, including alcohol, drugs must be highly fat soluble in order to enter the brain because they must diffuse across the cell membranes of the cerebral capillaries. Similarly, fat-soluble drugs typically cross the placenta of pregnant women to affect the fetus, and these same drugs are also found in the milk of lactating women.

This uneven distribution of a drug — that is, different concentrations of drug in different types of tissue — complicates efforts to find relationships between blood levels of a psychoactive drug and its behavioral effects, which are more closely related to drug concentrations in particular parts of the brain. While, in general, high drug blood levels are related to correspondingly greater behavioral effects than low levels, the relationship of blood concentration to intensity of effects varies from drug to drug.

---

[7]   The lymphatic system, composed of a network of glands and ducts, also plays a role in the distribution of certain drugs.

Because alcohol is water soluble, its distribution differs from that of most other psychoactive drugs. Alcohol crosses all barriers to distribute uniformly in total body water. There is no selective binding of alcohol to any tissue. Therefore, in the non-tolerant individual, blood levels are systematically related (i.e., highly correlated) with behavioral effects. The same relations also hold for some gaseous anesthetics and solvents.

Drug Metabolism (Biotransformation)

Drugs are generally eliminated from the body in both changed and unchanged states; that is, a part of the drug eliminated is chemically identical to that which was administered, and part has been chemically changed. The proportion of a drug dose eliminated in a particular state is determined by the chemical nature of the drug, its dose, its route of administration and the way the user's body functions (the user's physiological characteristics). As discussed in the section on excretion below, the excretion of unchanged psychoactive drugs through the urine or feces is generally inefficient because of their high fat solubility; the obvious exception is ethanol, which is water soluble. As a result, living organisms have evolved mechanisms for transforming fat-soluble substances into more water-soluble breakdown products that can be readily excreted by the kidneys and/or intestines. The processes by which a drug is changed to a different chemical state are called drug metabolism or biotransformation, and the new substances created by the process are called drug metabolites.

Drugs are biotransformed with the aid of specialized protein molecules called enzymes, which act as catalysts in the chemical reactions. Most drug metabolism occurs in the liver, although enzymes in the kidneys, gut (i.e., gastrointestinal tract), lungs, blood and, to a lesser extent, brain, may also aid in the process. Several types of liver enzymes are involved in the biotransformation of drugs, namely microsomal, mitochondrial and cytoplasmic enzymes.

Conversion of a fat-soluble drug to a substance that has sufficient water solubility for efficient excretion may involve several sequential chemical reactions, each of which produces its own "intermediate" product(s). Thus one parent drug produces many metabolites (for example, there are many known metabolites from tetrahydro-cannabinol, the main psychoactive ingredient of cannabis).

As the drug molecule is changed to progressively less fat-soluble substances through a sequence of biotransformation reactions, its ability to enter the brain (i.e., to cross the blood-brain barrier) is reduced. At the same time, the psychoactive potency of those drug metabolites that do reach the brain may be reduced or eliminated. For these reasons, drug metabolism was known previously as drug detoxification — a term that implies that the purpose of drug metabolism is to detoxify the drug; that is, to make it less harmful to the body.

Although most intermediate drug metabolites are less potent pharmacologically than the parent drug, and some have virtually no activity, others are quite active.[8] These typically produce the same sorts of pharmacological effects as the parent drug. For example, the anxiolytic drug diazepam is transformed to a large number of metabolites, including N-desmethyldiazepam, 3-hydroxydiazepam and oxazepam, all of which have pharmacological actions characteristic of the original drug. Occasionally a parent drug, such as chlorazepate (Tranxene®) for example, is inactive and must be metabolized in order to become effective.

Drug metabolites may differ from the original (or parent) drug not only in psychoactive potency, but also in toxicity. For example, methanol (methyl alcohol or wood alcohol) is metabolized to two very toxic metabolites — formaldehyde and formic acid. It is these metabolites that are considered responsible for damage to the optic nerve and disruption of the acid-base balance of the body, both of which pose serious problems in the case of methanol poisoning.

The microsomal and cytoplasmic enzymes that catalyze drug metabolism processes are *inducible* — that is, repeated drug exposure causes them to increase in number. This results in more rapid conversion of the ingested drug into its metabolites. This speeding-up of the process can result in increased intensity and faster onset of drug effects if the original substance was inactive and the metabolites active, or it can result in decreased intensity and duration of effect if the original drug was active and the metabolites inactive. This latter phenomenon is sometimes referred to as metabolic tolerance. When exposure to the inducing drug is stopped, the increase in drug-metabolizing activity (i.e., the metabolic tolerance) is gradually lost.

---

8   It is mainly products of the first or second biotransformation reaction that retain sufficient fat solubility.

Many drugs, including some medications prescribed by physicians, have the capacity to increase microsomal drug-metabolizing activity. Further, the enzymes induced by one drug will speed up the metabolism of the whole range of drugs that are metabolized by that process. Hydrocarbons in tobacco smoke, for example, are very strong inducers. Drugs that exhibit increased rates of biotransformation in smokers include heparin, propranolol and theophylline. When a heavy smoker stops smoking, his or her dose of such medications might need to be adjusted to avoid toxic side effects, as the activity of drug-metabolizing enzymes returns toward normal over a period of weeks or months following smoking cessation. Similarly, people who are stabilized on a particular medication may find that their dose is no longer adequate when they begin to take a new medication that induces drug-metabolizing enzymes.

Drug Excretion

Drugs of different chemical structures are excreted from the body by different routes following their absorption and distribution and, as relevant, their biotransformation. The excretory processes involve several major organ systems.

In humans, the major route of elimination of most drugs is in the urine. The kidney acts as a pressure filter through which the blood passes. On its way through the kidney, the blood is "filtered," and the filtrate or "primary urine" consists of a considerable amount of the blood's water together with all substances (including drugs) dissolved in this water. As the primary urine passes farther through the kidney tubules, the kidney reabsorbs most of the water and some of the dissolved substances. Substances that are fat soluble tend to be reabsorbed in this process. Consequently, the excretion of such substances (a category that includes all unmetabolized psychoactive drugs except ethanol) is inefficient.

The residual water and substances that have not been reabsorbed constitute the concentrated urine, which passes from the kidney into the bladder and is eliminated by urination. In addition, some substances (such as some penicillins) are transported directly into the concentrated urine by the cells of the kidney. This process is often referred to as active secretion.

The concentration of drugs and metabolites in the blood at the time of primary urine formation is reflected in the concentration of these substances in the primary urine because it is a filtrate of blood. However, the measured concentrations of drugs and drug metabolites in voided urine generally do not provide a valid basis for estimating the concentrations of these substances in blood at the time of urine collection. The differences between voided urine concentrations and blood concentrations at the time of voiding are determined by the chemical structure of the drug; the pH (i.e., relative acidity) of urine, which may be changed by disease conditions or administration of certain drugs or chemicals; the reabsorption process (and, where relevant, the active secretion process) in kidney tubules, which vary in efficiency among individuals; and the time elapsed between the formation of the concentrated urine that is stored in the bladder and the emptying of the bladder when the sample is collected for analysis.

Because alcohol is highly soluble in water, it is not preferentially reabsorbed from the primary urine. Therefore the concentration of alcohol in voided urine is a more consistent reflection of blood alcohol level at the time the concentrated urine was formed. However, the alcohol level in the voided urine sample is different from the blood alcohol level at the time of voiding because of the decline in blood level between the two events, which results from alcohol metabolism.

The intestines are a site of both drug excretion and drug absorption. Some drugs and drug metabolites have chemical characteristics that cause them to be actively secreted (or "pushed out") into bile as they pass through liver cells, and the drug-containing bile then empties into the intestines. This process is sometimes referred to as biliary secretion. The result of this process is that these drugs and metabolites may be excreted in the feces. However, similar to the situation in urinary excretion, fecal excretion may be greatly reduced by reabsorption of the fat-soluble compounds (including psychoactive drugs) into the bloodstream farther along in the intestines. When reabsorption occurs, the drugs will undergo the process of excretion all over again (enterohepatic cycling), and the drug effect may be prolonged.

Because of the reabsorption phenomenon, elimination of fat-soluble psychoactive substances by both the intestinal and renal (kidney) routes is often very inefficient. This explains the need for the chemical changes that occur in drug metabolism that decrease fat solubility and hence decrease reabsorption from the gut and kidney tubules.

Volatile drugs such as solvents (and volatile metabolites) are commonly excreted in the breath. For very volatile substances, such as general anesthetics, the breath may be the major route of elimination. For substances such as beverage alcohol, it is a minor route. Nonetheless, it is possible through stimulation of breathing to increase the loss of some drugs from the body. Since the amount of alcohol excreted in the breath can be reliably and validly related to the blood level, the concentration in the breath, as measured by the breathalyser test,[9] serves to estimate the blood level of alcohol.

All of the body's routes of elimination, including sweat and saliva (and, in lactating women, milk), play a role in drug elimination. Although the latter are minor routes, they can be important in forensic analysis. They also sometimes have major consequences. For example, elimination of drugs via mother's milk means ingestion of drugs by infants. Although transfer of drug across the placenta to the fetus may not usually be considered a process of "elimination," because no net loss of drug occurs from the pregnant woman's body, it is useful to recognize that it does involve the "loss" of drug from the maternal blood, and a "gain" of drug to the fetal circulation. This transfer process is most important for ethanol, which distributes through total body water because of its high water solubility, and for fat-soluble psychoactive drugs.

Drug Interaction with Receptors at the Site of Action

Drug Receptors

Although drug effects are often thought of as properties of the drug molecules themselves, most drug effects actually depend on the drug's interaction with specific tissue sites called receptors. As researchers have identified and examined more and more receptors, it has become clear that many types of receptors exist. They are typically three-dimensional areas of peptide, located within specific types of cells or on the cell surface.

The interaction between drugs and receptors, and the resultant formation of drug receptor complexes, occurs through various types of chemical bonds (e.g., electrostatic, hydrogen, pi and hydrophobic bonds). Like other chemical reactions, this

---

9   See CNS Depressants: Alcohols in Section 2 for more information.

binding requires a particular spatial relationship, a "good fit," between the drug (sometimes referred to as the "ligand") and the receptor. Consequently, each type of receptor is limited by its three-dimensional structure to binding with only certain types of drug molecules.

This relationship has often been likened to that of a lock and key, because of the importance of exact fit between the parts, the fact that their "engagement" produces a predictable result, and the fact that the drug and receptor are typically disengaged after their interaction and may re-combine repeatedly. However, the drug-receptor interaction actually differs from a traditional lock-and-key system in at least three important respects: first, most drug effects are produced only when many drug-receptor bindings have occurred; second, the interaction to form the drug-receptor complex may change the structure of the drug and/or the receptor; and third, the observed drug effect actually results from a chain or cascade of biochemical changes, which is triggered by the binding of drug and receptor.

It could hardly be imagined that the human body would contain a vast range of receptors that had no purpose until a particular type of psychoactive drug molecule was discovered or created to react with them. In fact, research has shown that many psychoactive drugs actually produce their effect by interacting with receptors that are "custom designed" to fit other molecules — chemicals such as serotonin, dopamine, norepinephrine and enkephalins — that exist naturally in the body and contribute to normal functioning of the central nervous system. Not surprisingly, each type of receptor is localized in particular areas of the brain, where it can fulfil its "normal" function. Therefore, to be effective, a drug must not only have the right structure to interact with a receptor, but it must also be distributed in the body in such a way that sufficient drug molecules are available in the area of the right receptor.

Although we speak of a given drug reacting with a particular receptor, the relationships of drug classes and receptor classes are more complex. It is clear that several types of receptors may interact with a certain family of drugs to produce the effects typical of that family. For example, at least three different families of receptors, designated μ (mu) κ (kappa) and δ (delta), interact with opioid drugs. Further, more than one type of receptor may contribute to a single drug effect. For example, the pain-relieving effect of morphine circulating in the body results primarily from the drug's interaction with μ receptors (specifically those known as μ_1), but morphine's interaction with κ receptors is also believed to contribute to its pain-relieving properties. Finally, opioids such as morphine, which exert their pain-relieving effect predominantly through interaction with μ receptors, produce a feeling of well-being or euphoria, while opioids relieving pain through interaction with κ receptors tend to produce the opposite effect, i.e., dysphoria and even hallucinations. This complexity of drug-receptor interactions provides real challenges for researchers attempting to design drugs with specific desirable effects, but without undesirable effects.

Receptor Affinity for the Drug

For most drugs, the process of drug binding to receptors can be viewed as a chemical reaction that is reversible. In this process drug molecules react with receptors to form drug-receptor complexes, which exist only momentarily and then dissociate so that both the original drug molecule and receptor are returned to their original state, and each may react again and again. When drug-receptor complexes are being formed at the same rate that they are dissociating (i.e., when the reaction is "in equilibrium"), the proportion of receptors "occupied" by drug depends on the strength of the binding (i.e., the receptor's "affinity" for the drug), and the numbers of drug and receptor molecules present. A high "occupancy level" of receptors under equilibrium conditions is generally associated with high drug "potency."

Since the various members of a given drug class (e.g., opioids or benzodiazepines) differ somewhat in chemical structure even though they share key structural features, it is not surprising that they differ in their binding characteristics to any particular type of receptor. Because of these binding differences, each requires a different concentration of drug at the receptor site to achieve the same "occupancy level." This, in turn, is reflected in their differing potency — those that require more drug present to achieve the given occupancy level are less potent.

Responsiveness of Receptors to Drugs — Intrinsic Efficacy

Although drug binding to receptors is an important contributor to the body's response to drugs, it is not the only contributor, for drugs that have similar binding properties may have quite different capacities to trigger a response. A drug's capacity to initiate a response, once it has bound to a receptor, provides a basis for categorizing drugs as agonists, partial agonists and antagonists.

Drugs considered to be agonists may differ from each other in the "strength" of response they initiate at a particular level of receptor occupancy. However, two drugs evoking different strength of response at the same level of occupancy may produce the same strength of response when more of the "lower-response" drug is available to bind to the receptors. Partial agonists are drugs that initiate a response that, regardless of the amount of drug present, is less than the maximal response produced by an agonist. Antagonists are drugs that bind to receptors, but fail to initiate a response.

For agonist drugs, therefore, drug potency is determined by both the receptor's affinity for the drug, and the drug's ability to trigger an "action response" (its intrinsic efficacy). The greater the efficacy of the drug, the smaller will be the level of "drug occupancy" of receptors required to produce a detectable drug effect. Based on these principles, it would be expected that agonist drugs of a particular chemical family, but varying somewhat in their chemical features, would have different levels of efficacy. Accordingly, for any given level of receptor occupancy, each would produce a different intensity of drug effect.

Drug-Receptor Interaction in the Presence of Other Molecules

In the preceding discussion it has been assumed that a single type of agonist drug molecule is available to interact with a particular type of receptor. However, in some circumstances two types of agonist drug molecules may be present, each with the ability to bind to the same receptor. In that case, the two types of drug molecules will compete for each receptor, and their relative success will depend on the receptor's relative affinity for each type of drug molecules. Accordingly, some proportion of receptors will bind with one drug, and some proportion with the other drug. The resultant intensity of drug effect is determined by these proportions and by the intrinsic efficacy of the two drugs.

However, when one drug is an agonist and the other is an antagonist, the same principles apply but the result may be quite different. Some proportion of the receptors will bind to the agonist, and some proportion will bind to the antagonist. These proportions will be determined by the receptor's different affinity for the two drugs, and the available concentration of each drug. However, in this scenario, the receptors bound to the antagonist drug will not contribute to the observed drug effect.

Therefore the intensity of agonist effect generated will be less than that produced by the same concentration of agonist in the absence of the antagonist.

From the principles presented above, it might be expected that the intensity of an agonist drug's effect, generated in the presence of an antagonist, could be altered by changing the relative amounts of the agonist and antagonist available at the receptors. In other words, if a high enough concentration of antagonist were present, the antagonist molecules might "monopolize" the receptors, so that few, if any, receptors would bind to the agonist drug, and therefore the intensity of the effect produced by the agonist would be close to zero.

This is precisely the principle on which the therapeutic use of opioid antagonists is based. The opioid antagonist naloxone is commonly used in the emergency treatment of heroin overdoses. Because naloxone molecules, present in sufficient concentration, will successfully compete with opioid molecules for opioid receptors, they (largely) prevent the formation of opioid-receptor complexes and the resultant opioid effects such as respiratory depression.

The same principles provide the rationale for using the opioid antagonist naltrexone in preventing relapse of patients who have ceased using heroin. As an antagonist, naltrexone does not produce the euphoric effects of heroin that users seek. Thus, when naltrexone is administered regularly, in sufficient doses to maintain an adequate concentration of naltrexone molecules around the opioid receptors, a large proportion of the opioid receptors will bind to naltrexone molecules, and few will be available to bind with heroin, should the patient relapse to heroin use. With few heroin-receptor complexes formed, the antagonist-treated patient who reverts to using heroin will experience little euphoria; that is, the antagonist will "block" the heroin effect. Consequently, the patient will not receive the expected "reward" for his or her heroin use, and will have little incentive to continue it.

The Body's Response to Drugs

The Relationship of Drug Dose and Effect

Anyone who is naive about the way drugs act might assume that doubling the dose of a drug would double its effect, tripling the dose would triple its effect and so on. This expected relationship of dose to effect is shown in Figure 1.

Figure 1.

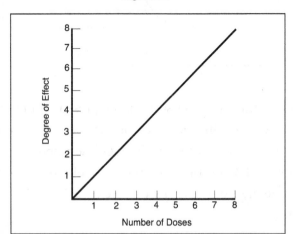

However, most North Americans are sufficiently sophisticated to appreciate that the actual relationship of dose to effect is not so simple. For example, while an initial drink of an alcoholic beverage may have little observable effect on the body,[10] each of the second and third drinks is likely to have a very noticeable effect. A person who has consumed three drinks, therefore, feels more than three times the effect of the first drink. This difference in effect can be interpreted in terms of a "threshold" level of drug. With a small dose, which doesn't reach the threshold concentration at the site of action, the drug's effects may not be observable, or even perceived by the user. However, when the drug concentration exceeds that threshold, each subsequent dose creates approximately the same size of effect up to an upper limit (sometimes called the ceiling or plateau). To show this concept graphically, the pharmacologist plots the intensity of drug effect against the logarithm of the number of doses (or the size of dose) to obtain a "log-dose response curve" (often abbreviated to the dose-response curve) that is typically S-shaped, as represented in Figure 2.

---

10   Unless the drinker is very light in weight and/or is drinking on an empty stomach.

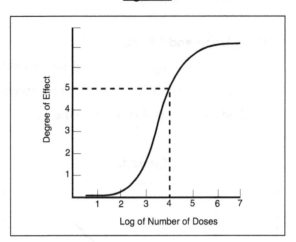

In the case of alcohol, the effect measured and represented in such a graph might be the number of mistakes made in a motor co-ordination test or the time taken to solve a problem. The exact characteristics of the log-dose response curve depend on the specific drug, its route of administration, the particular drug effect being considered and the degree of tolerance of the user (see Tolerance below).

Multiple (Poly) Drug Use

Problems in predicting the intensity of drug effects arise when someone uses two or more drugs that are interactive. For example, alcohol interacts with benzodiazepines, barbiturates and some antihistamines that also have CNS-depressant effects. Although one drink of alcohol *or* one dose of a particular antihistamine taken alone may produce almost no discernible psychoactive effect in a particular individual, one drink and one dose of the antihistamine taken close together by the same individual may impair his or her driving ability. Similarly, one dose of amphetamine combined with one dose of cocaine would be expected to produce a much more intense effect than one dose of either drug alone.

In both cases, the drug combination results in a quantitative change (i.e., a change in the amount or intensity) of effect — in these cases an increase. Pharmacologists recognize two subtypes of increased effect intensity — additivity (or addition) and synergism (or potentiation). Additivity refers to a drug interaction in which the identical (or very similar) effects of each of two (or more) drugs combine to produce a greater effect than either drug alone at the same dose. The intensity of the combined effect may be very similar to that of a double dose of one of the drugs alone. However, in other cases the intensity may be greater than that expected from a double dose. The size of change in the effect intensity will depend on the size of dose of each of the drugs in the combination, in relation to that drug's dose-response curve. In effect, combining the two drugs is equivalent to moving along the dose-response curve of either drug to a higher dose level.

Synergism, the other subtype of increased effect intensity, is used to describe the drug interaction when a combination of two drugs at specified doses produces a greater effect than could be accounted for by a proportional shift along the dose-response curve for either drug; that is, a greater than additive effect. The extra degree of effect could have many different biological explanations, some of which are suggested below.

In contrast, a combination of two drugs may result in a reduction in effect intensity relative to that produced by an identical dose of one of the drugs alone. Pharmacologists describe this phenomenon as "antagonism"; that is, the second drug cancels out some or all of the expected effects of the first drug. For example, the opioid antagonist naloxone greatly reduces — or, in sufficient doses, cancels — the effects of opioids when administered with, or shortly before or after, them. (See the discussion of drug-receptor interactions, above.)

Drug interactions may be generated as a function of pharmacokinetic and/or pharmacodynamic factors. *Pharmacokinetic* considerations relate to the way in which the body affects a specific type of drug — the processes of absorption, distribution, biotransformation and excretion. The presence of a second drug may alter one or more of these processes. For example, the absorption of alcohol from the intestine may be delayed if the alcohol is consumed by a person who is also using a drug that delays the movement of stomach contents into the small intestine. Another example of altered pharmacokinetics is the reduced rate of metabolism of methanol (wood alcohol) when beverage alcohol (ethanol) is also present. In fact, administration of beverage alcohol is an important treatment to prevent poisoning after methanol has been consumed, because the presence of ethanol slows the formation of formic acid and formaldehyde — the metabolites of methanol that produce methanol's toxic effects.

Pharmacodynamic considerations relate to the ways in which two or more drugs act together on a common physiological system. Such interactions occur when the mechanism of action of two drugs is the same. For example, two benzodiazepines, given together, will produce a more intense effect than either given separately, because they exert their effect by the same mechanism. Therefore the effect of the combination will be similar to having a higher dose of just one of the drugs present. However, pharmacodynamic interactions may also occur when the mechanisms of the drugs are different. For example, while both nicotine and amphetamine lead to increased blood pressure, they act on both different and common sites. Nicotine increases blood pressure by a combination of actions, including constriction of blood vessels and release of norepinephrine from the adrenal gland; norepinephrine, in turn, stimulates the heart to pump faster, thereby increasing blood pressure. Amphetamine also constricts blood vessels and causes the release of norepinephrine, but also has a direct stimulating effect on the heart, by its action on receptors in the heart tissue. Together, nicotine and amphetamine, acting by this combination of mechanisms, have a greater effect on blood pressure than either drug alone. However, the size of some effects produced by two drugs interacting pharmacodynamically may be smaller than anticipated because of the body's ability to compensate for drug-induced changes.

The Body's Adaptation to Drugs: Tolerance and Withdrawal

After regular exposure to some psychoactive drugs, especially at higher dose levels, the user's body is likely to change the way it functions, adapting to the presence of the drug. Two of the most important adaptations are tolerance and withdrawal.

Tolerance

Tolerance is the need for an increased amount of a given drug to achieve intoxication (or the desired effect) — or the reduction of a drug's effect with continued use of the same dose over time.

The magnitude of the body's response to a drug depends not only on its concentration at the site of action but also on the sensitivity of the target cells. This sensitivity is governed by innate (probably genetically controlled) factors and by adaptive changes that can occur in the body in response to chronic exposure to the drug substance. The result of these adaptive changes is often a progressive loss of sensitivity to the drug. This loss of sensitivity is called tolerance and can result from various mechanisms. Tolerance is an adaptation that, in turn, influences drug-taking patterns and behaviors.

The most important concepts in the area of tolerance include:

Metabolic (Dispositional) Tolerance: A person who uses a psychoactive drug usually wants the desired effect to last as long as possible. The process of drug metabolism or transformation, together with the process of excretion, limits the duration of action for most drugs. For many drugs, such as alcohol and phenobarbital, frequent exposure of the drug-metabolizing system to such a drug (as occurs in chronic use) may actually increase the metabolizing system's capability and efficiency. The result is that the drug is metabolized more quickly than it was previously, so that the duration, and often the peak intensity, of the desired effect are reduced. At this point a person is said to have developed metabolic tolerance to the drug. To regain the original duration and intensity of effect, the user may try to increase both the dosage and frequency of administration. However, the success of this strategy is likely to be short-lived as the rate of drug metabolism may be further increased with continuing use.

Metabolic (Dispositional) Cross-Tolerance: Metabolic cross-tolerance occurs when chronic use of one drug reduces the pharmacological effects of a second drug. The first drug, in the process of inducing its own increased metabolism, also induces increased metabolism of a second drug. Many drugs that affect the central nervous system are metabolized by the same enzymes. As a result, individuals who have developed metabolic tolerance to one type of sleeping medication, such as barbiturates, for example, may be metabolically tolerant to another. In contrast, barbiturates do not produce metabolic cross-tolerance to alcohol, because these two drug types are metabolized by different enzyme systems in the liver.

Central Nervous System Pharmacodynamic (Functional or Neurological) Tolerance: CNS pharmacodynamic tolerance (or functional or neurological tolerance) occurs when the CNS (or at least some part of it) adapts gradually to the action of a given drug in a way that reduces the effect that the drug in a given concentration will have on cells. Therefore a user who develops CNS tolerance to a drug typically uses doses of increasing size over time.

CNS pharmacodynamic tolerance to different effects of a drug does not develop at the same rate. In fact, it may not develop at all to some effects. For instance, tolerance develops rapidly to some effects of sedative/hypnotics, such as effectiveness in inducing sleep, but very slowly to the respiratory-depressant effect. The difference has important consequences for the chronic user of barbiturate-type sedative/hypnotics. As users increase their dose of these drugs, in order to overcome CNS tolerance and thus regain their sleep-inducing effect, they face a risk of respiratory depression and even respiratory arrest if the dose used is high enough. This situation arises because tolerance to the respiratory-depressant effect is much more limited than tolerance to the sleep-inducing effect.

Central Nervous System (Functional) Cross-Tolerance: CNS cross-tolerance occurs when the adaptive mechanisms developed in the user's brain in response to one drug similarly reduce the brain's response to some other drug that produces similar psychoactive effects. For example, a chronic heavy user of alcohol, which is a sedative, will require a higher dose of general anesthetic to reach the level of unconsciousness required for a surgical procedure than will a typical non-drinker. In fact, such individuals will experience less intensive effects from a given dose of most CNS depressants, including sedative/hypnotics, than would most non-drinkers, and more than they would have required before becoming heavy drinkers.

Tachyphylaxis: In contrast to drugs to which CNS pharmacodynamic tolerance develops, but that will continue to produce a certain intensity of effect if increasingly large doses are given, drugs such as LSD produce a type of CNS tolerance known as tachyphylaxis. Tachyphylaxis is characterized by a rapid reduction in the maximum achievable drug effect no matter how large a dose is used. Repeated doses of some tachyphylaxis-producing drugs over as few as four days may produce a state in which no drug effect is experienced, regardless of the size of the dose used. The user who wants to re-experience the effects of the drug must then abstain for several days in order to restore CNS sensitivity. This phenomenon leads to a pattern of episodic use of drugs such as LSD (e.g., "weekend tripping"). There is considerable cross-tachyphylaxis among LSD, mescaline and psilocybin, so that a switch from one of these drugs to another will not compensate for the overall reduction of response.

Behavioral Tolerance: Behavioral tolerance refers to experienced users' learned ability to compensate for a drug's effect by controlling their behavior. Individuals who have a great deal of experience using a particular drug, know how it affects them, and have experience with a particular task, may be able to learn how to compensate for the drug's effect so that their task-specific behaviors and performance appear unimpaired, or less impaired than would be expected for a given blood level of the drug.

Withdrawal

With chronic use of certain drugs, the body adapts physiologically to the continuing presence of the drug at a certain concentration in tissue. When the drug is abruptly removed, or the dose is significantly decreased, a dysfunctional state of "drug deprivation" develops. Individuals in this state experience withdrawal — that is, a cluster of distressing symptoms often accompanied by directly observable physical signs, which represent an unmasking of the body's adaptation to the drug's presence. Withdrawal can be viewed as the body's signal that it needs the drug at a certain level to maintain itself in its drug-adapted (or drug-dependent) state of functioning. If the user fails to return to use of the drug at the previous level, the body will gradually readapt to a decreased level or absence of the drug.

The nature, severity, onset and duration of withdrawal vary widely, depending on the nature of the drug that was used, the dose, frequency and duration of its use, and the characteristics of the user. For example, the individual experiencing withdrawal from heroin typically feels very distressed, unhappy and nauseous, and is likely to experience vomiting, muscle aches, as well as teary eyes and runny nose. The individual experiencing withdrawal from cocaine, however, may feel equally distressed and unhappy, but is likely to feel very tired, and have vivid unpleasant dreams and increased appetite.

Symptoms of drug withdrawal tend to be the opposite of the effects produced by the presence of the drug in the body. For example, barbiturates cause sedation, and withdrawal from barbiturates causes hyperexcitability. For heavy users of barbiturates, the levels of hyperexcitability produced by rapid withdrawal can be great enough to bring on fatal seizures. In the case of amphetamines, the reverse is the pattern: the normal effect of amphetamines is stimulation, while a principal withdrawal effect is fatigue and sleep. Longer-acting drugs tend to produce less intense withdrawal symptoms, since the drug effects on the body are reduced more gradually, giving the body more time to adapt to the diminishing amount of drug present.

The unpleasantness of withdrawal may be so severe that the individual fearing it (or experiencing it) may use the drug again just to avoid (or relieve) the symptoms.

Understanding Drug Use, Drug Dependence, Harmful Use and Drug Abuse

Drug Use

People use drugs because they gain something from their use. This gain may be the altered feelings produced by the drug's interaction with their brain chemistry, benefits of social interaction or simply the thrill of experiencing something new and possibly risky.

Some users enjoy the different feeling they get as a result of their drug use. For example, codeine and morphine may be used to relieve pain or withdrawal symptoms, alcohol to relax or temporarily escape from problems, amphetamines to achieve a sense of high energy and accomplishment, or LSD to experience heightened awareness and a unique relationship with the surroundings.

When unusually good feelings result from use of a drug, the drug use is more likely to be repeated. The ability of a drug to produce effects that make a user want to take it again is called "reinforcement." Many studies have shown a relationship between the strength of a drug as a "reinforcer" and the drug's ability to increase levels of neurotransmitters in critical areas of the brain. For example, cocaine, amphetamines, ethanol, opioids and nicotine, all of which are "feel-good" drugs for some users, are strong reinforcers and increase the concentration of available dopamine in a particular area of the brain. However, research suggests that the "feel-good" effects produced by these drugs are also related to changes in levels of other neurotransmitters, as well as the user's unique characteristics and expectations concerning the drug's effects.

Some users rarely use psychoactive substances when they are alone, but enjoy the benefits that such drugs bring in social situations. These benefits may include lowered inhibitions, which make some group activities more comfortable, the symbolism of sharing group values in religious or other ceremonies, or simply a feeling of belonging to a social group by engaging in the group's traditional practices. Finally, some users simply enjoy satisfying their curiosity about the effects of drugs or drug combinations they may have heard about but never tried.

In North American society, some of these reasons for use are generally approved, provided that societally imposed conditions are respected. For example, use of morphine for pain relief is generally accepted provided that the drug is prescribed for the user by a physician, obtained through legally regulated suppliers and used according to the prescriber's directions. Further, consumption of alcoholic beverages is accepted within traditional religious contexts, for celebratory toasts and as part of social gatherings, provided that the beverages are obtained from legally regulated suppliers and consumed in authorized settings, and that subsequent behavior meets societal standards — a constraint that precludes such practices as driving while intoxicated (and, in some jurisdictions, public drunkenness). In contrast, any (non-research) use of hallucinogenic drugs such as LSD is unacceptable in many segments of North American society where even possession of this drug may be illegal.

In short, society has complex rules for acceptable use of psychoactive substances, many encoded in legislation and regulation and reflecting consideration of potential risk and benefit to users and/or the community. Use that is not in accord with these rules, or the intent of these rules, may be viewed as a medical, legal and/or social problem.

Drug Dependence and Harmful Use as Substance Use Disorders

The current authoritative classifications of substance-related medical problems are provided by the *Diagnostic and Statistical Manual of Mental Disorders, Fourth Edition* (DSM-IV), published by the American Psychiatric Association, and the *ICD-10 Classification of Mental and Behavioral Disorders*, published by the World Health Organization (WHO). In both sources the general type of problem is described (e.g., dependence), and more detailed clinical criteria are included for each drug class. The brief descriptions below are adapted from these sources.

Drug Dependence

As suggested by the term "dependence," drug dependence involves a user's need for drug in order to feel and function in a way that the user considers acceptable. There are two commonly recognized types of drug dependence, reflecting the two spheres of drug effect on the body: physical dependence and psychological dependence.

- *Physical dependence* is a state in which the body has adapted to (or become dependent on) the presence of the drug at a particular concentration, so that when the drug concentration falls (because the user stops use or reduces the dose or frequency of use), the user experiences withdrawal signs and symptoms.

- *Psychological dependence* is a state in which stopping or abruptly reducing the dose of a given drug produces non-physical symptoms. Psychological dependence is characterized by emotional and mental preoccupation with the drug's effects and by a persistent craving for the drug. Craving is believed to be a major factor governing the continued self-administration of psychoactive drugs. It was once believed that the sleep disturbances and irritability that occur when heavy users stop their drug use were of psychological origin, but these symptoms are now widely believed to be subtle withdrawal effects associated with physical dependence.

The essential feature of substance dependence, described by the DSM-IV is *a cluster of cognitive, behavioral, and physiological symptoms indicating that the individual continues to use the substance despite significant substance-related problems...a pattern of repeated self-administration that usually results in tolerance, withdrawal, and compulsive drug-taking behavior.*[11]

Although this description includes tolerance and withdrawal as usual features of substance dependence, the DSM-IV notes that neither one is necessary for a diagnosis of substance dependence. For example, cannabis-dependent individuals typically show a pattern of compulsive use without any signs of tolerance or withdrawal. Conversely, some patients who have received high doses of opioids for pain relief over a prolonged period may show tolerance to opioids and experience withdrawal symptoms, without showing signs of compulsive use, and would not be deemed opioid-dependent according to this definition.

---

[11]   Reprinted with permission from the *Diagnostic and Statistical Manual of Mental Disorders*, Fourth Edition (DSM-IV). Copyright 1994 American Psychiatric Association.

Compulsive use associated with dependence is further described in the DSM-IV in terms of the following criteria:

- *The individual may take the substance in larger amounts or over a longer period than was originally intended.*
- *The individual may express a persistent desire to cut down or regulate substance use. Often there have been many unsuccessful efforts to decrease or discontinue use.*
- *The individual may spend a great deal of time obtaining the substance, using the substance, or recovering from its effects. In some instances… virtually all of the person's daily activities revolve around the substance [and] important social occupational or recreational activities may be given up or reduced because of substance use.*
- *The individual may withdraw from family activities and hobbies in order to use the substance in private or to spend more time with substance-using friends. Despite recognizing the contributing role of the substance to a psychological or physical problem… the person continues to use the substance.*[12]

Addiction

The term "addiction" is an older term that has been largely discarded in medical circles. It referred to dependent patterns of drug self-administration, including compulsive drug use, and was once popularly interpreted to include an overtone of moral weakness. Although once a useful term to refer to the situation of chronic users of a specific drug class such as opioids, it is problematic when applied to chronic users of various drug classes, because individuals "addicted" to different drugs have different profiles of physical and psychological dependence. Therefore it has been essentially replaced by the term "drug dependence," often with specific descriptive modifiers indicating the type of drug involved (e.g., amphetamine dependence), and/or the type of criteria met (e.g., physiological dependence).

It is still common, however, to refer to the "addiction liability" of a drug, which describes the propensity of a drug to produce psychological or physical dependence in those who use it. In this book, the term "addiction liability" has been replaced by the term "dependence liability" (see below).

---

[12]   Reprinted with permission from the *Diagnostic and Statistical Manual of Mental Disorders*, Fourth Edition (DSM-IV). Copyright 1994 American Psychiatric Association.

Harmful Use

The ICD-10 describes harmful use as:

> *A pattern of psychoactive substance use that is causing damage to health. The damage may be physical (as in cases of hepatitis from the self-administration of injected drugs) or mental (e.g., episodes of depressive disorder secondary to heavy consumption of alcohol). The diagnosis requires that actual damage shoud have been caused to the mental or physical health of the user.*

This focus on the user's health reflects the diagnostic focus of this definition. However, "harmful use" in its diagnostic sense must be distinguished from the more colloquial use of the term. This is emphasized by the ICD-10 as follows:

> *Harmful patterns of use are often criticized by others and frequently associated with adverse social consequences of various kinds. The fact that a pattern of use or a particular substance is disapproved of by another person or by the culture, or may have led to socially negative consequences such as arrest or marital arguments is not in itself evidence of harmful use [in the diagnostic sense].* [13]

Drug Abuse — Medical and Social Perspectives

"Drug abuse" appears to be a recently coined phrase, not entering the English language until the early 20th century. The earliest instances of its application (in the United States) appear to have been racially motivated and pejorative in the extreme: first, pertaining to the use of cocaine among southern black Americans and then to the use of opium among Chinese Americans. In both cases, unfounded fears, hatred and economic motives were behind the condemnation by the white majority of "drug abuse" among these visible minority groups. After the passage of the Harrison Narcotic Act in the United States in 1914, the non-medical use of heroin and morphine was also referred to as drug abuse. Since then, the phrase has been applied to an ever-increasing number of drugs and drug-use situations.

Drug abuse remains a highly complex, value-laden and often excessively vague term that does not lend itself completely to any single definition. Its meaning can differ from one society to another, and within the same pluralistic society a number of

---

[13]   Reprinted with permission from the *ICD-10 Classification of Mental and Behavioral Disorders*. Copyright 1992 World Health Organization.

meanings may be advanced by various subcultural groups with different values, norms and lifestyles. In addition to its many culturally based meanings, drug abuse may be defined from legal, medical, ethical-religious and various other perspectives.

For example, Jaffe (1980) observed that any use of LSD in North American society is far more likely to be viewed as drug abuse than certain occasions of "gross intoxication" with alcohol. Injecting street-purchased heroin is viewed by many as definitely drug abuse, but it has been argued that the controlled (i.e., non-destructive, non-excessive) use of heroin or any other illicit psychoactive drug on an occasional basis does not necessarily constitute drug abuse. Conversely, smoking a package of cigarettes per day is rarely referred to as drug abuse, despite the fact that such behavior poses potentially lethal consequences for the smoker, and an increased risk of health problems for non-smokers who share the smoker's environment.

The difficulty in drawing a firm line between use and abuse is further complicated by the practice in some countries of prescribing heroin on a continuing basis (i.e., maintenance therapy) for individuals who are heroin dependent. It is difficult for many people to consider such patients' injection of their prescribed heroin as legitimate use, but these same patients' use of supplementary heroin from the street as drug abuse. In fact, the difficulties in adequately defining drug abuse led the Government of Canada in 1969 to avoid the term in establishing terms of reference for a national commission of inquiry into substance use issues. Instead the so-called Le Dain Commission[14] was charged with addressing the "non-medical" use of various drugs.

Despite the problems of defining drug abuse, readers may benefit from considering some of its more widely embraced definitions, selected from both medical and social orientations. The authors recognize that none of the definitions chosen may be entirely satisfactory, but they are helpful in understanding how the term "drug abuse" is used in our society.

Medical Perspectives on Drug Abuse

In 1994, the American Psychiatric Association's (APA's) DSM-IV defined substance abuse as including the following features:

- *a maladaptive pattern of substance use manifested by recurrent and significant*

---

14   Officially, the Commission of Inquiry into the Non-Medical Use of Drugs.

> *adverse consequences related to the repeated use of substances. There may be a repeated failure to fulfil major role obligations, repeated use in situations in which it is physically hazardous, multiple legal problems, and recurrent social and inter-personal problems. [and]*
>
> - *the symptoms have never met the criteria for Substance Dependence for this class of substance.*[15]

This description stresses patterns of drug use resulting in impairment of functioning and/or in socially unacceptable behavior, without demonstrating the characteristics of substance dependence, and without necessarily damaging the user's physical or mental health, as required for harmful use. Thus a diagnosis of substance abuse is most likely in individuals who have only recently started using a substance, although some individuals continue to experience substance-related problems over the long term without developing evidence of substance dependence. Further, this definition is not considered applicable to caffeine or nicotine.

Given its diagnostic orientation, this DSM-IV statement is narrower than the following definition of drug abuse, proposed in 1988 by a task force of the American Medical Association:

> *any use of drugs that causes physical, psychological, economic, legal, or social harm to the individual user or to others affected by the drug user's behavior (Rinaldi, Steindler et al., 1988).*

The key element of this definition is the causing of harm, but the definition of harm is exceedingly broad, including the harm to the user or to others. This reflects a much broader perspective on drug abuse than earlier medical models that focused on harm to the user, and suggests convergence of medical and social perspectives on drug abuse.

Social Perspectives on Drug Abuse

In contrast to the medical-pharmacological model, the social deviance model of drug abuse generally addresses permissible (i.e., socially acceptable) and impermissible (i.e., socially unacceptable) drug use within a given society. Such judgments tend to be based on custom and tradition, coupled to varying degrees with expert opinion.

---

[15]   Reprinted with permission from the *Diagnostic and Statistical Manual of Mental Disorders*, Fourth Edition (DSM-IV). Copyright 1994 American Psychiatric Association.

Jerome Jaffe's socially based definition of drug abuse is often quoted in the North American drug abuse literature. It is thoughtfully constructed and straightforward, and generally avoids arbitrary pronouncements.

> *Drug abuse refers to the use, usually by the self-administration, of any drug in a manner that deviates from the approved medical or social patterns within a given culture. The term conveys a notion of social disapproval, and is not necessarily descriptive of any particular pattern of drug use or its potential adverse consequences (Jaffe, 1980).*

When this definition is applied to our society, all of the following can be thought of as meeting the minimum criteria for drug abuse:

- the use of any prohibited (i.e., illicit) drug
- the use of any therapeutic drug[16] for other than its intended purpose(s)
- the intentional taking of any therapeutic drug in amounts greater than prescribed and/or the self-administration of any drug by routes other than medically approved
- the excessive use of licit social drugs (such as alcohol, caffeine and tobacco)
- the taking of two or more intoxicating substances in combination in order to obtain a more pleasurable or intense "high."

The traditionally narrower medical model and the social model complement each other while serving essentially different purposes. The medical model tends to focus on diagnostic features, the user's behavior, risks and problems: failure to fulfil role obligations, use in situations in which there is risk to physical health (such as driving a motor vehicle), legal problems, and continuing use despite persistent or recurring problems. Thus, it is possible for a person to abuse drugs under a variety of conditions set out in the social deviance (i.e., socially unacceptable use) model without qualifying as a drug abuser according to the criteria of the medical model. On the other hand, virtually all circumstances of drug abuse identified in our society by the medical model fall within the scope of the social deviance model.

While the traditional medical model of drug abuse has been criticized as too restrictive, the social deviance model (as applied in our society) is thought by some to be excessively inclusive. Superficially, the social deviance model, which assesses drug

---

16   Including over-the-counter medications.

abuse from a societal perspective (i.e., what is in the best interest of both society and its collective membership), may appear to be nothing more than a series of societally imposed "dos and don'ts" that arbitrarily divides drug-taking into two fixed categories: drug abuse and acceptable drug use.

However, labelling the unsanctioned use of many psychoactive substances as socially deviant is based on awareness of the broad scope of potential harm from psychoactive substance use — harm not only to the individual, but also to the community. The consequences of drug dependence and damage to health may be considered narrowly, for some drugs, to affect only the user. However, the reality is that drug dependence and damage to the user's health will likely have adverse effects on society, such as excessive use of health care services, family dysfunction, and the user's reduced capacity to function in productive employment or volunteer activity. Therefore our society has chosen to protect the societal interest by restricting, or even banning completely, access to most psychoactive substances that have the potential to produce such adverse outcomes. A breach of such restrictions is commonly considered as drug abuse.

However, when applying a social deviance model of drug abuse to a given culture, it is not always necessary to provide evidence that a particular drug is undoubtedly damaging to health or likely to produce dependence. Some drug-intoxicated users violate or threaten widely accepted norms of behavior and social functioning within a given culture. For example, in our society, the use of alcohol is widely accepted when it is confined to amounts that do not lead to intoxication. However, drinking that results in grossly intoxicated behavior is commonly viewed as deviant, and therefore meets the criteria for abuse of alcohol.[17] Furthermore, consumption of smaller quantities of alcohol, which may not cause gross intoxication, may be considered deviant, and labelled abuse, if the resultant behavior increases the risk of harm to the community — for example, driving shortly after consuming as little as one or two drinks.

Further, the use of certain drugs may be banned completely in some cultures primarily because they can cause temporary psychological and behavioral changes that are seen

---

[17]   In fact, alcohol use and drinking to intoxication by adolescents are noteworthy anomalies to these general statements. Alcohol use by adolescents, even in small quantities, is not sanctioned in most Canadian provinces or U.S. states; yet most North American adolescents report some alcohol consumption. Paradoxically, many adolescents who drink alcoholic beverages routinely do so with the express intent of becoming intoxicated. Thus, both "underage drinking" and drinking to intoxication are deviant by the standards of the general community reflected in legislation, but not necessarily deviant in relation to the adolescent sub-population.

to be inherently harmful for at least some users. For example, the temporary but extreme loss of psychic control created by certain hallucinogens, as well as certain psychosis-mimicking effects (sensory distortions, hallucinations), were key reasons in many societies (particularly those that emphasize personal responsibility for control over one's behavior and emotions) for labelling as deviant any use of these substances. However, not all societies have reacted so negatively to the effects of hallucinogens. Many of these substances have been used ceremonially by a number of cultures throughout history, specifically to induce the very effects that other cultures have proscribed.

These examples underscore the importance of appreciating the traditions and behavioral norms of a particular culture before attempting to apply a social deviance model of drug abuse. Indeed, unlike the medical model of drug abuse, which attempts to adopt a fixed set of criteria for universal application, the social deviance model is of greatly diminished value when culture-specific variables are not considered.

Abuse Potential

The concept of "abuse potential" as used in this book involves three main contributors — the intrinsic dependence liability of a drug (i.e., the drug's fundamental propensity to produce physiological or psychological dependence), the availability of the drug within society, and its inherent harmfulness with respect to the direct physical and psychological effects it produces in the user. The actual abuse potential of any given drug will depend on the degree to which these various factors interact to promote or limit widespread abuse.

Dependence Liability

The dependence liability of a drug, i.e., the tendency of a drug to produce physical and psychological dependence, varies from one drug to another and depends on three drug factors: the intrinsic pharmacological nature of the specific drug (i.e., the pharmacological activity of the drug molecule itself), the route by which it is administered and the amount of the drug used.[18]

---

18   Of course, susceptibility of the individual user is also a factor in both physical and psychological dependence.

Nature of the Drug: Both animal and human experiments have shown that drugs are natural reinforcers in much the same way as food, water and sex. That is, the pleasurable effects produced by a drug increase the probability that it will be taken again. Drugs vary dramatically in their intrinsic reinforcing properties. For example, heroin and cocaine, which produce intensely pleasurable effects, have a very high intrinsic dependence liability, whereas anxiolytics (e.g., diazepam) have much less intensely pleasurable properties and, as a result, a significantly lower intrinsic dependence liability.

The intrinsic dependence liability of new drugs is typically determined in animal studies, because the strength of a drug's reinforcing properties in animals is a good predictor of its reinforcing properties in human beings, and the drug preferences demonstrated by animals are similar to those in human beings. For example, the highly addictive nature of cocaine in humans is reflected in a strong preference of animals for this drug relative to many other classes of drug. In fact, cocaine has such intense reinforcing properties that animals will prefer it even when food, water and sex are available as alternatives and even when exercising their preference leads to death. Because of this similar human/animal response, animals are used in drug-screening procedures to ensure that new substances being considered for release as legitimate medications do not have an unacceptably high dependence liability.

Route of Administration: Drugs that can be administered by routes that produce rapid effects have greater abuse potential than drugs that can be taken only by the slower routes. For example, drugs that are taken by sniffing, inhalation or intravenous injection are generally more abuse-prone than those of equal intrinsic dependence liability that can be taken only orally, since the former routes allow for more rapid and intense gratification.

Amount Used: For any psychoactive drug that can produce intense gratification, the probability of developing dependence increases with an increase in the frequency of administration and the size of dose used. However, the contribution of frequency of use is limited by the development of tolerance with regular use.[19] With alcohol beverages, for example, occasional consumption involving low to moderate amounts is unlikely to create a state of dependence in the user. However, frequent high-dose use of alcoholic beverages greatly increases the probability of dependence.

---

19   See the discussion of tolerance earlier in this section.

Availability

Availability of the drug within society is a major factor determining the level of use/abuse of psychoactive drugs — the more widespread and abundant the supply, the more they are likely to be abused. Alcohol, for example, which has only moderate intrinsic dependence liability, is nonetheless the most highly abused psychoactive substance in our society, in large part because of its widespread availability. In contrast, heroin, which has very high intrinsic dependence liability, has traditionally posed a much lower overall social risk in North America because of the restrictions placed on its availability. Legislation and law enforcement activity severely curtail heroin's legal and illegal manufacture, possession, distribution and importation. This is an example of the powerful social impact of availability: the more available a psychoactive drug is, the greater will be the number of people using it at higher dose levels. Therefore, it often becomes necessary to restrict access to a drug of even low to medium dependence liability.

Inherent Harmfulness

Inherent harmfulness or "toxicity" refers to the body damage or even death that a drug has the potential to produce. If a drug is perceived as a serious risk to health or life, even at low doses, large numbers of people are unlikely to use it, even if it is widely available and can produce desirable effects in addition to its toxic effects.[20]

Methyl alcohol (methanol) and isopropyl alcohol (isopropanol) are two examples of drugs that are widely available and that can produce inebriating effects similar to those produced by ethyl alcohol (ethanol, beverage alcohol). However, both methyl alcohol and isopropyl alcohol have a high degree of toxicity. Methyl alcohol, consumed even in small doses, may cause blindness and death, while isopropyl alcohol (often found in rubbing compounds and other non-drinkable commercial products) is believed to produce severe liver and kidney impairment when consumed regularly in very small amounts, and in higher doses it can also be fatal. However, since both are known to have a very high degree of inherent harmfulness, they have a very low abuse potential.

---

[20]   The determination of which effects should be considered toxic is somewhat arbitrary and in part depends on the viewpoint of the observer. Obviously, drug-induced carcinogenesis (e.g., lung cancer) would be considered toxic by virtually everybody. On the other hand, a cannabis-induced "high" might be desirable to the adolescent user, but the disruption of short-term memory and concentration that occurs as part of the intoxication would be thought of as harmful by the user's teacher.

Background Reading

Alksne, H. (1981). The social bases of substance abuse. In J.H. Lowinson & P. Ruiz (Eds.), *Substance Abuse: Clinical Problems and Perspectives*. Baltimore: Williams and Wilkens.

American Psychiatric Association. (1994). *Diagnostic and Statistical Manual of Mental Disorders, DSM-IV* (4th edition). Washington: American Psychiatric Association.

Jaffe, J. (1980). Drug addiction and drug abuse. In A.G. Gilman, L.S. Goodman & A. Gilman (Eds.), *The Pharmacological Basis of Therapeutics*. New York: Macmillan.

O'Brien, C.P. (1996). Drug addiction and drug abuse. In J.G. Hardman, L.E. Limbird, P.B. Molinoff, R.W. Rudden & A.G. Gilman (Eds.), *Goodman and Gilman's The Pharmacological Basis of Therapeutics* (9th edition). New York/Toronto: McGraw-Hill Health Professions Division.

Pratt, W.B. & Taylor, P. (Eds.) (1990). *Principles of Drug Action. The Basis of Pharmacology* (3rd edition). New York: Churchill Livingston.

Rinaldi, R.C., Steindler, E.M., Wilford, B.B. & Goodwin, D. (1988). Clarification and standardization of substance abuse terminology. *Journal of the American Medical Association, 259 (4)*, 555–557.

World Health Organization. (1992). *ICD-10 Classification of Mental and Behavioral Disorders. Clinical descriptions and diagnostic guidelines*. Geneva: World Health Organization.

Zinberg, N.E., Harding, W.M. & Apsler, R. (1978). What is drug abuse? *Journal of Drug Issues, 8*, 9–35.

2

Major Drug Classes

CNS DEPRESSANTS: ALCOHOLS

See the chapters in Section 3 on ethyl alcohol (ethanol, beverage alcohol), disulfiram (Antabuse®), methyl alcohol (methanol, wood alcohol) and isopropyl alcohol (2-propanol). Section 5 includes brief notes on acamposate (calcium acetylhomotaurinate) and calcium carbimide (Temposil®).

Alcohols such as ethyl alcohol (ethanol, beverage alcohol), methyl alcohol (methanol, wood alcohol) and isopropyl alcohol are members of the chemical family sometimes called low molecular weight aliphatic alcohols. Because of their similar chemical structures they share many properties in pure form, for example, they are clear, colorless liquids that are completely miscible with water (i.e., mix completely with water in all proportions), they evaporate quickly at skin temperature, and when they are mixed with water the resulting solution freezes at a lower temperature than pure water (so that they are useful in various types of antifreeze products). Further, they can be chemically oxidized: methyl alcohol to formaldehyde (and later, formic acid); ethyl alcohol to acetaldehyde (and later, acetic acid); and isopropyl alcohol (less readily) to acetone. These oxidation reactions of alcohols occur both in the chemical laboratory and in the body where they are catalyzed by enzymes such as alcohol dehydrogenase (and, in the case of methanol and ethanol, aldehyde dehydrogenase).

Given these similarities, it is not surprising that these alcohols are similar in some of their drug actions. In other drug actions — and in their toxicity — however, they are dramatically different, with the result that they have very different uses. One important similarity is their central nervous system (CNS)-depressant effects.[1] All three depress the functions of the brain and other parts of the central nervous system, although the potency of methyl alcohol is much less than that of ethyl alcohol and isopropyl alcohol. Also, both ethyl alcohol and isopropyl alcohol have antiseptic properties, killing a wide range of micro-organisms upon contact. However, these alcohols are markedly different in their toxicity. These differences in toxicity reflect, to a considerable extent, the different rates at which they are oxidized in the body and the different products they form as a result of the oxidation processes. Because of its metabolism in the body to formaldehyde and formic acid, which are more toxic, methyl alcohol acts as a poison for both humans and animals, and should not be used either internally or on the skin. Its use is restricted to household and industrial solvents that require warnings about their poisonous nature. Isopropyl alcohol is less rapidly oxidized in the body, but its oxidation produces acetone, which also has CNS-depressant activity[2] and is harmful to the body in large quantity. As a result, in medicine isopropyl alcohol is restricted to external uses, in which it is applied to the skin in rubbing compounds and as an ingredient in some lotions. In contrast, ethyl alcohol is metabolized most rapidly, and the products of its metabolism are much less toxic to humans or animals. Therefore ethyl alcohol is widely used both internally and externally: in a wide range of alcoholic beverages; as a solvent in a wide range of medicines prepared for oral use (including many cough syrups and mouthwashes) or for application to the skin; with denaturants[3] in rubbing alcohol preparations; and in many cosmetics.

---

[1]   Depression here refers to a slowing/reduction in function rather than to mood or emotional depression.

[2]   As a result, the CNS depression caused by isopropyl alcohol is longer lasting than that of ethyl alcohol.

[3]   Denaturants are substances that are added to ethyl alcohol to make it unpalatable for consumption as a beverage. A manufacturer requiring ethyl alcohol as an ingredient in products for external medicinal use, cosmetics or other non-beverage preparations, normally purchases ethyl alcohol to which an approved denaturant has been added, in order to avoid paying an excise tax on the alcohol or storing it under stringent security and complying with strict documentation requirements concerning its use in manufacturing.

Ethyl Alcohol as Beverage Alcohol[4]

Ethyl alcohol is the oldest known sedative/hypnotic and intoxicant. The use of fermented alcoholic beverages dates back to at least 6400 BC, when beer and berry wine were introduced; indeed, some historians trace alcohol use even further back to 8000 BC, when mead was prepared from honey. The date of the discovery of distillation remains uncertain; however, many experts believe the process was used in Arabia in about 800 BC. The word "alcohol" is derived from an Arabic word meaning "finely divided spirit," and originally it referred to that part of the wine collected through distillation — the essence of wine. References to distillation at about the same time in China and India have also been found.

Brewing and wine-making are based on the biochemical process called fermentation. Undoubtedly the earliest fermented beverages were accidental discoveries. Fermentation occurs when certain kinds of yeast act on sugar in the presence of water, with the yeast deriving energy from the sugar by converting it into ethyl alcohol. However, when the alcohol concentration reaches about 15 per cent, fermentation stops.[5]

Distillation is the process whereby higher alcohol concentrations can be obtained from the crude fermentation product. The product, containing both water and alcohol, is heated, and the vapors are then collected and condensed into liquid again. Alcohol has a boiling temperature of 78.3 C and water 100 C. Because of this difference in boiling points, the vapor produced by heating the original fermentation product contains a higher concentration of alcohol than the original fermentation mash and, when the vapor is cooled, the resulting liquid is similarly enriched in alcohol. Repeating the process increases the alcohol concentration of the distillate further — up to a theoretically possible concentration of 95 per cent.[6] However, modern distilled beverages usually contain a substantially lower concentration of alcohol.

---

4   In the remainder of this chapter the term "alcohol" is used to refer to ethyl alcohol unless otherwise noted, and the term "alcoholic beverage(s)" is used to refer to beverage(s) containing ethyl alcohol.

5   Another factor that may limit the concentration of alcohol in the final fermentation product is the availability of sugar in the yeast mixture (mash); that is, smaller amounts of sugar in the initial mixture produce lower concentrations of alcohol.

6   Production of 100 per cent pure alcohol (i.e., absolute alcohol) requires use of different techniques.

Proof scales are widely used measures of alcohol concentration in various beverages.[7] The two widely used modern proof scales, the American and British, differ in certain respects. The U.S. proof strength (also used formerly in Canada) is twice the percentage of alcohol in the beverage. Absolute alcohol, by this measure, is 200 proof, and a distilled spirit that is 40 per cent alcohol by volume is 80 proof. In the more complex long-standing British system, 100 proof is 57.15 per cent alcohol by volume at a temperature of 15.6 C, and concentrations are expressed as degrees over and under (100) proof.

Alcohol has become one of the most popular and widely used psychoactive drugs, and it has an important role in the social behaviors of most cultural groups, although some (such as the followers of Islam) expressly forbid its consumption. Traditionally, it has been used for three major purposes:

- in medicinal use, as an anesthetic and for its sedating and sleep-inducing (i.e., sedative-hypnotic) properties[8]
- for religious and other celebratory occasions and rites, including sacramental use among Christians and Jews
- for recreation.

Virtually all cultures that have permitted recreational use of alcohol have also recognized the potentially harmful (and even hazardous) effects of heavy acute and chronic consumption. Accordingly, each has developed its own complex pattern of social and legal sanctions to discourage alcohol abuse and/or punish those abusers whose behavior harms, or presents a risk of harm, to others in the community.

Ethyl Alcohol as a CNS Depressant

Like most drugs classed as sedative/hypnotics, alcohol can produce a spectrum of CNS-depressant effects ranging from mild sedation and relaxation to anesthesia,

---

[7]   The term "proof" is believed to originate from a rough test used until the 17th century to determine the quantity of alcohol in a given liquid. Gunpowder and a sample of the liquid alleged to contain alcohol were mixed and fire applied. If the liquid contained a sufficient proportion of alcohol, the powder would ignite. Thus, gunpowder ignition was "proof" of the alcohol content.

[8]   The traditional use of an alcoholic beverage before meals was based on ethyl alcohol's relaxant (CNS depressant) effect and/or stimulation of gastric secretion, and in some cases the alleged digestive benefits of certain herbal principles contained in the beverage. Recent evidence of alcohol's effect in reducing risk of death from cardiovascular disease for low level drinkers has caused some individuals to use alcoholic beverages for this purpose, in some cases with the concurrence of their physician.

coma, and death from respiratory arrest. In the past, ethyl alcohol was widely used as an anesthetic. However, doses necessary to produce anesthesia also produce dangerous and uncontrollable depression of those brain centres responsible for respiration and circulation, as well as unpredictable involuntary muscle movements and, in some individuals, erratic and possibly highly aggressive behavior.

In a drug-free state of wakefulness, the brain receives a constant barrage of stimuli from the environment; normally, these stimuli generate a level of excitation that we associate with alertness. More intense or greater numbers of stimuli produce uncomfortable levels of excitation that we usually experience as anxiety or tension. At low doses, alcohol and other sedative-hypnotic drugs depress the central nervous system, raising the threshold for normal stimulation. As a result, fewer stimuli reach the higher brain centres, and those that do are reduced in intensity. The effects of low doses experienced by an individual user are affected by setting and user expectations, particularly the user's reason for consuming the alcohol. Typically reduced levels of excitation and alertness are experienced as relaxation or sedation. In some users the most noticeable effects are drowsiness, mildly to moderately impaired motor co-ordination (e.g., swaying) and some clouding of mental functions. A tired individual, or one who is particularly sensitive to the effects of alcohol or who already has a CNS-depressant drug present in body tissues, may become very drowsy and fall asleep.

A normal person consuming a low dose of an alcoholic beverage on a social occasion is likely to experience a period of mild release of inhibitions, which often passes as a pleasant state of stimulation. This is the basis for alcohol's widespread recreational use. However, alcohol does not exert true stimulant effects; rather, "[the] apparent stimulation results from the unrestrained activity of various parts of the brain that have been freed from inhibition as a result of the depression of inhibitory control mechanisms" (Ritchie, 1975). This effect is termed "disinhibition." Some users experience euphoria; others experience decidedly dysphoric reactions such as feelings of hostility or depression. As behavioral disinhibition increases with higher doses, hostile feelings may be translated into action. Anger, aggression and even physical violence, for example, are a common result of consumption of high doses of alcohol in our society.

Moderate doses of alcohol taken by healthy adults do not ordinarily exert harmful respiratory or cardiovascular effects. However, mild respiratory depression and a small drop in blood pressure often occur. This reduction in blood pressure results, at least in part, from dilation of capillaries at the surface of the body; this capillary dilation is evident in the familiar flushing and sensation of warmth experienced by many drinkers, (i.e., loss of heat to the environment). Although these may be pleasant sensations under some circumstances, the combination of heat loss and CNS depression may be fatal for people who are alcohol-intoxicated and remain outdoors without adequate clothing under extremely cold conditions.

At sufficiently high doses alcohol may be fatal. Death may result from the direct effects of alcohol on the central nervous system. However, other effects of alcohol may be contributing factors: for example, alcohol-intoxicated individuals may vomit and inhale (aspirate) their vomit, with resultant damage to the lungs. (For more detailed information, see the chapter on ethyl alcohol in Section 3.)

Abuse of Ethyl Alcohol — Problems for Users, Families and Society

Alcohol and tobacco are unique among the psychoactive drugs that pose serious health,[9] social and legal problems in our society — unique because adults can obtain them without a physician's prescription. Moreover, alcohol's easy availability, its high degree of social acceptability, and the popularity of its psychoactive effects are factors that, in combination, all too easily allow abuse. The consequences are often harmful for both the abuser and others. In fact, the incidence of socially deviant behavior resulting from abusive drinking is undoubtedly far greater than that caused by all other drugs of abuse combined.

Violent Behavior toward Others

Alcohol depresses the inhibitory/emotional control centres of the brain. Although there are substantial individual variations in the type and intensity of response, the likelihood of greater emotional disinhibition generally increases with the amount of alcohol consumed within a given period. In most cases, external controls, as well as a lifetime of training, are sufficient to dissuade most people from engaging in violence. However, many studies have found that in most violent crimes, the attacker, the victim, or both have consumed alcohol. Aggressors and victims also are often known to each other or are related. In fact, clinicians working with the families of male alcoholics find that the large majority of the subjects' partners have been the victims

---

9   Health problems associated with alcohol abuse and dependence are discussed in the chapter on ethyl (beverage) alcohol in Section 3.

of physical abuse by their spouses at least once, and frequently more often. The same applies to the children of alcoholics, irrespective of the sex of the drinking parent.

Although a history of alcohol-related violent behavior is the best predictor of future violent behavior, it is very rare to find an individual who behaves violently on all drinking occasions. Rather, violence tends to be relatively infrequent, given the total number of drinking episodes in the lifetime of the sometimes violent drinker. Also, given the enormous number of drinkers in our society, only a very small fraction behave violently at any time in their lives, even after heavy alcohol consumption.

Alcohol-related violence is a complex interpersonal phenomenon. For the aggressor, high doses of alcohol can impair judgment, lower the frustration tolerance threshold and the effectiveness of personal controls, increase the likelihood of risk-taking behavior and often produce inflated confidence. These effects tend to create some of the conditions conducive to violence. So-called "senseless" violence — violence without any apparent motive and without serious psychological disturbance — is relatively infrequent with the use of alcohol.[10]

In instances of alcohol-related violence, the behavior of the victim need not be hostile in order to provoke the aggressor, although mutual hostility is not unusual when both aggressor and victim have been drinking. Attempts by the victim to avoid a confrontation may actually provoke hostility from the aggressor. Avoidance may be interpreted by the drinking aggressor (often correctly) as fearfulness, which has been shown to increase the probability of aggressive and attack behavior in humans (and many animal species) even when alcohol is not involved.

Self-Destructive Behavior

Many people resort to using alcohol to relieve emotional depression. Unfortunately, however, its disinhibiting effects can exacerbate their depression. Moreover, it increases the possibility of impulsive behavior and in large doses can severely impair judgment. This combination of effects has often resulted in suicidal action in clinically depressed people.

---

[10]   By contrast, for example, in the case of violence perpetrated by someone in a state of amphetamine-induced psychosis, the actions are based on an internal delusional system that results in a highly impaired ability to interpret reality correctly.

Drug overdose is the most common means of suicide attempt. Alcohol taken alone can produce lethal results if very large quantities are rapidly consumed (e.g., 600 to 800 mL, or 20 to 30 oz., of spirits (40 per cent alcohol by volume) within an hour or less). However, most successful suicides, as well as many accidental deaths, involving alcohol overdose also involve concurrent overdose of other drugs, usually other sedative/hypnotics or anxiolytics. Despite their relative safety, large amounts of benzodiazepines can dangerously increase the respiratory-depressant effects of large amounts of alcohol. When high doses of alcohol are combined with such potent sedative/hypnotic drugs as barbiturates, the lethal risk is much greater, as both agents can profoundly depress the respiratory control centres in the brain.

Drinking and Driving

Driving a car is a complicated task; the addition of alcohol makes it even more complex. Driving involves three elements: skill (the ability to perform), processing (making judgments while performing a number of tasks) and attitude. It should be noted that the factors considered in the following discussion of driving apply also to flying airplanes, driving boats and snowmobiles, and handling any motorized vehicle or complex machinery.

The relationship between the blood level and impairment of driving skills is not a simple one. At low blood levels there can be a slight improvement of performance, possibly due to relaxation. This is followed at higher levels by a significant deterioration. In general we can say that well-learned tasks are less affected by alcohol than are newly learned tasks, and the tasks akin to natural movement are also less affected. However, driving is not just a composite of individual tasks such as stopping or starting. Its related tasks involve the brain's ability to process information and to make judgments, and alcohol has a much greater and more deleterious effect on processing information than on physical skills.

Driving is a "divided-attention task." That is, it involves several simultaneous tasks. Impaired drivers whose physical driving skills may not be adversely affected by relatively low blood alcohol levels may nevertheless become involved in accidents because they cannot integrate quickly enough the many pieces of information that must suddenly be considered in an emergency or in a suddenly complicated driving situation.

Possibly the most dangerous effect that alcohol has on driving, however, is on the driver's attitude. It has been found to increase willingness to engage in risk-taking behavior. Obviously, increased risk-taking increases the probability of accidents. This alteration in the risk-taking threshold is not related to ability to perform the necessary manoeuvres or to process information.

An often-cited example of the increased risk-taking threshold is a British experiment carried out in the 1950s (Cohen, Dearnaley & Hansel, 1958). Bus drivers, after drinking, were asked to drive through a gap between a pair of light standards. Some drivers received no alcohol, others received 2 oz. (57 mL) of whisky, and a third group received 6 oz. (170 mL) of whisky. Drivers were asked to indicate the narrowest gap through which they thought they could always drive their buses, and the width of gap through which they were willing to try. Finally, drivers had to attempt to actually drive through the gap. Both the control group and the group that consumed 2 oz. of whisky thought they could always drive their buses through a gap of 8 ft. 1.5 in. (2.89m). (This figure and the following are averages.) The control group was able to get through a gap of 8 ft. 8.5 in. (2.60m), and the other group through a gap of 8 ft. 7 in. (2.62m). After they had drunk 6 oz. of whisky, the third group thought they could always get through a gap of only 7 ft. 10.5 in. (2.40m), but actually got through a gap of 8 ft. 7.5 in. (2.63m). It is also interesting to note that three of the drivers who had consumed only 2 oz. of whisky were willing to attempt to drive through a gap that was actually 14 inches (0.36m) narrower than their buses.

The ability to drive may also be impaired by other CNS-depressant drugs, even those taken for therapeutic reasons, such as anxiolytics and barbiturates. When these are taken in combination with alcohol, the resulting impairment is likely to be significantly increased. Certain other drugs may also adversely affect driving performance. For example, many antihistamines have side effects that include drowsiness and sedation, and when they are taken in conjunction with alcohol, the impact of these side effects on driving ability is likely to be even more pronounced. In fact, if a driver has consumed any drug that may produce such CNS-depressant side effects, no quantity of alcohol can be safely consumed.

Breathalyser Measurement of Blood Alcohol Level

Most modern societies have established laws that permit the police in certain circumstances to demand a measurement of blood alcohol levels from those whom they suspect to be impaired at the wheel of a car. These laws are a response to the large number of deaths and disabling accidents that are associated with drinking and driving. Though there are various ways of measuring blood alcohol levels, the most common official method currently in use is the breathalyser, a machine that allows rapid and accurate measurement of blood alcohol levels by analysis of breath samples. The technique works because alcohol is volatile at body temperature.

Breath analysis allows accurate determination of blood alcohol levels for the following reason. After alcohol is absorbed into the bloodstream, it is rapidly delivered to the lungs, where it equilibrates with air in the little sacs known as alveoli. (That is, the amount of alcohol in the air in the lungs is directly proportional to the concentration of alcohol in the blood passing through the lungs.) Because of the equilibrium between lung air and lung blood, a measure of alcohol in lung air is an accurate reflection of the lung blood alcohol level. In human beings, at equilibrium, 2.1 litres of air contain as much alcohol as 1 mL of blood. This ratio is constant in all humans and has been confirmed and officially certified as a standard by the U.S. National Safety Council's Committee on Alcohol and Drugs. The breathalyser measures the alcohol concentration in the lung air with great accuracy.

Three steps are involved in using the breathalyser. First, a deep lung breath sample is collected by having the subject blow into a piston constructed to retain the air last expelled from the lungs. The apparatus (piston) is then heated so that water vapor in the breath does not condense. (If the water were allowed to condense, the alcohol would dissolve in it, and the analysis of the breath would give much lower alcohol value than was really representative.) In the second step, the retained air is bubbled into a mixture of potassium dichromate and sulphuric acid plus a catalyst. This solution converts the alcohol into acetic acid and some of the potassium dichromate into chromic sulphate. The final step consists of measuring the concentration of the converted products. The potassium dichromate is yellow in solution, and the chromic sulphate is green. The amount of color change is directly related to the amount of alcohol converted. The whole procedure, then, is a matter of measuring the decrease in concentration of the yellow color. The less yellow the solution, the more alcohol existed in the original breath sample. The machine is designed so that this decrease can be read directly as blood level in a matter of minutes without calculation. This final conversion step is independent of outside factors and is not influenced by significant concentration differences in the solution components because only a change in color is measured. The most important variable is the dimension of the vial of solution used. The dimension of each is checked with a template provided with the machine.

Being able to measure blood alcohol in this way is important pharmacologically. Alcohol levels are related to lung blood, which, after a short trip through the heart, goes directly to the brain. Thus lung blood alcohol levels correspond very closely to levels in the brain, and it is the brain level of alcohol that determines the degree of impairment.

The breathalyser is particularly valuable from a legal perspective because it delivers the sample for analysis directly into the machine. There is no question of the sample being lost or mislabelled. However, if the subject is unable to be brought to a machine, a breath sample can be collected in a plastic bag and stored for 48 hours; it is then analysed in the normal manner and, if proper procedures have been followed, will yield the same results as if it had been tested at the same time as collected. Users of the machine have a checklist of steps that, if followed closely, result in very high accuracy and replicability of blood alcohol level readings.

If alcoholic beverages or oral preparations containing alcohol (e. g., some mouth-washes and cough medicines) are consumed just before a breathalyser measurement, there will be a falsely high reading; however, this misleading effect will disappear in fewer than 15 minutes. It is standard procedure, therefore, to observe subjects to ensure that they take nothing containing alcohol by mouth for at least that period. The same delay is also necessary following vomiting.

Other factors make a slight but not significant difference to the blood alcohol measurement. Foods that have a strong odor, such as garlic and onions, have no appreciable effect on the determination. The acetone on the breath of diabetics is not a significant factor in the apparent blood alcohol levels, nor are the increased amounts of acetaldehyde excreted by the lungs of people using Antabuse®.

Non-beverage alcohols (e.g., isopropyl alcohol) and paraldehyde will react to the breathalyser in the same way as ethyl alcohol. However, the presence of these materials can be detected either by odor or by other means and can easily be differentiated from ethyl alcohol by their different rates of reaction. For ethyl alcohol, the measurement will be the same at 90 seconds as at 120 seconds after the reaction with dichromate. For these other substances, the 120-second reading will be appreciably higher.

Blood alcohol values can be expressed in a variety of ways, but the level is usually given as a percentage indicating alcohol weight in grams per 100 mL of blood volume. The legally prohibited blood level for drivers in Canada, for example, would be more than 80 mg (of absolute ethyl alcohol) per 100 mL (80 mg/100 mL). In Europe, however, the level is generally given in grams per litre; thus the same impairing value would be expressed as more than 0.8 g/L. In a third system, the level is given in grams per 100 mL, and the same value would be expressed as 0.08g/100 mL.

Although there are varying legal blood alcohol level values in different jurisdictions (ranging from 50 to 150 mg/100 mL), the purpose in all cases is the same. Blood alcohol levels serve as a legal benchmark and constitute reliable evidence for prosecution of drinking drivers.

While it is generally true that people with higher-than-legal blood alcohol levels are impaired, it has been argued that a person may exceed these levels and drive as well as someone else with a lower blood alcohol level. However, the traffic system operates on a societal level of competence. The already difficult traffic situation would become impossible if people drove at their minimum level of competence. Like legal speed limits, legal blood alcohol levels are not foolproof predictors of whether any single individual is driving better or worse than the mean response of the population of all drivers. What these levels really indicate is that people who exceed them are at greater-than-acceptable risk of impairment of their driving skills.

For a simple overview of blood levels, we can say that below a blood alcohol level of 50 mg/100 mL most but not all drivers are reasonably safe from alcohol-induced impairment. (This assumes that a driver has not consumed any other drugs that could add to impairment.) As the level approaches 80 mg/100 mL, the drinker moves progressively into the area of impairment. Blood alcohol levels of 150 to 250 mg/100 mL clearly indicate intoxication. At blood levels approaching 400 mg/100 mL and higher, the person is usually "dead drunk." Levels of 500 mg/100 mL and higher are potentially lethal.

The question of concern to many people is how many drinks are required to produce the above levels. The answer to this question depends on many factors, including:

- the amount of alcohol in each drink
- the rate of absorption, which is largely determined by the contents and condition of the individual's stomach and small intestine
- the rate at which alcohol is metabolized
- the individual's weight, sex and body composition.

For further information, see the chapter on ethyl alcohol in Section 3.

Some drinkers may become both legally and behaviorally impaired at levels of consumption that would not cause a normal person any difficulty.

Alcoholism, Problem Drinking and Alcohol Dependence

Alcoholism is a traditional term that has been largely replaced in clinical circles by terms with more specific definitions. The World Health Organization (WHO) defined alcoholism as an impairment resulting from alcohol abuse that can be manifested in "a noticeable mental disturbance or an interference with...bodily and mental health, interpersonal relations, and...smooth social and economic functioning." Jellinek, a pioneer in the field of alcoholism in the 1940s and '50s, essentially agreed with the elements of this definition, but also proposed that alcoholism is a distinct disease. He contended that a true state of physical dependence occurs in the large majority of alcoholics and that most alcoholics cannot control their intake. Since Jellinek's time, the pendulum has swung in both directions. Some researchers have come to believe that alcoholism is primarily a psychological rather than a medical disorder, while genetic studies have given support to the illness model of alcoholism. While our understanding of alcoholism continues to develop, it is clear that Jellinek's illness concept was largely responsible for challenging the widely held belief that alcoholism is a state of moral degeneracy.

Today it is recognized that alcohol problems occur along a spectrum of severity. "Problem drinkers" drink above the guideline limits for "low-risk" drinking (see the chapter on ethyl alcohol in Section 3) and may have one or more alcohol-related problems, but do not have the clinical syndrome of alcohol dependence. They outnumber alcohol-dependent individuals by a ratio of at least four to one, and as a result, the bulk of alcohol-related illness and death occurs in the problem drinking group. Such individuals often respond to brief advice and reduced drinking strategies.

Alcohol dependence is a clinical syndrome recognized by the American Psychiatric Association, with criteria specified in its Diagnostic and Statistical Manual (DSM-IV). Consistent with the DSM-IV's generic criteria for substance use dependence, alcohol dependence is characterized by "a cluster of cognitive, behavioral, and physiological symptoms indicating that the individual continues to use [alcohol] despite significant [alcohol-related] problems," and a pattern of use that usually results in tolerance, withdrawal and compulsive use. Clinically alcohol-dependent individuals are often seen to engage in continued drinking despite severe physical,[11] employment, family or social consequences. They are often preoccupied with alcohol, neglectful of their responsibilities, and unable to moderate their drinking, and often experience both physical and psychological dependence.

Drinking Patterns

Drinking patterns, and therefore associated types of alcohol problems, vary from one culture to another. A well-known Southern European style of drinking involves the everyday consumption of wine. If large enough amounts are consumed on each occasion, this style of drinking is characterized less by drunkenness than by a high rate of alcohol-related disease and deaths.

A contrasting drinking style common in North America is weekend drinking. A significant percentage of North Americans drink irregularly and modestly throughout the week but indulge in heavier drinking, mostly of beer and distilled spirits, on the weekends (i.e., weekend binges). Other "binge" drinkers may abstain for extended periods and then engage in extremely abusive drinking for several days and in some cases for much longer. All forms of binge drinking are likely to be severely harmful to the drinker and may jeopardize both his or her family and social circle, and often other innocent members of society.

In North America, there are also other widely recognized stereotypes of alcohol-dependent individuals. Two of the most visible of these are skid-row drinkers and more socially integrated drinkers who nonetheless drink large quantities of alcohol every day or on most days. Drinkers in the latter group, after their first drink, usually lose control over their alcohol consumption and tend to drink until they are intoxicated or fall asleep.

---

11   A discussion of health problems associated with chronic high dose alcohol use is presented in the ethyl alcohol chapter in Section 3.

The Bases of Alcoholism and Alcohol Dependence[12]

Our understanding of alcoholism is still in the theoretical and speculative stage, and there are many different theories or models that attempt to explain its roots or causes. Over time there appears to be increasing recognition that this complex problem has multiple roots.

Some genetic/biological theories propose that alcohol dependence results from inherited (i.e., genetically determined) metabolic abnormalities such as an atypical form of enzyme or an enzyme deficiency or an endocrine imbalance. Such theories stem, in part, from the fact that a much higher rate of alcoholism occurs among the children of alcoholics than of non-alcoholics. However, no specific genetic abnormality has yet been found to occur in all alcohol-dependent individuals. Furthermore, some critics have suggested that the higher rate of dependence among children of alcoholics may be due to behavioral coping styles learned at an early age.

Many researchers in the field of personality theory have stressed a psychodynamic cause for alcohol dependence. Considerable attention has been directed toward the search for common personality characteristics and abnormalities underlying alcoholism, that is, a search for the "alcoholic personality." However, researchers have concluded that no currently available measure of personality can discriminate accurately between dependent and non-dependent users.

Other investigators have proposed a behavioral model of alcoholism. In this scheme, alcohol is viewed as a drug that can rapidly reduce tension and anxiety, replacing unpleasant feelings with a state of relaxation, disinhibition and pleasurable intoxication. For some drinkers, the too-frequent association of alcohol consumption with tension reduction and the pleasurable effects of drinking has several negative implications. Such drinkers:

- resort to alcohol in an ever-increasing variety of stressful situations, even when the stress is relatively mild
- drink with increasing frequency under non-stressful conditions to achieve desired alcohol effects
- may ultimately drink alcohol in part to relieve the stress produced by its absence in the body.

---

12   Many of the studies that inform our understanding of problem drinking and alcohol dependence involved subjects who met the criteria for alcoholism of that time.

Finally, many observers believe that sociocultural factors play an important role as determinants of alcoholism. They correctly note that the rate of alcoholism is the highest in those cultures that have a permissive attitude toward regular alcohol use and in those cultures in which alcohol is the most freely available.

It must be stressed that none of these possible factors is totally incompatible with any of the others. Alcoholism appears to be very complex, with a number of factors contributing to the development of this pervasive problem.

Alcoholism and the Family

For more than 30 years there has been increasing interest in the effects of alcoholism on the spouse and children of the alcoholic. Particular emphasis has been placed upon whether unique behavior patterns or certain psychological disorders are more likely to develop in alcoholic as opposed to non-alcoholic families. The risk of emotional problems for the children of alcoholics is considerably greater than for children in the general population, although not greater than for the children of parents with other serious psychiatric disorders. One pioneering author, Margaret Cork, on the basis of her own clinical impressions, reported that 92 per cent of offspring she studied who had at least one alcoholic parent were assessed as being from "fairly" to "very seriously" emotionally damaged. Subsequent research has generally substantiated her findings.

No unique behavior patterns have yet been uncovered for the partners of male alcoholics, and even less is known about the partners of female alcoholics. Their strategies or coping styles range from attack to withdrawal, depending on their own predispositions and the behavior of the drinking spouse. Nevertheless, clinical observations consistently find female partners to be hostile, despairing and resentful of their life situation. Suicidal gestures or attempts to leave the alcoholic partner are not uncommon, and the majority appear to need professional counselling.

Treatment for Alcohol Problems

A wide array of psychosocial, sociobehavioral and pharmacological therapies have, at one time or another, been used with alcohol-dependent individuals. These include psychoanalysis, Gestalt therapy, insight-oriented therapy, hypnosis, LSD, various types of counselling and cognitive-behavioral strategies, combinations of these treatments in specialized inpatient and outpatient programs, and the use of so-called "protective" (or alcohol deterrent) drugs such as disulfiram (Antabuse®; see the chapter on disulfiram in Section 3), calcium carbimide (Temposil®; see Section 5), and acamposate (calcium acetylhomotaurinate) to deter patients from drinking or to reduce craving. Among the more recent developments are self-directed recovery programs using self-help manuals, in some cases complemented by telephone consultation with trained therapists. Further, the worldwide self-help/mutual support model of Alcoholics Anonymous[13] has stimulated the development of other self-help/mutual support programs.

Success rates vary considerably, with the variation appearing to depend somewhat on the definition of successful treatment outcome. For example, those studies that define success in terms of total abstinence from alcohol have had substantially lower success rates than those that define success in terms of improved control over drinking. Another key factor is the personal profile of the alcoholic client. For example, those who have an intact marriage, a good work history and a stable place of residence tend to be more successful than those who do not. Indeed, some researchers question whether the type of treatment employed matters at all. Certain large-sample studies have found the type of treatment used by the therapist to be unrelated to treatment outcome. These findings, however, have not been universally accepted, and continue to be the subject of intense debate.

During the past two decades, one of the most lively debates in the addictions field concerns whether individuals who have become alcohol-dependent can learn to drink in a controlled manner. Several researchers have reported that such a goal is appropriate and achievable, but many others (as well as many individuals associated with Alcoholics Anonymous) disagree. Several studies support each point of view. However, it may be that both can be effective and that success depends on quite specific (but not yet sufficiently defined) patient characteristics; some patients may respond positively to the controlled drinking approach, but for others abstinence is the only reasonable recourse.

---

13   Complementary programs for spouses and adolescent children of alcoholics are provided by Alanon and Alateen.

Background Reading

American Psychiatric Association. (1994). *Diagnostic and Statistical Manual of Mental Disorders. DSM-IV.* (4th edition). Washington: American Psychiatric Association.

Cohen, J., Dearnaley, E.J. & Hansel, C.E.M. (1958). The risk taken in driving under the influence of alcohol. *British Medical Journal, 2,* 1438–1442.

Klaassen, C.D. (1996). Nonmetallic Environmental Toxicants. Air Pollutants, Solvents and Vapors, and Pesticides. (Chapter 67). In J.H. Hardman, L.E. Limbird, P.B. Molinoff, R.W. Rudden, & A.G. Gilman, (Eds.), *Goodman and Gilman's The Pharmacological Basis of Therapeutics,* (9th edition). New York/Toronto: McGraw-Hill Health Professions Division.

Motto, J.A. (1980). Suicidal risk factors in alcohol abuse. *Suicide and Life-Threatening Behavior, 10 (4),* 230–238.

Ritchie, J.M. (1975). The aliphatic alcohols. In L.S. Goodman and A. Gilman (Eds.), *The Pharmacological Basis of Therapeutics,* (pp. 137–151). New York: Macmillan.

World Health Organization. (1968). *Public Health Paper No. 35, Prevention of Suicide.* Geneva: WHO.

CNS DEPRESSANTS:
OPIOID ANALGESICS
AND ANTAGONISTS

See the chapters in Section 3 on the following drugs: buprenorphine, codeine, fentanyl (Sublimaze®), heroin, hydromorphone (e.g., Dilaudid®), meperidine (e.g. Demerol®), methadone, morphine, naloxone (e.g., Narcan®), naltrexone (ReVia®), oxycodone (e.g., Supeudol®), pentazocine (e.g., Talwin®), and propoxyphene (e.g., Darvon®). See Section 4 for chapters on anileridine (e.g., Leritine®), butorphanol, diphenoxylate (e.g., Lomotil®), hydrocodone (e.g., Hycodan®), LAAM (i.e., l-alpha-acetylmethadol), levallorphan (Lorfan®), MPPP and MPTP, and opium. Section 5 includes brief notes on alfentnil, alphaprodine, clonidine, cyclazocine, dextromoramide, dihydrocodeine, kava-kava, laudanum, levorphanol, metopon, nalbuphine, nalmephene, nalorphine, noscapine, oxymorphone, phenadoxone, phenazocine, pholcodine, remifentanil, sufentanil citrate and TMF.

The terms "opioid" and "opioid antagonist" have become standard terminology in drug abuse circles in recent years. "Opioid" is a term used to describe drugs with morphine-like activity, whether they occur naturally, or are produced semi-synthetically or synthetically. This term has largely replaced the term "narcotic analgesics," which was used to describe drugs with pain-relieving properties similar to morphine and codeine (see below). In contrast, the term "opioid antagonist" describes substances that block the receptors with which opioids react, and therefore block the effects of opioid drugs.

One subgroup of opioids is the family of opiates — substances that occur naturally in opium or are produced in the laboratory by changing the structure of substances that occur naturally in opium (i.e., semi-synthetics). The naturally occurring opiates (notably morphine and codeine) are obtained by refining opium, the crude tar-like material scraped from slits made in the unripe pods of the poppy *Papaver somniferum*, a flowering plant found in many areas of southern Asia, including Thailand, Laos and Afghanistan. Among the approximately 20 alkaloids of opium, only morphine and codeine have pain-relieving properties; morphine comprises typically 10 to 15 per cent of the raw opium and codeine, one to two per cent. Some of the semi-synthetic opiates such as heroin and hydrocodone are considerably more potent than the naturally occurring opiates from which they are derived.

A second subgroup of opioids includes substances that have some opiate-like chemical features but are synthesized in the laboratory without using a naturally occurring opiate as a starting material. This subgroup includes the drugs methadone and meperidine.

The third subgroup of opioids includes substances with a peptide structure (i.e., a structure composed of several amino acid units). Some of these opioid peptides are produced naturally in the human body. These are known as endorphins, and include three subtypes: the enkephalins, the dynorphins and the ß-endorphins (beta-endorphins). Other members of this subgroup have been produced synthetically.

The terms "narcotic" and "narcotic analgesic," long used by pharmacologists to describe pain-relieving drugs similar to morphine, are now used primarily in legal contexts. However, such terms have different meanings when used in pharmacological and legal circles. Pharmacologists originally used the term "narcotic" to refer to drugs such as morphine, which relieve pain by interfering with pain perception (i.e., "deadening the pain," as suggested by the Greek prefix *narco*, meaning to deaden or benumb) and produce sedation or sleep (as suggested by the name morphine, derived from the name of the Greek god of dreams, Morpheus). In contrast, in Canadian legal circles, the term "Narcotic" (usually capitalized) has long been used to refer to any substances regulated under Canada's *Narcotic Control Act*, legislation that was recently replaced by the *Controlled Drugs and Substances Act*.[1] The *Narcotic Control Act* regulated substances as pharmacologically different as morphine, cannabis and cocaine.

Although the pharmacological use of the term "narcotic analgesic" emphasizes pain-relieving and sleep-inducing properties, many of the substances in this class have a long tradition of medical use for other purposes. For example, tincture (i.e., an alcohol or alcohol-water extract) of opium has long been used to control diarrhea, and codeine continues to be used as a cough suppressant. Other substances, notably methadone, are used to manage physical dependence on other opioids. Because of these different medical uses, which extend well beyond pain control, "opioid" has become the preferred term to describe the diverse family of drugs that are related in structure, action and/or effects to the opium alkaloids morphine and codeine.

---

1   Canada's *Controlled Drugs and Substances Act* controls not only drugs previously regulated under the *Narcotic Control Act*, but also those previously falling under the *Food and Drug Act*.

Chronic use of any of the opioids at sufficient doses can result in physical and psychological dependence. Unfortunately, at present no known alternative is as effective in relieving moderately severe to severe pain without also posing a significant risk of dependence for the user.

As their name suggests, opioid antagonists are substances that interact with opioid receptors to block the action of opioid drugs, thus preventing an opioid drug from producing its usual effect. Some antagonists, such as naloxone, are useful in the emergency treatment of individuals who have taken a potentially lethal overdose of the opioid, because the antagonist prevents the opioid dose from having its full effect. Another antagonist, naltrexone, has been used to "protect" individuals who were formerly physically dependent upon opioids but are now drug-free. While they are taking naltrexone, these individuals will not experience opioid effects if they once again try using an opioid.

Some drugs, such as pentazocine and buprenorphine, have both opioid agonist and antagonist (i.e., mixed) properties. That is, they have a combination of morphine-like and morphine-antagonizing properties. Such drugs are thought to react at more than one type of receptor, exerting a different effect through each.

History of Use

"Opium" is derived from the Greek word *opion*, meaning poppy juice. Opium has been used for its pleasurable (and possibly medicinal) effects for several thousand years. The first known written reference was in a Sumerian text (c. 4000 BC), in which the written representation for the poppy was *hul* ("joy") combined with *gil* ("plant"). The first unequivocal reference to poppy juice was found in the writings of Theophrastus in the third century BC. Ancient Greek writers were aware of the effects of opium and wrote of the symptoms of habituation and withdrawal. During the Middle Ages, Arab physicians were quite familiar with opium and frequently prescribed it for sedation, pain relief and the management of dysentery. It is believed that opium was first introduced to Asia by Arab traders.

Opium made its way across Europe during the Renaissance and was one of the first drugs to be used in calming manic conditions. The great German physician Paracelsus (1493–1541) was credited as the first to compound laudanum — a name initially designating any of the many opium preparations but now restricted exclusively to tincture of opium. Within a few decades, during the mid-16th century, laudanum became widely used throughout Europe to treat various physical and mental illnesses.

In 1803, a young German pharmacist, Sertürner, isolated an alkaloid from opium and named it morphine. (Codeine was isolated 30 years later.) Although morphine was in general use as a painkiller in the 1830s, its enormous potential was not realized until after the perfection of the hypodermic needle in 1853 by the Scottish physician Alexander Wood. Its significantly more rapid action and greatly enhanced potency when administered by injection soon led to morphine's extensive and invaluable (but often excessive) use among the wounded in the American Civil War and later in the Franco-Prussian War. The practice resulted in the physical dependence of literally tens of thousands of soldiers. In fact, physical dependence on morphine (sometimes termed "morphinism") was so widespread among the wounded that it was often referred to as the "soldier's disease."

Historically strategies for treating morphine dependence included the use of other psychoactive drugs. In the 1880s, cocaine was briefly believed to be effective in treating "morphinism." But as scholars and physicians increasingly reported that cocaine was not only ineffective but also addictive in its own right, its use for this purpose was discontinued. Heroin, first synthesized in 1874, also enjoyed brief, but considerable, popularity with physicians at the end of the 19th century. It was considered to be both a possible analgesic substitute for morphine (possessing three times morphine's analgesic potency) and a possible cure for morphine addiction. However, the harmfulness of heroin was subsequently recognized by the medical profession, as is observed in the following passage:

> In reviewing the very remarkable history of the rapid increase in the use of this drug, its wide popularity as a therapeutic agent, the acclaim with which it was received by the medical profession, and the persistence with which manufacturers advertised its virtues, both in technical and lay publications, it is astonishing that physicians were so slow to recognize its dangers and that for six or eight years of its employment there were only a few among the large number who proposed its employment in an ever increasing number of conditions, and who appreciated the harm that was being done (Terry and Pellens, 1928).

In the early decades of the 20th century, highly restrictive legislation regarding production, importation, distribution, trafficking, possession and medical uses of these drugs was introduced in North America and Europe. This legislation was the result of several key factors:

- the alarming failure of the medical profession to comprehend fully the dangers and widespread abuse of the highly addictive heroin
- the large numbers of morphine addicts on both continents[2]
- the easy availability of opioids in various preparations, many of which were sold without a prescription
- what some observers regarded as growing hysteria in the United States and Canada over continued, uncontrolled use of opium among the ethnic Chinese (in the notorious "opium dens"), which was viewed as a menace to the "American way of life." (At the same time there were also widespread but ill-founded fears that wholesale cocaine-induced[3] crimes of violence would be perpetrated by blacks against whites.)

Although law enforcement officials continued to be frustrated in their attempts to extinguish the steady flow of illicit opioids in North America and Europe, they did greatly reduce it. However, a serious outgrowth of their efforts was a unique criminal subculture of opioid (mainly heroin-using) addicts. Not only was the possession of these drugs now made illegal in many countries, but their reduced availability also led to higher prices. This, in turn, meant that many users could afford the drug only by participating in criminal activities. Meanwhile, the inflated prices of this illicit market encouraged the development of increasingly sophisticated but clandestine drug distribution chains, extending from the producers in parts of Asia, through a host of go-between buyers, chemists, wholesalers, smugglers and "cutters"[4] to a pecking order of dealers (many of whom also "cut") and ultimately the street consumer.

Scientists, too, met with frustration as they searched for a cure for morphine and heroin dependence as well as for a potent analgesic alternative without significant dependence-producing properties. Efforts directed toward the development of synthetic products were given a major impetus when, in World War II, Germany was unable to import much-needed morphine. Methadone, which possesses an analgesic

---

[2]   However, their numbers were dwarfed by the enormous population of opium addicts in China, the result of over a century of large-scale opium trafficking by British and to a lesser extent European, American and Chinese nationals, many of whom amassed huge fortunes.

[3]   In Canada, cocaine, like opioid drugs, was classified as a narcotic (i.e., controlled under the *Narcotic Control Act*) until the recent introduction of the *Controlled Drugs and Substances Act*, despite the fact that it is pharmacologically a CNS stimulant.

[4]   "Cutting" is a street term for diluting.

76   **Drugs & Drug Abuse**

potency approximately equivalent to morphine, was synthesized and introduced into medical care in wartime Germany. It is generally recognized as the first widely used synthetic opioid. Meperidine (e.g., Demerol®) had been synthesized earlier (1939), but was initially employed only as an anti-spasmodic agent until its analgesic effects were later recognized. However, hopes that these agents and subsequent synthetic opioids would not produce physical dependence when they were used chronically were not realized. In fact, these opioids became drugs of abuse themselves. Nevertheless, some of them produce less severe withdrawal symptoms than heroin or morphine do when chronic use is abruptly terminated.

Endorphins (Endogenous Opioids)

Endorphins are opioid peptides produced naturally in the human body. In the early 1970s, specific receptor sites for opioid molecules were identified in the brains of experimental animals and of humans. This discovery caused scientists to question not only the nature and function of these receptors but also the reason for their existence. Most concluded that it was highly unlikely that so many species of animals would have independently evolved a set of receptors to bind compounds synthesized in a species of poppy growing only in some parts of the world. Rather, they theorized, the opioids such as codeine and morphine just happened to interact with receptors that already existed in the brain to mediate the effects of some unknown endogenous substance(s) (i.e., substance[s] produced within the body).[5]

These theories were borne out in 1975 with the isolation of endogenous substances that could bind specifically to opioid receptors. Further research revealed other families of compounds capable of binding to these receptors. In total, three families were identified: enkephalins, dynorphins and β-endorphins. These three groups of endogenous peptides are known collectively as endorphins (a term derived from "endogenous morphine"). Each group is distributed differently, not only in the various parts of the brain and spinal cord, but also in certain other parts of the body. Endorphins seem to act in a way similar to the opioid drugs, producing their effects by means of several different mechanisms. In some parts of the brain, they appear to act as neurotransmitters; in others, they serve as regulators of neuronal function or as hormones.

---

[5]   Current evidence supports the view that morphine and some related compounds occur naturally in bound form in mammalian tissue.

Endorphins are believed to play an important role in many aspects of brain function. Like the opioids, they affect the perception of, and emotional response to, pain and other stressors. Acupuncture is believed to relieve pain by causing their release from nerve endings. Endorphins also appear to influence mood, and are thought to be an important component of the reward pathway of the brain. A disruption in their function has been associated with certain psychiatric disorders. Intake of food and water appears to be modulated by the endorphins, as are many other important physiological functions.

The role of the endorphins in the development of drug dependence is still unclear. If, as has been suggested, these substances act by enhancing the impact of pleasurable stimuli (such as food) and decreasing the responsiveness to negative ones (such as pain), it can be easily understood why opioids, which act on the same receptors, are so highly reinforcing. It has also been suggested, based on research with animal models, that other drugs such as alcohol may work indirectly via the opioid system. It is hoped that future research will clarify the relationship between endorphins and the reinforcing properties of certain psychoactive drugs.

Changes in endorphin regulation are also implicated in the development of tolerance to and physical dependence on opioids. Recent evidence suggests that endorphin balance is also altered after chronic administration of seemingly unrelated substances (such as alcohol). Slow recovery of this system may explain some of the symptoms reported by users of these drugs long after their use has been discontinued.

Pharmacological Properties

Absorption, Distribution and Elimination

Although opioids are generally absorbed adequately from the gastrointestinal tract, heroin and morphine are best known as injection drugs. Injecting morphine avoids the loss of active drug that occurs when morphine absorbed from the gastrointestinal tract after oral administration passes immediately through the liver and is subject there to extensive biotransformation before reaching its action sites in the brain. The result of this biotransformation is that much of the original dose is changed quickly to less active or inactive metabolites. It has been estimated that only 25 per cent of an orally administered dose may actually be available to the target tissues. Because heroin is rapidly transformed into morphine in the stomach, it too suffers the same fate. By contrast, when injected into veins and muscles or under the skin, these drugs initially bypass the liver and are therefore metabolized much more slowly than when taken orally. Administration by injection also provides the drug with more rapid access to the bloodstream and hence to the brain, where the desired effects are initiated. Intravenous administration (injection of the drug directly into the bloodstream) produces the most immediate and intense effects.[6] Therefore, heroin and morphine users who have a limited supply of their costly drug, and want to experience as intense a drug effect as possible from a small dose, will prefer to administer it by injection (or sometimes, in the case of heroin, by "snorting" it).

Despite the loss of active morphine that occurs with its oral administration — that is, the "first-pass effect" — morphine is administered orally in certain clinical situations, notably as a constituent of tincture of opium for the control of diarrhea, and increasingly to control pain in patients with advanced cancer. Although the oral route of administration results in a less intense effect than that provided by the same dose given by injection, it has the advantage of easy administration by the patient or caregiver in the home setting. Less commonly, morphine or some other opioid analgesic is administered rectally in a suppository form.

However, even when these drugs are injected intravenously, a substantial proportion is distributed by the blood to other tissues and never reaches the brain. Opioids travel in the bloodstream partly in protein-bound and water-soluble salt forms that do not readily penetrate the blood-brain barrier. In general, this barrier permits only gradual and incomplete passage of these drugs into the brain, thereby restricting the amount that can reach those specific brain target sites where the main actions of opioids are initiated. After the drugs have been distributed from the bloodstream to tissues throughout the body, the concentration of these opioids may be much lower in the brain than in other organs such as the lungs, kidneys and liver. Since heroin is much more fat-soluble than morphine, it penetrates the blood-brain barrier more quickly. This difference is believed to account for the higher potency and the more intense "rush" of heroin, as compared with morphine, after intravenous administration.

---

6   Although intravenous administration of opioids produces the most rapid onset of action and greatest intensity of effects, some opioids are highly effective even when taken by mouth; these include hydromorphone (e.g., Dilaudid®), hydrocodone (the opioid present in Novahistex DH®), and oxycodone (the opioid present in Percodan®). Because oral consumption of these drugs does not present the risks associated with chronic needle use, they are highly desirable to some opioid abusers.

These drugs are largely metabolized by the liver before being excreted in the urine.[7] In the case of most opioids, metabolism is quite rapid and (with a few exceptions such as methadone) the duration of action after a single injection or typical oral dose is therefore brief — typically three to five hours. However, sustained-release tablets of morphine sulphate have a considerably longer duration of action — up to 24 hours.

Analgesia

The primary pharmacological effect for which morphine and many other opioid drugs are administered is their ability to reduce sensitivity and emotional response to pain. Although some of the commonly used opioids have other applications, all possess this attribute in varying degrees. At the weaker end of the scale are drugs such as codeine and propoxyphene (e.g., Darvon®), which are used for mild to moderate pain. Drugs such as meperidine (e.g., Demerol®) and anileridine (e.g., Leritine®) are used to treat moderately severe pain. At the most potent end of the scale are heroin, hydromorphone (e.g., Dilaudid®) and oxymorphone (e.g., Numorphan®), which are ordinarily used only for severe pain.

When considering the analgesic effects produced by opioids, it is useful to think of two interacting components of pain: the sensation of pain, and the affective, or emotional, reaction to that sensation. In the case of the former, research evidence indicates the presence of specific opioid receptor sites in cells located in certain ascending pain pathways of the spinal cord and brain. It is believed that the opioid drug molecule must bind to these sites in order to produce its analgesic effect. The distribution of the receptors in the central nervous system suggests that they may allow the drug to interfere with the transmission of impulses from pain-stimulus receptors before these impulses can reach the higher brain centres responsible for perception and awareness of pain.

Of considerable interest is the high density of the opioid receptors in certain sub-cortical brain structures (i.e., brain structures other than the cerebral cortex), collectively referred to as the limbic system. Although certain limbic structures also play a role in many other functions, they have been shown to be involved in the production of emotional sensations. For example, when particular limbic regions in experimental

---

[7]   For example, morphine is inactivated in the liver largely through conversion to its 3-monoglucuronide metabolite. Up to 90 per cent of morphine and its metabolites are then excreted in the urine and the remaining 10 per cent chiefly in the feces.

animals are electrically stimulated, a fright reaction similar to that produced by a painful stimulus is observed. As well, stimulation of other limbic areas will cause animals to work very hard in order to receive further stimulation. These so-called "pleasure-producing" structures have also been shown to be present in humans. This evidence comes from patients' reports when implanted electrodes are stimulated prior to psychosurgery. While much remains to be learned about the opioids' mechanisms of analgesic action, it appears that the emotional components of pain are dampened, at least in part, by the interaction of opioids and the limbic receptor sites.[8] This may explain the reduction in emotional reaction to pain and the concurrent euphoria typically experienced by patients treated with opioids.

Effects Other than Analgesia

Initial experiences with opioids are usually not exclusively euphoria-producing. In fact, some users experience anxiety or depression during their first few drug-taking episodes.[9] Many inexperienced users, both medical and non-medical, suffer from common side effects such as nausea and vomiting. However, in most cases these unpleasant effects either are transitory or disappear with a reduction in dose. Thus, inexperienced heroin users may continue to use the drug despite its early effects rather than because of them. Often users must develop tolerance to these undesirable effects before they are fully able to appreciate the desired effects of heroin.

Many opioids are powerful cough-reflex suppressants (antitussives), and agents such as codeine, hydrocodone and hydromorphone are widely used in cough-control medications. Hydrocodone and hydromorphone, among the more potent opioids with respect to both cough suppression and euphoric action, are popular among street abusers. Both can produce physical dependence (as can codeine) when they are chronically abused. For this reason, considerable research effort has been directed toward developing a drug with satisfactory cough-suppressant properties without physical-dependence-producing properties. Dextromethorphan, a cough suppressant with potency approximately equal to that of codeine, generally meets these criteria when used in therapeutic doses. Dextromethorphan is present in many cough products marketed in North America, some of which include the letters DM in the product name to indicate the presence of this ingredient.

---

8   Those treated with opioids often report that they still perceive the painful stimulus but are no longer bothered by it.

9   Others may never experience euphoria; many of these are medical patients who nevertheless experience pain relief from these drugs.

All opioid analgesics possess strong anti-diarrheal properties. Morphine and opium have been invaluable in regions where amebic dysentery is a major problem, since morphine's ability to produce constipation prevents the development of profound and possibly fatal dehydration. However, morphine is the drug of choice only for very severe conditions. Otherwise even the opioid diphenoxylate (e.g., Lomotil®), which possesses no analgesic action at therapeutic doses, is adequate in controlling diarrhea.

Another action of opioids is depression of the brain centres responsible for a range of biological processes including breathing and heart function. Breathing is typically depressed before heart functioning.[10] Therefore, death from overdose nearly always results from respiratory arrest. Hence, management of overdose includes artificial support of respiration until the drug is adequately eliminated from the body, or the use of opioid (or narcotic) "antagonist" drugs that promptly reverse the depressant effects of overdose.

Opioid Agonists and Antagonists

In theoretical considerations of the intensity of a drug's action, two major characteristics of the drug are considered — its affinity for specific receptor(s) and its efficacy. Affinity refers to the ability of the drug to bind to an appropriate site of action (i.e., a specific receptor). Efficacy refers to the ability of the drug, having bound to the receptor, to produce its effect(s) — that is, its ability to function as an agonist. A drug that has high affinity, but little or no efficacy, not only does not produce an effect of its own, but also has the potential to block other drugs from accessing these receptors, so that they cannot produce their effect. Such high-affinity, no-efficacy drugs function as pure antagonists. In addition to pure agonists and pure antagonists, a group of drugs exists that is best described as mixed agonist-antagonists. Such drugs may function as an agonist at one type of receptor and an antagonist at another, or have high affinity but low efficacy, so that they block the effect of more potent opioids, while producing a very limited effect of their own.

Three classes of opioid receptors have been identified in the central nervous system and designated μ (mu), κ (kappa) and δ (delta). Each type of endorphin, along with each clinically useful opioid analgesic, antagonist and mixed agonist-antagonist, has a characteristic affinity profile for these receptors. For example, β-endorphins have a high affinity for μ receptors; dynorphin A also binds to μ receptors, but not as strongly

---

10   However, at very high opioid blood levels, the heart may stop beating.

as to κ_1 receptors; and the enkephalins bind to both μ and δ receptors. Most of the clinically useful opioid analgesics and opioid antagonists such as naloxone and naltrexone have a high affinity for μ receptors but some also bind to other receptors. For example, morphine also binds to some extent to κ receptors, while the agonist etorphine and the antagonists naloxone and naltrexone are thought to bind to μ, κ and δ receptors. Within each class of receptors, different subtypes may be responsible for different effects of a single drug. For example, morphine's analgesic effect at the level of the brain is attributed to its action on μ_1 receptors, while its respiratory depression and constipating effects have been attributed to its action on μ_2 receptors. Mixed agonist-antagonist agents (e.g., nalorphine) typically interact with more than one type of receptor, generally functioning as an agonist at one receptor, but an antagonist at another.

Agonists, antagonists and mixed agonist-antagonists have all been used to treat opioid dependence. Opioid drugs act at a finite number of receptor sites in the brain, and the net effect produced at these sites at any time will depend on what proportion of the receptors are occupied by an agonist, an antagonist or a mixed agonist-antagonist. When two or more of these drug types are present, they may be considered to occupy the receptors in a "musical-chairs" fashion, with the molecules "sitting down on" and "leaving" the receptors very rapidly in competition with each other. Therefore, the proportion of the receptors occupied by any one of these drug types at any one time will be related to (1) the number of drug molecules of that drug type in the environment of the receptor sites as compared with the number of molecules of the other drug types, and (2) the relative efficiency of the various drug types in "sitting down on" the receptor (i.e., their affinity).

If morphine is the only drug administered to a patient, the patient will experience the full effects of the morphine dose because only morphine molecules will occupy the receptor sites. If increasing amounts of a potent antagonist such as naloxone are then injected, the drug effects of morphine will diminish as the naloxone molecules crowd out the morphine molecules. At some point, as more naloxone molecules become available, the morphine effect will become effectively zero even though some morphine molecules are still present. If large amounts of morphine are then administered, the characteristic morphine effect will be re-established.

The use of antagonists entails some risk in drug-dependent persons. If both agonist and antagonist are administered to a person who is not drug-dependent, the antagonist functionally displaces the agonist from its sites of action, and thus returns the person to a normal drug-free state. In contrast, the drug-dependent person's body functions comfortably only when some opioid molecules are interacting with opioid receptors. Such a person, if reduced to an effectively drug-deficient state because of the action of an antagonist, will show withdrawal symptoms. This type of response forms the basis for the use of opioid antagonists in the clinical assessment of the degree of a patient's physical dependence on opioid drugs. In practice, one should never administer morphine without having the antagonist (e.g., naloxone) available, nor should one administer an antagonist without having an agonist (e.g., morphine) present, in case there is a sudden need to reduce the intensity of the patient's reaction to the first drug administered.

Medical Uses

In all of the above-noted medical uses for opioid analgesics, their function is in symptom management rather than modification of the underlying pathology (i.e., the cause of the pain, diarrhea, cough and so on).

Several factors should be considered in the physician's choice of an opioid analgesic for a specific clinical purpose. These factors include differences in potency, specific side effects and certain properties such as duration of action and dependence liability. Consideration must also be given to size of dose, route of administration and anticipated duration of use. For example:

- Morphine is a powerful antitussive and anti-diarrheal agent, as well as an effective analgesic, but because it poses a very high risk of dependence, and because other antitussive and anti-diarrheal agents with lower dependence liability are available, morphine is not used for these purposes except in extreme cases.
- Drugs such as meperidine, oxycodone and methadone retain a substantial degree of their analgesic efficacy when administered orally (in contrast to morphine), and are often preferred for pain relief when an oral dosage form is desired.
- Under some conditions (e.g., in the case of the later stages in the terminally ill patient with severe pain), the relative comfort of the patient is of justifiably greater concern to the physician than the dependence liability of a particular drug. Therefore the physician will typically prescribe the most potent analgesic that does not have side effects disturbing to the patient, regardless of its dependence liability.

In this last case, there remains the important issue of daily dosage. For many years, the medical community has recognized that the risk of drug dependence is not a relevant issue in controlling the pain of terminally ill patients, and few physicians have invoked this concern as justification for prescribing dose levels insufficient to keep the patient comfortable. Today, health care professionals find that it is the patient or a family caregiver who is more likely to want to keep the dose level low out of an inappropriate concern for acquired tolerance, i.e., the fear that the patient will ultimately need larger doses of the opioid to control pain than can be provided without risk of fatal respiratory depression.

Analgesic Comparisons

The following table indicates the dose levels of various opioids that have approximately the same analgesic potency as 10 mg of morphine used intramuscularly.

Table 1: Approximate Analgesic Equivalency of Opioid Analgesics [11]

Drug	I.M. Dose (mg)	Oral Dose (mg) except as noted	Examples of Trade Names
Anileridine	25	75	Leritine ®
Codeine	120	200	
Fentanyl	0.1 - 0.2	N/A [ii]	Sublimaze ®
Heroin (Diamorphine)	5-8	10-15 [i]	
Hydromorphone	1.5	7.5	Dilaudid ®
Morphine	10	20-30	
Oxycodone	N/A	10-15 [iii]	Percodan ® [iv] Percocet ® [v]
Oxymorphone	1.5	5-15 [vi]	Numorphan ®
Pethidine (Meperidine)	75	300	Demerol ®
Propoxyphene	50	100	Darvon-N ® [vii]

[i] Use not recommended.
[ii] No data available.
[iii] For oxycodone in combination with ASA or acetaminophen.
[iv] Contains ASA.
[v] Contains acetaminophen.
[vi] Suppository.
[vii] As the napsylate salt.

Other Issues Pertaining to Pain

Evidence indicates that sharp, localized pain is usually poorly relieved by the opioid analgesics. In contrast, these drugs tend to control duller, less well localized, and more chronic pain very effectively. There appear to be distinct pathways conveying each form of pain to higher perceptual centres, and the distribution of receptors along the pathways may be quite different.

Pain resulting from certain types of tissue inflammation (e.g., arthritis) may be adequately controlled by acetylsalicylic acid (ASA; e.g., Aspirin®) alone. However, opioid analgesics alone are not effective for this purpose. When moderate to moderately severe pain results partially or largely from inflammation, but is not controlled by ASA alone, opioid-ASA combination products that take advantage of ASA's anti-inflammatory property may be used effectively (e.g., oxycodone with ASA in Percodan®; codeine with ASA in 292s®).

Because of the risk of physical dependence with chronic administration, it is generally agreed that, unless otherwise clearly indicated, treatment for symptomatic relief from pain should be initiated with non-opioid analgesics.[12] The appropriateness of adding an anxiolytic to deal with the emotional components of pain depends on each patient's situation. Avoidance of opioid analgesics is particularly essential for chronic conditions accompanied by mild to moderate pain, such as certain types of headache and back pain, where psychological factors are thought to contribute. Also, the premature and continued administration of opioids could likely mask both the underlying pathology and treatment progress in the case of those disorders where pain is a primary symptom. However, it should be stressed that, under the close supervision of a physician, relatively short-term or occasional use of opioids for relief from moderate to severe pain does not ordinarily produce physical dependence and can be justified in the case of recurring conditions.

Methadone Maintenance and Withdrawal

Until the mid-1960s, North American society's basic response to heroin-dependent individuals was to incarcerate them and compel them to undergo total withdrawal ("cold turkey") followed by forced abstinence. This approach was sometimes

---

12   The same principle applies to the choice of a non-opioid cough medication and an anti-diarrheal preparation.

supported by adjunctive psychotherapeutic, social service and/or institutional care. Generally, even with the most humane and concerned treatment, the rate of rapid relapse continued to be extremely high, and complete recovery was the exception rather than the rule. However, some therapeutic communities (such as Synanon in Santa Monica, California, and Daytop Village, in New York) that rely on "cold-turkey" withdrawal, with prolonged post-withdrawal residence and support, have reported a high success rate among long-term residents, although early dropout rates are also high.

Because the dependent heroin user was typically viewed as beginning heroin use as a pleasure-seeking activity and having a highly deviant lifestyle, he or she was commonly viewed as a moral degenerate. This view influenced legislation, which provided harsh penalties for illegal possession of opioids geared to removing the abuser from society. Until the 1960s, little attention was directed toward developing treatment programs with any reasonable prospects for rehabilitation. Indeed, some observers have suggested that the "cold-turkey" withdrawal experienced by incarcerated users constitutes additional punishment.

Recognizing that this traditional approach was clearly ineffective in resolving opioid dependence problems, the New York City Health Council granted funds in 1963 to Dole and Nyswander to develop a methadone maintenance pilot project for heroin addicts. This approach to treatment, which usually continues over a period of years, provides the opioid-dependent individual with an individualized daily dose of the opioid methadone sufficient to prevent the development of withdrawal symptoms. In effect, the legally prescribed methadone substitutes for the dependent individual's usual opioid. It thus provides the physiological stability that allows the opioid-dependent individual to stop the daily search for drugs and to engage productively in psychosocial treatment and employment, education or training.

Among the available opioid drugs, methadone has the following advantages that have made it the preferred choice in North America for maintenance treatment:

- Cross-dependence occurs between methadone and other powerful opioid analgesics, such as heroin and morphine. That is, when provided in sufficiently high doses methadone can fully prevent withdrawal symptoms that would otherwise occur in physically dependent users after abrupt abstinence from these other drugs.

- When administered orally, methadone retains much of its efficacy in reducing "drug hunger" without renewing euphoria.
- Because of methadone's long duration of action, only a single daily administration is required.
- Cross-tolerance between methadone and other opioids also occurs. Therefore, patients maintained on large daily oral doses of methadone will not experience the euphoric or other desired effects of heroin (or any other opioid analgesic) even when the latter is intravenously injected. Since the desired effects of injected opioids are no longer achieved, opioid-injecting behavior may soon cease in the regular methadone user.
- Long-term maintenance of opioid-dependent individuals on therapeutic doses of methadone does not appear to produce serious health problems.

The appropriate daily dose of methadone for treatment of opioid dependence is one that provides relief of withdrawal symptoms and cravings, but does not cause drowsiness or other side effects that interfere with the individual's effective functioning. Typically the initial dose provided to new clients is quite low, often 15 to 30 mg. Doses at this level present a low risk of harm, even if the client has developed little tolerance to opioids, but are unlikely to prevent withdrawal symptoms or craving in most clients. Therefore the daily dose is usually increased fairly quickly to a more effective level. The maintenance dose range varies considerably across clients and across programs. Some patients do well on daily doses as low as 20 to 30 mg, but most find comfort at doses in the 50- to 120-mg range. Research evidence suggests that clients receiving daily doses greater than 60 mg (and possibly 80 mg) are more likely to remain in the treatment program and reduce or eliminate their use of illicit drugs.

In most maintenance programs methadone is taken under supervision, usually in a small serving of fruit-flavored drink, at the clinic or an officially designated methadone-dispensing site (which, in some jurisdictions, may be a community pharmacy or physician's office). However, as the client becomes functionally stable, methadone "carries" (i.e., take-home doses) may be permitted.[13] Some programs allow the client to take home initially one or two doses for a weekend, and later up to six doses so that the client returns to the clinic only weekly. Since methadone is typically dispensed in an orange-flavored drink that must be refrigerated, program clients receiving carry doses must be made aware of the importance of storing their

---

13   In some programs methadone "carries" are permitted only when urine monitoring has provided evidence that the client is no longer using illicit opioids.

take-home supply safely out of the reach of children and other adults who might not recognize it as medication.

Research has shown that clients receiving methadone maintenance treatment, even without counselling or with very little counselling, are more likely to be free of heroin, less likely to be involved in deviant and criminal behavior, and more likely to be employed than individuals receiving no treatment or only assisted withdrawal. Further, methadone maintenance clients are more likely to continue in treatment than those not receiving methadone, and a longer duration in treatment is associated with better outcomes. These findings, together with evidence that outcomes are improved when a broader array of treatment modalities is included, have encouraged the continuing improvement of methadone maintenance programs. It is important to remember that methadone maintenance is not a cure for opioid dependence — in fact, the client continues to be dependent on the opioid methadone.[14] Nevertheless, after three decades, methadone maintenance treatment has been demonstrated to reduce significantly the rate of relapse to illicit drug use and the associated problems for the user and the community.

It was perhaps inevitable that, when methadone maintenance programs were established on a large scale, some clients would attempt to use the legally dispensed methadone in ways that were not intended by treatment staff. In particular, there is ample evidence that some clients with "carry" privileges attempt to divert at least part of their take-home supply to other individuals, and some have attempted to inject the liquid intended for oral administration.

Various strategies have been used to minimize the risk of methadone injecting. These include providing the methadone in dilute solution of as much as 100 mL (approximately 3 oz.) of orange-flavored drink. A second strategy designed to reduce the risk of methadone being injected is the use of special dosage forms that combine methadone with another non-drug or drug ingredient. One experimental methadone product, for example, included a substance that produced a thick liquid when water was added, so that the methadone could not be drawn up into a syringe. Another approach was to include an opioid antagonist such as naloxone in the methadone preparation. The theory behind this approach is that, when taken orally, the

---

14   Clients may be withdrawn from methadone by gradually tapering the dose level, if and when they want to become drug free. However, most find such withdrawal very difficult, particularly when the dose level of methadone is reduced below 10 to 15 mg.

naloxone in this preparation is absorbed and then metabolized so rapidly on its "first pass" through the liver that it should have no effect on opioid receptors in the brain, while the methadone, which is less rapidly metabolized, would have its desired effect. However, if the combination is administered by injection, both drugs should reach the receptors in the brain together, and the naloxone should diminish or completely block the effects of the methadone. It was further suggested that the amounts of the two drugs used in the product could be calculated so that the naloxone effects would predominate, and the needle user would experience a withdrawal reaction if the combination was injected. Such formulation strategies would make these methadone products unattractive to the illicit market.

In some jurisdictions, and particularly in some correctional settings, methadone-assisted withdrawal has been considered a preferred alternative to indefinite methadone maintenance. Methadone withdrawal programs involve substitution of methadone for the illicit opioid and gradual reduction of the daily dose of methadone, usually over a period of several weeks or months, until a drug-free state has been achieved. Although this approach produces moderately unpleasant symptoms, they are not nearly as severe as those of "cold-turkey" withdrawal. However, critics have pointed out that while gradual withdrawal is more humane, clients of withdrawal programs are much less likely to remain in treatment and free of illicit drugs than are clients in methadone maintenance programs.

Other important considerations regarding methadone therapy include the following:
- Methadone can produce or maintain profound physical dependence; withdrawal may be lengthy and painful if the drug has been used at high daily doses and is then abruptly terminated.
- The first-year dropout rate for many methadone maintenance programs is reported to be quite high — sometimes more than 50 per cent; many dropouts return to illicit drug abuse.
- Many patients abuse drugs other than opioids while participating in methadone maintenance programs. The other drugs most often recorded in these instances are stimulants such as amphetamines and cocaine, cannabis, and depressants such as benzodiazepines, barbiturates and alcohol.
- In some jurisdictions, where methadone maintenance programs are accessible only (or mainly) in certain types of communities, such as large metropolitan centres, program clients may find themselves unable to pursue employment or access to supportive living arrangements because the location would prevent them from reporting daily to their program clinic.

European Responses to Opioid Dependence

Prior to 1961, there were fewer than 500 known opioid-dependent individuals in the United Kingdom. These were mainly middle- and upper-middle-class persons, most of whom were also middle-aged. All were believed to be iatrogenically addicted (i.e., as an inadvertent result of medical treatment). They were maintained, usually on morphine, by their personal physicians, who were encouraged but not required to report them to the Home Office. In the early 1960s, the number of heroin addicts increased at an alarming rate. These newer addicts differed from the known chronic group in that they were substantially younger, were mainly drawn from the lower social classes, and often had a history of criminal behavior. By 1968, almost 3,000 opioid addicts were known to the Home Office. Several theories were offered in attempting to account for this almost sixfold increase in such a brief period. Factors that seemed most likely to account for this phenomenon included excessive prescribing by a few London practitioners whose addict patients either sold or gave away their excess supply; the increasing willingness of young people to engage in socially deviant drug-using behavior during the 1960s; and expansion of the international drug trade, leading to greatly increased drug availability. In 1968, legislation was passed requiring addicts to register with the government in order to obtain heroin or another opioid exclusively for addiction maintenance.

Over the subsequent two decades, methadone maintenance programs were developed in Europe, but more slowly than in North America, particularly in France and Germany, where development has been largely a phenomenon of the 1990s. In the United Kingdom, much of the methadone dispensing continued to occur in physician practices, rather than in specialized clinics. As in North America, increasing awareness of AIDS risks and the role of needle-sharing in HIV transmission stimulated development of innovative services for populations at risk. In the Netherlands, the "low-threshold" methadone program was developed for less highly motivated opioid-dependent individuals. In this model, methadone is provided to clients from a mobile dispensary, without requiring participation in counselling or urine testing.

The continuing threat of AIDS in the late 1980s and 1990s resulted in harm reduction (as opposed to regulation, law enforcement and abstinence-oriented treatment) becoming the dominant philosophy shaping European public policy towards injection drug users. Harm reduction is a public health approach based on the principles that safer drug use is possible, and that public policies can be developed that reduce harm to drug users and the public. The harm reduction philosophy is evident in the development of needle/syringe exchange services, the expansion of methadone substitution programs, and readily available condom supplies for injection drug users. Such services are designed to reduce users' risk of HIV, hepatitis and other infections resulting from the sharing of contaminated needles and syringes and unprotected sexual activity. A further harm reduction strategy, taken in some European centres, was the provision of safe environments for injection drug use.

Perhaps the most publicized harm reduction strategy was the provision of heroin maintenance for heroin-dependent users. Physicians in the United Kingdom have long had more flexibility in their prescribing for drug-dependent patients than have physicians in North America. Some recently developed U.K. programs have incorporated the principle of providing the user's primary drug, administered by the user's primary method. Heroin has also been provided to dependent users in a Swiss program. In the Netherlands, pilot projects have been conducted using morphine maintenance and other injectable opioids. In 1997, the Dutch government announced a planned trial of the provision of free heroin to a limited number of heroin-dependent users, beginning in 1998. The purpose of the trial is to provide a more attractive alternative than methadone to users with a street-based lifestyle including criminal involvement.

Abuse of Opioid Analgesics

The euphoria produced by opioid analgesics is not only a key component in overall relief from pain but also the primary reason for their abuse. Indeed, the greater the euphorogenic (euphoria-producing) potential of a given opioid analgesic, the more likely abusers will value it. Generally, those opioids that possess the greatest analgesic potency (traditionally heroin and morphine) also tend to produce the greatest euphoria. This is consistent with the evidence that euphoria and analgesia, as well as respiratory depression, miosis and reduced gastrointestinal motility, are produced through the interaction of the drug with μ receptors.

Several factors, in addition to the properties inherent in the particular drug, influence the degree of euphoria experienced by users of opioid analgesics. The most significant factors include:
- the size of dose administered

  • the route of administration
  • the innate and acquired tolerance of the user to opioid analgesics
  • whether the opioid analgesic is taken in combination with some other drug(s).

Size of Dose

The intensity of euphoria of opioids is dose-related, so that a given degree of euphoria is produced by smaller doses of the more potent drugs. Many of the drugs that are less potent in producing euphoria nevertheless have side effects comparable in intensity to the more potent euphoria-producing opioids. Therefore, while larger quantities of the less potent opioids can produce a degree of euphoria comparable to smaller doses of the more powerful substances, these high doses can produce serious adverse effects. For example, very high doses of both codeine and propoxyphene can produce seizures.[15]

Route of Administration

As noted earlier, users seeking the euphoriant effects prefer administration by injection to oral administration because the effects are experienced more rapidly and because the intensity of euphoria is much greater, for the same dose level. In general, intravenous injection ("mainlining") is the preferred method, because only through this route can the user achieve a "rush," an immediate intense orgasmic sensation in the abdomen. However, not all heroin users experience this phenomenon. Although it is most often associated with intravenous injection of heroin and morphine, even propoxyphene can produce such a "rush" when taken intravenously.[16] Because the highly pleasurable "rush" occurs so rapidly after injection, the two events become associated. Eventually, for the chronic injection user, the act of injection itself tends to produce powerful secondary gratification; that is, the very act of injecting a substance even when it is not psychoactive can become highly rewarding.

---

[15]   Regular opioid analgesic abusers tend to resort to these weaker drugs only when their preferred drug is not available.

[16]   The occurrence of a rush is not exclusive to opioid analgesics. Intravenous users of methamphetamine and cocaine report a similar phenomenon.

Advantages of Oral Administration

All of the opioid analgesics lose some of their euphoric potency when orally ingested. Nonetheless, legally produced potent opioid analgesics intended for oral administration[17] have several advantages for the street user:

- The quality (purity) of street drugs such as heroin is variable: often it is quite poor, at other times heroin of unusually high purity increases the risk of over-dose. By contrast, there is very high consistency of quality in the opioid analgesics produced by the legitimate pharmaceutical industry.

- Because these opioid analgesics are designed and formulated so as to retain sufficient potency when taken orally, they can provide a level of euphoria and tranquillity acceptable to many regular street users.

- Most licit oral preparations of opioid analgesics are available at local pharmacies, where an abuser can obtain them by theft, by forged prescription or often by legitimately written prescription.[18]

- By taking oral preparations a user avoids the discomforts and health hazards associated with chronic injecting and non-sterile equipment.

- If the user obtains the drugs from a pharmacy (by whatever means), the risk of being "burned" (cheated) on the street is avoided. For many, the likely result of being "burned" is the onset of withdrawal sickness.

- The user is not at the mercy of either the often extreme fluctuations in the price of street heroin or, even worse, the periodic complete "drying-up" of street sources.

Combination Drug Abuse

Many street heroin users acknowledge experience with several other drugs of abuse. Many who have tried a combined "hit" (intravenous injection) of heroin mixed with cocaine or methamphetamine claim that it produces an even greater "rush" than when each is administered alone, and the increased availability of cocaine in recent years has enabled more users to experience this combined effect. However, the intensity of the combined drug effects depends on the proportions of the two drugs and the extent to which the combination product has been diluted. Administering a potent "speedball" (heroin plus either of these stimulants) is more a fantasy than reality for many users.

---

17   For example, oxycodone, hydromorphone, hydrocodone and meperidine.

18   Many abusers are highly adept at duping some physicians into prescribing opioids by pretending to have symptoms and complaints associated with medical problems for which an opioid analgesic is indicated.

However, research suggests that heroin users who also use cocaine are less likely to become heroin-free as a result of methadone treatment than non-users of cocaine.

Addiction in Health Care Workers

The prevalence of opioid analgesic abuse among health care workers, especially physicians, nurses, pharmacists and dentists, has long been of interest to regulatory bodies that encounter substance-abusing professionals from time to time. Surveys over several decades have suggested that abuse of and dependence on opioids is greater in the health professions than in the general population. Some observers have noted that the availability of such drugs in hospitals and medical clinics is the most important contributor to this problem. Availability and accessibility differ across different work settings and across the professions because of rules and procedures concerning drug orders or prescriptions, storage, delivery to sites of use, record-keeping and audits.

In a recent self-report study of Canadian professionals, Brewster (1994) found very low levels of opioid use: hydrocodone and meperidine were the opioids (other than codeine) most frequently used by physicians and pharmacists; meperidine use was also reported by lawyers, but hydrocodone was not; and more pharmacists were occasional or regular users of codeine (either by prescription or otherwise) than were physicians or lawyers. It is important to recognize that these findings reflect use, not abuse. However, feelings of dependence on opioids were reported with low frequency by physicians and pharmacists, but not by lawyers. While these results tend to support the view that availability may be a contributing factor to health professionals' use, including self-medication, personal factors appear to be important in precipitating abuse.

Possible misconceptions about opioid analgesics may also play a role in abuse, even among physicians. It has been suggested that the lower analgesic potency of meperidine may give rise to some mistaken beliefs, including:
- that it possesses a very much lower dependence liability than morphine
- that the probability of physical dependence on orally administered opioids (frequently the route of administration for meperidine) is quite low
- that the "habit," even after protracted use, would not be difficult to break because meperidine is so widely and safely used with patients.

None of these beliefs is valid.

Effects of Opioid Abuse

The following factors must be considered when evaluating the possible effects of opioid analgesics on the abuser:
- the pharmacological actions of this class of drugs
- the tendency toward chronic injection of the drugs
- the deviant lifestyle often associated with opioid abuse.

Drug Effects and "Needle" Effects

Most opioid analgesics do not produce serious adverse consequences with chronic use, except for the development of physical dependence. Common symptoms include constipation, pupillary constriction (which may result in impaired night vision) and blurred vision, reduced libido, menstrual irregularity and mood instability. The last symptom is due mainly to the relatively short period of action of most opioids. It should be noted, however, that opioid analgesics cause respiratory impairment, which may contribute to some respiratory tract problems.[19] Chronic high-dose abuse of a few opioid analgesics, such as meperidine and propoxyphene, differs from abuse of most other opioid analgesics in that these drugs may also cause such adverse CNS-stimulant effects as persistent muscle twitches and tremors, hyperactive reflexes, startle responses, agitation, and occasionally seizures and/or toxic psychosis.

Harmful effects directly related to actual chronic needle administration include abscesses, other local irritation and infections at the sites of administration, collapsed veins and potentially serious diseases such as viral hepatitis, AIDS and systemic bacterial infections, including tetanus, resulting from the use of non-sterile equipment.

Lifestyle

Virtually all opioid analgesics (except codeine) are available to the dependent street user in North America only through illicit means or, in the case of drugs available by prescription, by deception of a physician.[20] Further, because procuring the necessary

---

[19]   The incidence of both pneumonia and tuberculosis is significantly higher among opioid-dependent individuals than the general population; however, this may reflect primarily the living conditions of some opioid users.

[20]   Some low-dose codeine combination products are available in Canada without a prescription.

funds to buy the drugs (or procuring the drugs themselves) often involves theft, prostitution and other illegal activities, criminal behavior may be a regular part of the dependent user's daily life. Crimes of violence are not unusual within the drug subculture. However, unlike the situation with "speed" (methamphetamine) and cocaine, the pharmacological effects of the opioid analgesics do not directly cause violent behavior.

The life of the street user may be described as characterized by a sense of urgency, frequently heightened by attempts to avoid withdrawal symptoms. For needle users, obtaining funds for a buy is only part of their daily concern. As noted earlier, those who purchase their drugs mainly on the street are presented with a number of risks (such as being "burned," buying drugs of unknown quality, or being faced with a dramatic escalation in cost or the complete drying-up of street supplies).[21] In recent years, as some drug users have tried to protect themselves against HIV infection from shared needles and sexual relations, obtaining clean needles, syringes and condoms has also become a daily concern. All users of illicit drugs also face the ongoing fear of arrest.

Many heroin-dependent individuals have observed that they ultimately want only one source of security — a continuous supply of their drugs. In desperate times, in the face of withdrawal symptoms, drug-seeking behavior is usually self-centred and drugs may be stolen from even a partner or close friends. Social relations are therefore typically erratic and significantly dictated by drug availability.

Researchers consistently report that illicit opioid users of all ages (particularly needle users of heroin) have significantly higher rates of generally poor health, serious illness and mortality than their contemporaries in the general population. In addition to the health problems already discussed, the following variables also contribute:
- Street addicts spend most of their money maintaining the habit, typically leaving little for adequate nutrition, housing or medical care.
- Needle users are afraid that their drug habit will be easily detected because of the "track marks" clearly visible on their arms and other parts of the body. For this reason, they likely will avoid medical attention until illness becomes quite serious.[22] However, this reluctance may result in the development of

---

[21]   The last two are most likely to occur after a large quantity of drugs has been confiscated by the authorities. Addicts point to this as a "panic" situation.

[22]   By contrast, the oral abuser may see as many as a dozen physicians per week, complaining, for example, that a "chronic cough" is not adequately relieved by weaker preparations.

serious health problems because lung disorders and sexually transmitted diseases, which have a particularly high incidence in this group, are conditions that require early diagnosis and treatment. The high incidence of complications in pregnancy among dependent women is related to lifestyle factors and inadequate prenatal care.

- Chronic high-dose users rapidly acquire tolerance to the euphoric effect of the weak heroin available on the streets in some jurisdictions. Some therefore often resort to other drugs (which can also produce dependence) to achieve a pleasurable "high." However, multiple drug abuse can have serious results. Because opioid analgesic users ordinarily do not suffer serious adverse effects resulting directly from the actions of these drugs, such users often mistakenly assume that they can continue to take large quantities of other drugs with the same degree of safety. Many deaths among heroin addicts have been attributed to overdose of drugs other than heroin, such as barbiturates and other sedative/hypnotic drugs.[23]

Tolerance and Dependence

Tolerance

Tolerance develops to the euphoric, analgesic, sedative, respiratory-depressant and emetic (nausea-producing) effects of opioids but not to their pupillary and only slightly to their constipating actions. (Typically chronic users must use laxatives regularly.) The result may be, in the long term, that a tenfold or greater increase in the daily dose is needed to produce the desired intensity of effect.

Tolerance to Respiratory Depression Effects — Death from Overdose: In contrast to the situation with barbiturates and some other sedative/hypnotic drugs, substantial tolerance to respiratory-depressant effects does occur with opioid analgesics. However, most deaths resulting from opioid analgesic overdose, even among heavy regular users, are due to respiratory arrest. Many experts believe that sudden death in dependent users (particularly of heroin) following intravenous injection is usually due to a much greater dose of drug than that to which they are accustomed. Instead of getting their usual dose of heroin from a street product of low concentration, they

---

[23]   However, the most common cause of death among heroin addicts is, in fact, from heroin or other opioid analgesic overdose: see Tolerance and Dependence.

unknowingly got a much higher dose — with respiratory depressant effects beyond their level of tolerance — from a product with a much higher heroin concentration. However, sudden death may also result from other respiratory or cardiovascular complications.

Tolerance to Pleasurable Effects: To compensate for acquired tolerance to the subjectively pleasurable effects of opioid analgesics, users periodically increase their daily dose. Eventually, with chronic use, they can reach a dose plateau beyond which no amount of opioid analgesic can produce the desired intensity of effects.[24] Typically drug-taking continues daily at the plateau dose level, despite the loss of pleasurable effects, but now the motivation is primarily to avoid withdrawal. Desired levels of pleasurable effects can be restored only after withdrawal and, generally, several weeks of abstinence.

Cross-Tolerance: Once users have become tolerant to a particular effect produced by one opioid analgesic at a given daily dose, they will also be tolerant to that same effect of all other opioid analgesics at comparable doses. This phenomenon is known as cross-tolerance. For example, 10 mg of morphine provides approximately the same analgesic effect as 100 mg of meperidine when each is administered by subcutaneous injection. A user who has acquired tolerance to the analgesic effect of the 10 mg of morphine will also be tolerant to the analgesic effect produced by 100 mg of meperidine.

Dependence

Physical Dependence: Chronic use or abuse of opioid analgesic drugs can produce physical dependence, and abrupt abstinence from these drugs can result in withdrawal sickness. The kinds of symptoms, as well as their severity and duration, are affected by (1) the particular drug; (2) the chronicity and pattern of use; (3) the typical daily dose; (4) the concurrent use of other drugs; (5) the general health status of the user; and (6) the chosen route of administration (oral versus injection).

---

24   This pattern assumes that users are able to obtain sufficient amounts of their drug to increase the dose at will. For most street heroin addicts such good fortune is unlikely; for them, their maximum daily dose is ordinarily restricted by limited availability of heroin and by its high cost. Indeed, some impoverished heroin "addicts" cannot support a daily habit.

Contrary to popular belief, opioid analgesic withdrawal (unlike sedative/hypnotic withdrawal) is rarely a life-threatening medical problem in otherwise healthy adults. In fact, although withdrawal can cause considerable suffering, several of the main symptoms resemble those of a moderately severe bout of influenza.[25] It is quite unusual for symptoms to include the seizures that often accompany sedative/hypnotic withdrawal. For many years, most street heroin available in North America, particularly in the United States, was so highly diluted that the dependent user was likely to experience relatively mild symptoms during withdrawal, compared with users in other parts of the world whose heroin was of higher concentration. In recent years, however, the concentration of North American street heroin has increased considerably, so that withdrawal symptoms may be more severe.

The peak intensity of withdrawal symptoms in a physically dependent user commonly occurs between 48 and 72 hours after the last administration. However, early withdrawal symptoms may begin within a few hours. Morphine users, for example, often experience withdrawal symptoms within six hours or less after the last drug administration. It is therefore not surprising to find users taking drugs three, four or five times a day, with each administration being preceded by some degree of early withdrawal discomfort. Since methadone is excreted more slowly than other opioid analgesics, withdrawal symptoms appear and reach a peak later in methadone users.

Psychological Dependence: The issue of duration of withdrawal reactions is in dispute. Some evidence suggests that withdrawal reactions can persist six months to a year after the last drug-use episode. However, there is a very real problem in distinguishing between psychologically based abstinence signs and biologically based abstinence signs, and this problem complicates assessment of the duration of withdrawal reactions. There is clear evidence in the case of amphetamine-like drugs that sleep disturbances last for several months following termination of drug use. While for opioid analgesics the case is not nearly so clear, the possibility of prolonged physical withdrawal should not be dismissed in favor of an explanation entirely in terms of psychological factors.[26]

---

[25]   It should be kept in mind that North Americans usually experience rather mild forms of influenza.

[26]   Symptoms that may last for extended periods after the classical phase of opioid analgesic withdrawal is completed can include depression, anxiety (sometimes with periods of severe agitation), insomnia, loss of appetite and a persistent craving for opioid analgesics.

Cross-Dependence: Some drugs can suppress the withdrawal symptoms produced by abstinence from another drug of the same class. This phenomenon is known as cross-dependence, and it has been demonstrated to occur generally among opioid analgesics. For example, as noted earlier, methadone is a highly potent drug capable of suppressing even heroin withdrawal (if administered in sufficient quantities). The less potent opioid analgesics, such as codeine and propoxyphene, also can suppress withdrawal resulting from abrupt abstinence from more powerful opioid analgesics. The doses required may be so great, however, that they produce potentially serious side effects.

Neonatal Drug Dependence

When a mother is physically dependent on opioid analgesics during pregnancy, she faces an increased risk of premature delivery and a low birth-weight infant, and therefore an increased risk of infant death. At birth, the infant undergoes an abrupt termination of the drug supply to which he or she has become accustomed via the mother's circulation and a resulting withdrawal reaction, characterized by irritability and sleep disturbances, tremors, poor feeding, vomiting and, occasionally, seizures. It is not known whether the period of fetal dependence has any predisposing effect on later drug-seeking behavior.

Methadone-treated mothers are likely to receive better prenatal care and are less likely to experience opioid withdrawal during the pregnancy; therefore, their infants are less likely to be born prematurely and at a low birth weight. However, such infants experience opioid withdrawal symptoms, which begin typically within 72 hours of birth and last for several weeks or months.

Background Reading

Brands, B. (Ed.), (1997). *Methadone Maintenance: A Clinician's Manual.* Toronto: Addiction Research Foundation.

Brewster, J.M. (1994). *Drug Use Among Canadian Professionals. Executive Summary of Final Report.* Ottawa: Health Canada.

Drucker, E. (1995). Harm reduction: a public health strategy. *Current Issues in Public Health,* 1, 64–70.

Hartel, D.M., Schoenbaum, E.E., Selwyn, P.A., Kline, J., Davenny, K., Klein, R.S. & Friedland, G.H. (1995). Heroin use during methadone maintenance treatment: The importance of methadone dose and cocaine use. *American Journal of Public Health, 85(1)*, 83–88.

McLellan, A.T., Arndt, I.O., Metzger, D.S., Woody, G.E. & O'Brien, C.P. (1993). The effects of psychosocial services in substance abuse treatment. *Journal of the American Medical Association, 269 (15)*, 1953–1959.

Reisine, T. & Pasternak, G. (1996). Opioid analgesics and antagonists. In J.G. Hardman, L.E. Limbird, P.B. Molinoff, R.W. Rudden & A.G. Gilman (Eds.), *Goodman and Gilman's The Pharmacological Basis of Therapeutics* (9th edition). (Chapter 23). New York/Toronto: McGraw-Hill Health Professions Division.

Riley, D. (1993). *Pragmatic Approaches to Drug Use from the Area between Intolerance and Neglect.* Ottawa: Canadian Centre on Substance Abuse.

Saxon, A.J., Wells, E.A., Fleming, C., Jackson, T.R. & Calsyn, D.A. (1996). Pre-treatment characteristics, program philosophy and level of ancillary services as predictors of methadone maintenance treatment outcome. *Addiction, 91*(8), 1197–1209.

Single, E. (1995). Defining Harm Reduction. *Drug and Alcohol Review,14*, 287-290.

Terry, C.E., & Pellens, M. (1928). *The Opium Problem.* New York: The Committee on Drug Addictions in Collaboration with the Bureau of Social Hygiene, Inc.

Veale, J. (1994). Harm reduction and the community. *International Journal of Drug Policy, 5(2)*, 115–119.

CNS DEPRESSANTS:
SEDATIVE/HYPNOTICS
AND ANXIOLYTICS

See the chapters in Section 3 on antihistamines, barbiturates and benzodiazepines. See Section 4 for chapters on buspirone, chloral hydrate, meprobamate and dimenhydrinate. Section 5 includes brief notes on bromides, ethchlorvynol, flumazenil, flunitrazepam, glutethimide, methaqualone, methyprylon, paraldehyde and zolpedem. See also the chapters on CNS Depressants: Alcohols in Section 2 and on ethyl alcohol (ethanol, beverage alcohol) in Section 3.

The sedative/hypnotics and anxiolytics are a chemically diverse group of substances that cause depression of the functions of the central nervous system. Depression here refers to a slowing or reduction in function rather than to mood or emotional depression. The term "sedative/hypnotic" refers to drugs that are used to induce sleep. The term "anxiolytics" refers to drugs that are used to allay anxiety. The older term "minor tranquillizer" was somewhat misleading, since the pharmacological actions of these drugs are qualitatively rather than quantitatively different from those of the "major tranquillizers," which are now called "antipsychotics." In fact, anxiolytics are generally ineffective in modifying psychotic symptoms, irrespective of the size of the dose taken. The same chemical types of drugs are used as sedative/hypnotics and anxiolytics — whether a specific drug is used as a sleeping pill or an anti-anxiety agent has to do with its particular features such as speed of onset or duration of action.

The most important drugs used as sedative/hypnotics and anxiolytics are the benzodiazepines (e.g., diazepam) and barbiturates. Beverage alcohol (ethyl alcohol), which may also be classified as a sedative-hypnotic, it is discussed in separate chapters in Sections 2 and 3. Certain over-the-counter sleep aids contain antihistamines, which are not classified as sedative/hypnotics but produce drowsiness and sedation as side effects to their main actions. Additionally, although they are not generally recognized as sedative/hypnotics, many industrial and commercial solvents, as well as certain aerosol propellants, produce a similar range of effects when inhaled. (See the chapter on volatile solvents in Section 3.)

Depending on the size of the dose, the effects produced by many sedative/hypnotics and anxiolytics range from mild sedation and hypnosis (i.e., sleep induction) to general anesthesia and, in severe overdose, death from respiratory arrest. Usually these drugs, especially the older agents such as the barbiturates, are abused for their pleasurably intoxicating and inhibition-releasing properties. The benzodiazepines are much less problematic because of their wide margin of safety and their substantially lower propensity to produce physical dependence.

History of Use

The first agents to be introduced into clinical medicine specifically as sedative/hypnotics were bromides, in the mid-19th century. Prior to that, ethyl alcohol and various herbal preparations were used to aid sleep. Bromides were also found to effectively control certain types of seizures. Unfortunately, however, the chronic use of bromides often produced serious side effects. Because they are slowly metabolized and excreted, bromides accumulate in the body and eventually give rise to a toxic state known as "bromism"; this syndrome is characterized by mental and neurological aberrations, a skin rash that can cover the entire body, and gastrointestinal disturbances. Several drugs with sedative/hypnotic properties but without these side effects were subsequently introduced. Two of these, paraldehyde and chloral hydrate, are chemical derivatives of aldehydes.

Paraldehyde is a polymer of acetaldehyde, a product of the oxidation of ethyl alcohol. Paraldehyde was considered for many years to be an exceptionally safe sedative/hypnotic; however, it does give rise to tolerance and dependence. It also tends to decompose when stored; if then consumed, the resultant products of decomposition induce a state of intoxication that is clinically complex and difficult to manage. Paraldehyde also tastes unpleasant and leaves a disagreeable breath odor. For these reasons, it is now rarely used.

Chloral hydrate is a substance formed by the chemical reaction of trichloroacetaldehyde (chloral) with water. Chloral hydrate produces satisfactory sedative/hypnotic effects; however, it too presents tolerance and dependence problems and causes gastrointestinal irritation in some users. Although the medical use of chloral hydrate rapidly declined after the introduction of the barbiturates, this drug is still used as a sedative/hypnotic under certain circumstances.

In the past, people suffering from anxiety and tension states were treated with such CNS-depressant drugs as opium, alcohol and the early sedative/hypnotics (e.g., paraldehyde and bromides). None of these substances were satisfactory, as all produce a number of unwanted side effects as well as significant tolerance and dependence problems.

Following the rapid advances made in organic chemistry in the late 19th century, a great many new drugs were synthesized. In 1903, the first barbiturate, barbital, was introduced and marketed under the trade name Veronal®. The origin of the name barbiturate is unknown. One version suggests it was named after Saint Barbara to mark its discovery on that saint's day. An alternative and colorful theory proposes that its discoverer, von Baeyer, named it after a girlfriend named Barbara. Barbituric acid, the parent compound of the barbiturates, is a condensation product of malonic acid and urea. Although barbituric acid itself lacks sedative/hypnotic properties, many active analogues of this acid, which represent only slight variations of its chemical structure, are potent sedative/hypnotics.

Barbiturates are prescribed for sedation, induction of sleep, anesthesia and the management of certain types of epileptic seizures. Although once widely believed to be safe, barbiturates are now recognized as having several significant liabilities. Chief among these are depression of the respiratory control centres in the brain (causing life-threatening toxicity in overdose), the rapid production of tolerance as well as physical and psychological dependence, and the potentially life-threatening effects of sudden unsupervised withdrawal. These problems prompted the search for new sedative/hypnotic compounds that might prove to be safer. The result has been a number of compounds with similar sedative/hypnotic effects (e.g., glutethimide [Doriden®], methyprylon [Noludar®], methaqualone [e.g., Tualone®, Quaalude®] and ethchlorvynol [Placidyl®]). Likewise, meprobamate was introduced in the mid-1950s as an anxiolytic. Most of these drugs did not represent any significant advance in terms of the inherent liabilities posed by the barbiturates. Each time one of these new drugs was initially marketed, researchers and practitioners claimed that it was effective and less harmful than the barbiturates. Unfortunately, these endorsements proved to be premature.

The first compound belonging to the benzodiazepine family of drugs was experimentally synthesized in 1933. However, the anxiolytic effects of the benzodiazepines were not recognized until the late 1950s. At that time a new compound, chlordiazepoxide (e.g., Librium®), was discovered to have a taming and quieting effect on animals at doses much lower than those needed to induce sleep. Chlordiazepoxide was introduced into clinical medicine in 1961. Diazepam (e.g., Valium®) was introduced in 1963. Since then, several other members of the benzodiazepine family, such as oxazepam (e.g., Serax®), lorazepam (e.g., Ativan®) and alprazolam (e.g., Xanax®), have been marketed in North America. The benzodiazepines are effective sedative/hypnotics and after over 30 years of clinical use, there is substantial evidence that they do not possess serious drawbacks to the same degree as the other sedative/hypnotic and anxiolytic drugs. These drugs have a wide margin of safety; even when they have been taken in very large quantities, death resulting solely from benzodiazepine overdose is rare. However, when overdoses are taken with other CNS depressants, the probability of lethal results increases.

More recent efforts have produced two newer agents. Zopiclone (e.g., Imovane®) is a hypnotic that is chemically unrelated to the benzodiazepines but has a similar pharmacological profile. Buspirone (e.g., Buspar®) is an anxiolytic agent that is very different from previous agents — in fact, it does not demonstrate cross-tolerance with the other drugs. It may be beneficial to those patients suffering from less severe generalized anxiety.

Pharmacological Actions and Medical Uses

Sedative/hypnotic and anxiolytic drugs can produce a spectrum of CNS-depressant effects ranging from mild sedation and relaxation to anesthesia, coma and death from respiratory arrest. The doses necessary to produce a given effect vary greatly from one drug to another. For example, for most people, 1 mg of the benzodiazepine lorazepam is sufficient to induce sleep, whereas the typical amount of chloral hydrate necessary to produce essentially the same result is 500 times greater. However, since lorazepam is available as 1-mg tablets and chloral hydrate as 500-mg capsules, the difference in potency is not clinically important. It is important to know that the "strengths" of different sedative/hypnotics and anxiolytics cannot be compared directly. Sedative/hypnotics vary widely in their duration of action. It is now recognized that there are wide variations among users with regard to the elimination half-life of a given drug. Also, because of the distribution of drugs to the brain and other areas of the body, the elimination half-life of many of these drugs does not necessarily correspond to their duration of action.

Insomnia and Its Treatment

A brief discussion of the known highlights of the normal drug-free sleep process is necessary to understand the action of these drugs. It is generally agreed that sleep is biologically essential, and that under most conditions a sleep-deprived person experiences adverse and sometimes drastic psychological consequences. Using electroencephalograms (EEGs), which measure electrical activity in various areas of the brain, and also using measures of sleep activity, researchers have found that two distinct phases recur in cycles during normal sleep. These are often referred to as REM (rapid eye movement) and non-REM sleep. The non-REM phase, which normally accounts for 75 per cent of total sleep time, comprises four stages, and the depth of sleep (i.e., the difficulty in wakening the sleeper) increases as the sleeper progresses from stage one to stage four. Relatively little dreaming occurs during the non-REM sleep phase, although night terrors and sleepwalking (somnambulism), when they occur, do so during stage four non-REM sleep. Throughout non-REM sleep, there are frequent slow, rolling eye movements, and muscle tone tends to be only slightly below that of the relaxed awakened state. About 90 minutes after the onset of sleep, there is a transition from the fourth stage of non-REM sleep to REM sleep. During REM sleep, the sleepers' eyes constantly oscillate beneath the eyelids; the sleepers' skeletal muscles are completely relaxed; and sleepers who are wakened at this time usually report that they were dreaming. Anxiety dreams, nightmares and other vivid dreams are more likely to occur during REM rather than non-REM sleep. REM sleep episodes, which account for approximately 20 to 25 per cent of total sleep time, last for 20 to 30 minutes each. After the completion of REM sleep, the entire cycle is repeated throughout an uninterrupted night of sleep.

Insomnia has been categorized into three types. Transient insomnia lasts only two or three days and is usually caused by a brief situational stressor. Short-term insomnia lasts for fewer than three weeks and may be caused by an ongoing stressor such as grief or job problems. Long-term insomnia lasts for more than three weeks and may have a number of possible causes. For example, it may be due to a psychiatric or medical illness, it may be a conditioned disorder (i.e., in which patients become anxious about falling asleep and associate the bedroom with wakefulness rather than sleep), it may be related to drug or alcohol use or it may be due to shift- or night-work. The most appropriate starting point for helping these individuals is first to identify the cause of the problem accurately, then to provide advice about non-pharmacological approaches to improve sleep, and finally to recommend pharmacological treatment if required.

Non-pharmacological approaches include instruction on "sleep hygiene." Good habits include waking up and going to bed at the same time each day (even on weekends), not using the bed for activities other than sleep and sex (e.g., reading, watching television or working), leaving the bed if sleep is delayed, avoiding napping, exercising and regulating intake of caffeine and nicotine.

The decision whether to prescribe a drug to combat a sleeping problem, as well as which drug to prescribe and for how long, depends not only on the symptom but also on the cause. For example, if the onset of sleep is interfered with by a painful medical condition, an analgesic rather than a sedative/hypnotic is likely to produce the desired result. In the case of emotional depression, sleep dysfunctions often improve with the use of antidepressants. In the case of insomnia created by temporary and emotionally stressful conditions, sedative/hypnotics are an appropriate short-term intervention in conjunction with good sleep hygiene.

Older sedative/hypnotics such as barbiturates, glutethimide and meprobamate are no longer recommended for the treatment of insomnia, due to the availability of safer agents (e.g., benzodiazepines, zopiclone).

The size of dose necessary to produce sleep varies from one sedative/hypnotic to another and from one user to another. While sedative/hypnotics can initially induce sleep and increase the number of hours of continuous sleep, they can also affect important aspects of normal sleep. Benzodiazepines reduce slow-wave, non-REM sleep and, to a lesser extent, REM sleep. The full importance of these changes in sleep patterns is not known.

During an extended period of nightly sedative/hypnotic administration, tolerance can develop, leading to a decrease in effectiveness. This may produce a "rebound" insomnia when use is abruptly discontinued. Although this temporary state constitutes a simple withdrawal reaction from the drug, the person experiencing it may interpret it as the return of the original sleep disturbance. It is important that physicians prescribing a sedative/hypnotic inform the patient of the possibility that this type of problem will occur for a few nights after the drug has been abruptly discontinued. Since sedative/hypnotics can cause decreases in cognition, long-acting agents can produce symptoms of confusion the day following night-time administration; this increases the risk of falls, for example, in the elderly. Shorter-acting agents may cause rebound day-time anxiety. If the decision is made to discontinue regular use of a sedative-hypnotic, it should be gradually tapered rather than abruptly stopped.

Anxiety and Its Treatment

In a drug-free state of wakefulness, the brain receives a constant barrage of stimuli from the environment; normally, these stimuli generate a level of excitation that we recognize as alertness. More intense or greater numbers of stimuli produce uncomfortable levels of excitation that are usually experienced as anxiety or tension. Like insomnia, anxiety is a disturbing symptom of many psychiatric and medical illnesses. Again, the most appropriate treatment addresses the underlying cause. Anxiolytics are appropriately used as adjuncts to primary treatment, in order to treat the anxiety directly, or as primary agents if a cause cannot be identified. At low doses, anxiolytic drugs raise the threshold for normal stimulation so that fewer stimuli get through to the higher brain centres, and those that do are reduced in intensity. The result is reduced levels of excitation and alertness, which the individual experiences as relaxation or sedation.

Benzodiazepines are the most commonly used agents for treating anxiety. While some antidepressants have been found to be effective in treating panic disorder, and buspirone is effective for treating less severe generalized anxiety, benzodiazepines are effective in the treatment of acute anxiety states. The recommendations for long-term regular use of benzodiazepines in the treatment of anxiety are less clear. Concerns over the potential for dependence and over-prescribing of these agents have been raised; however, there is also evidence that the level of use of these agents is consistent with the incidence of anxiety disorders in the population. It has even been suggested that some physicians may under-treat anxious patients. As is the case with most pharmacotherapy, benzodiazepine use must be viewed as an adjunct to other treatment measures and the risk/benefit profile for an individual patient evaluated carefully.

Anesthesia

General anesthesia is a drug-induced state of unconsciousness so profound that no external stimuli can rouse the patient to consciousness. With general anesthesia, therefore, even the greatest levels of pain, such as those during surgery, are not experienced. Many substances, including the sedative/hypnotics, can induce this degree of CNS depression; however, very few drugs in this class are clinically used as anesthetics. At doses high enough to produce anesthesia, most sedative/hypnotics would also produce dangerous and uncontrollable side effects. These include respiratory depression and, to a lesser extent, cardiovascular depression; death might result from respiratory arrest. A few ultrashort-acting barbiturates, such as thiopental, can be administered intravenously in doses sufficient to induce general anesthesia i.e., 100 to 200 mg) without normally producing harmful side effects. Unconsciousness follows as rapidly as 10 to 20 seconds after the initial dose. The ultrashort-acting barbiturates can be employed either alone in brief surgical procedures (usually those taking less than 15 minutes) or, in more lengthy procedures, to initiate anesthesia before the anesthetist switches to a maintenance drug, such as a gaseous anesthetic.

Other Medical Uses

At one time, phenobarbital was the most commonly used drug for the management of certain types of epileptic seizures, such as generalized tonic-clonic and partial seizures. Although most barbiturates have anti-seizure activity, phenobarbital is one of the few that is effective for this purpose at doses lower than those needed to produce hypnosis. However, phenobarbital is prescribed less frequently for this purpose than in the past because of the introduction of anti-convulsant drugs such as phenytoin (e.g., Dilantin®). Phenytoin is effective in controlling seizures without causing general CNS depression. The benzodiazepines also have a place in the treatment of certain other types of seizures. For example, clonazepam is useful for absence seizures and myoclonic seizures in children, although tolerance does develop. Diazepam and lorazepam are used in the treatment of status epilepticus.

Because of cross-tolerance, benzodiazepines are clinically useful in reducing the severity of symptoms associated with acute alcoholic withdrawal. These drugs are also used in relieving muscle spasms associated with certain types of physical disorders, such as cerebral palsy.

Abuse of Sedative/Hypnotics and Anxiolytics

The benzodiazepines have a low potential for abuse. None of the benzodiazepines generates the high level of euphoria associated with the barbiturate-like drugs. As a result, benzodiazepines are much less desirable to potential abusers. Nonetheless, doses of diazepam beyond the therapeutic level can produce a degree of pleasurable intoxication great enough to be attractive to street drug abusers. This drug is popular with heroin addicts and with patients in methadone maintenance programs, many of whom have been known to take large quantities of diazepam, either alone or with other drugs, to achieve a pleasant "high." Many abusers of hallucinogens and of stimulants also use benzodiazepines, mainly to combat the agitation and overstimulation caused by the former drugs.

Barbiturates and the older sedative/hypnotics have a high potential for abuse. They are much more likely to produce a pleasurable euphoria. This is one of the key reasons their medical use has declined substantially since the introduction of benzodiazepines.

Buspirone has a very low potential for abuse. It is very different from the other sedative/hypnotics and anxiolytics; it generally does not cause psychomotor impairment to the same extent and does not show cross-tolerance with the other agents.

Tolerance and Dependence

With regular use, tolerance to the effects of most sedative/hypnotics develops as rapidly as within a few weeks. Higher doses are then required to maintain the original level of effectiveness. With occasional use, however, tolerance does not ordinarily develop. Tolerance to different effects may develop at different rates. For example, tolerance to sleep induction may develop rapidly. However, tolerance to the barbiturates' anti-convulsant action does not appear to develop, nor does appreciable tolerance to the respiratory-depressant effects. Tolerance to the anti-convulsant effects of benzodiazepines does seem to occur.

A high degree of cross-tolerance appears to develop among sedative/hypnotics; once tolerant to the effects of one of these drugs, the user will also be tolerant to a dose equivalent in effectiveness of most others, including alcohol. Pre-tolerance sensitivity is usually restored after a few weeks of complete abstinence from all of these drugs. The exception to this phenomenon is the anxiolytic agent buspirone, which does not show cross-tolerance.

Psychological dependence on any sedative/hypnotic may develop with chronic use, irrespective of daily dose. In such an instance, the drug acquires a central role in the person's life and there is a persistent craving for its effects. Psychological dependence is not necessarily manifested as a need for daily use.

Chronic use of barbiturates can produce physical dependence so severe that if use is abruptly terminated, the ensuing withdrawal syndrome may be life-threatening. There is a high risk of delirium and tonic-clonic seizures. This is another important reason for the decline in barbiturate use.

Potentially severe withdrawal symptoms also occur after the protracted use of excessively high doses of benzodiazepines is abruptly terminated. These symptoms may occasionally include delirium and tonic-clonic seizures; however, the risk of these occurrences is much lower than that associated with barbiturates. Some patients maintained on therapeutic doses of benzodiazepines for a long period become physically dependent. Symptoms of withdrawal may include agitation, abdominal discomfort, sweating, tremors, unusual sensory perceptions, insomnia and other sleep dysfunctions, and loss of appetite. Rather than abruptly ending long-term use of benzodiazepines, slow tapering of the dose of the drug is recommended in order to reduce the number and severity of withdrawal symptoms. If an older person has been taking a benzodiazepine regularly for a very long period, the discontinuation may be a long and difficult process. If the decision is made to leave the patient on the medication, regular assessments of daytime side effects should be made.

Background Reading

American Society of Health-Service Pharmacists. (1991). *American Hospital Formulary Service (AHFS) Drug Information 1991.* Bethesda, MD: American Society of Health-Service Pharmacists.

Dundee, J.W. & McIlroy, P.D.A. (1982). The history of the barbiturates. *Anaesthesia, 37,* 726–734.

Fauci, A.S., Braunwald, E., Isselbacher, K.J., Wilson, J.D., Kasper, D.L., Hauser, S.L. & Longo, D.L. (Eds.) (1988). *Harrison's Principles of Internal Medicine.* (14th edition). New York/Toronto: McGraw-Hill Health Professions Division.

Gillin, J.C. & Byerley, W.F. (1990). The diagnosis and management of insomnia. *New England Journal of Medicine, 322 (4),* 239-248.

Hardman, J.G., Limbird, L.E., Molinoff, P.B., Rudden, R.W. & Gilman, A.G. (Eds.) (1996). *Goodman and Gilman's The Pharmacological Basis of Therapeutics.* (9th edition). New York/Toronto: McGraw-Hill Health Professions Division.

McKim, W.A. (1997). *Drugs and Behavior — An Introduction to Behavioral Pharmacology.* (3rd edition). New Jersey: Prentice-Hall, Inc.

HALLUCINOGENS

See the chapters in Section 3 on cannabis, LSD (lysergic acid diethylamide), mescaline, PCP (phencyclidine), and psilocybin, and on stimulants such as MDA (methylenedioxyamphetamine) and MDMA ("ecstasy"). See Section 4 for chapters on amanita muscaria (fly agaric mushroom), anticholinergic agents, DMT (dimethyltryptamine), harmaline and harmine, ketamine, morning glory seeds, nitrous oxide, nutmeg and peyote, as well as stimulants such as PMA (paramethoxyamphetamine), STP (DOM; 2,5-dimethoxy-4-methylamphetamine) and TMA (trimethoxyamphetamine). Section 5 includes brief notes on AMT, angel's trumpet, bufotenin(e), catnip, DET, ibogaine, methysergide, nabilone, PCE and PHP.

Hallucinogens include a wide variety of drugs that are structurally dissimilar. These range from wholly synthetic products to substances that occur naturally in many plant species throughout the world.[1] Typical doses of most hallucinogens can produce a spectrum of vivid sensory distortions and markedly alter mood and thought. Users most frequently experience visual distortions, but any of the other senses (hearing, smell, taste, touch) can also be intensely affected. Furthermore, the individual's perception of time, of the external world and even of self can be changed dramatically.

The effects produced by any hallucinogen and the subjective reaction to those effects can differ significantly among individual users and may range from ecstasy to terror. In fact, during any one hallucinogenic episode a user is likely to experience various psychic and emotional reactions. Any hallucinogen, taken in exactly the same dose by the same user, can also induce widely varying experiences from one drug-taking episode to the next.

In addition to the pharmacological properties of any hallucinogenic substance, other variables that can influence the user's response include the size of the dose taken; the user's personality, attitudes and expectations; the user's previous experiences with hallucinogens; the setting or context in which the drug is taken; and the user's emotional state at the time of drug-taking. Therefore, it is difficult to predict accurately a given user's response during a specific drug-taking episode. Even a regular user with a highly positive attitude and a history of pleasant drug use can, on occasion,

---

1   Most naturally occurring hallucinogens can also be synthesized in laboratories.

experience unexpected and intensely unpleasant effects. These factors make it more difficult to generalize about hallucinogen experiences than about experiences with any other class of psychoactive drugs.

History of Hallucinogen Use

The earliest recorded use of hallucinogenic substances for their intoxicating effects is found in India's ancient Vedic writings, dating back to approximately 1600 BC. Use of the mysterious and supposedly divine "soma" is celebrated in the hymns of the Rig Veda; these hymns, written in Sanskrit, are among the earliest foundations of the Hindu religion. One in 10 of the more than 1,000 hymns directly refers to and deifies a plant able to produce altered states of consciousness; this plant is now believed to be the fly agaric mushroom, *Amanita muscaria*.[2]

A similar ancient tradition of religious (and in this case also therapeutic) use can be traced for *Cannabis sativa* and its derivatives, marijuana and hashish. Evidence of cannabis use for its mood-altering properties was recorded in ancient China and is also found in the works of the early Greek writer Herodotus (5th century BC). Researchers in the field of hallucinogens R. Gordon Wasson and Albert Hofmann (1978), and the scholar of classical Greece Carl A.P. Ruck, also present compelling arguments concerning the secret ritual use of lysergic acid alkaloids (obtained from ergot-infected grain) in ancient Greece.

Various plants of the *Solanaceae* (potato) family[3] containing one or more of the hallucinogenic alkaloids atropine, scopolamine and hyoscyamine have been used for centuries. They were used in ancient cultures such as those of Greece, Rome, Assyria, Persia, Egypt, Hindu India and China — not only in religious rituals but also in medicine, sorcery and magical applications, probably for prophecy and divining, and not infrequently as poisons. These substances were used in Europe during the late medieval period and the Renaissance — times of widespread witchcraft and demonology. The strange visions and bizarre behavior induced by them were taken as proof of contact with Satanic forces.

---

[2]   Some researchers have speculated that fly agaric was probably in use before recorded history; in fact, it continues to be used in rituals in such remote areas as northeastern Siberia.

[3]   Including several species of the genus Datura, *Atropa belladonna* (the belladonna plant), several species of Mandragora (including *Mandragora officinarum*, the mandrake plant), and *Hyocyamus niger* (the henbane plant).

In contrast to the Eastern Hemisphere, where only about a dozen species of plants contain hallucinogenic alkaloids, there are over 90 such species (known) in the Western Hemisphere. Evidence suggests that many Indian tribes of North and South America and the West Indies used hallucinogens mainly for ritual and medicinal purposes long before the intrusion of the Europeans. Huge carved "sacred mushroom" stones have been discovered in a remote area of Guatemala; the stems appear to be the head, and in some cases the entire figure, of a god. Archeologists believe these stones to be over 3,000 years old, greatly predating the Mayan civilization in this area. Chroniclers of Columbus's second voyage wrote of a snuff widely used by the natives of the West Indies that was alleged to induce visions and was used on purely social occasions as well as in religious ceremonies. It is believed that this snuff was obtained from the plant *Piptadina peregrina*, which contains the moderately potent hallucinogen DMT (dimethyltryptamine).

Some cultures, such as the Mayan and Aztec, not only used hallucinogens but also cultivated plants that had hallucinogenic properties. Among these was the vine-growing morning glory *Rivea corymbosa*, the seeds of which contain the alkaloid d-lysergic acid amide.[4] Other cultivated plants included "sacred mushrooms" (belonging to the genus Psilocybe), which contain the hallucinogens psilocybin and psilocin, and such varieties of the peyote cactus as *Lophophora williamsii*, in which mescaline is found.

Unlike Pizarro and his successors, who permitted the conquered natives of Peru to continue using coca leaves (the source of cocaine), the conquistadors in Mexico attempted to eradicate all use of hallucinogens by the Mexican people. However, despite severe treatment by the Spanish invaders, secret Indian sects continued to use hallucinogens in their rituals. In the 19th century, raiding Mescalero Apaches adopted the peyote ritual from northern Mexican tribes. Its use then rapidly spread to other Indian tribes in the western United States and even in Canada.

In 1918 the Native American Church was incorporated, with a following composed entirely of members of Indian tribes. After several court battles, peyote use by members of this church, in religious sacraments, was recognized legally. This was the only legally approved use of any major hallucinogen in North America outside of research.[5]

---

4   Many of the effects of this substance (LSA) are similar to those produced by LSD, although the potency is different.

5   Although there are branches of the Native American Church in Canada, the legal right of its members to use peyote has not been established.

However, a 1990 decision by the U.S. Supreme Court gave individual states the right to prohibit such religious use.

Among other North Americans and Europeans, hallucinogens did not achieve broad popularity until the last half of the 1900s. Several theories have been advanced to explain the dramatic discovery and subsequent widespread use among young people of these substances during the 1960s, when LSD and cannabis were in the vanguard and achieved the greatest popularity of the hallucinogenic drugs. The beginning of the 1960s to the early 1970s was a period of deep division in American (and to a lesser extent Canadian) society between large segments of the youthful and adult populations. Many young people rejected traditional values in favor of experimentation with new ideas and values; among these ideas was experimentation with various hallucinogenic drugs, a practice generally disdained by the adult population. However, many folk heroes of that time — including pop singers and some respected intellectuals, notably Harvard professors Timothy Leary and Richard Alpert — gave open support to the use of hallucinogens. That these drugs are also illegal probably served as an additional incentive to many young people in their defiance of the older generation. Nonetheless, it should be kept in mind that only a minority of young people regularly used hallucinogens.

More recently, surveys have tracked a lengthy period of decline in adolescent drug use during the 1980s, but a resurgence in the 1990s.[6] A recent analysis of U.S. survey data from 1988 to 1992 found that "past-year" hallucinogen use was highest at the age of 19 and that the first occasion of hallucinogen use was most likely to occur between the ages of 15 and 19. However, the most recent Ontario student survey found that the first use of cannabis by current Grade 7 students occurred earlier than for older students. Among adults, the notable trend has been continuing aging of cannabis users; "past-year" use by Ontario adults aged 30 to 49 years increased from 15.4 per cent in 1977 to 46.5 per cent in 1997.[7]

---

6   The Addiction Research Foundation's 1997 Ontario Student Drug Use Survey, which includes students in Grades 7 through 13 (or the Ontario Academic Credit [OAC] year), found that overall drug use showed no further increase between 1995 and 1997; however, use of hallucinogens such as mescaline and psilocybin continued to increase significantly. Use of cannabis and other hallucinogens within the preceding year was reported by 24.9 per cent and 10 per cent of the survey sample respectively.

7   This suggests that those who began using cannabis as adolescents in the 1970s and 1980s are continuing their cannabis use as adults.

Hallucinogenic Actions

Class Designations Derived from Drug Actions

The terms "hallucinogen," "psychotomimetic" and "psychedelic" have often been used interchangeably as designations for most or all of the members of this class of drugs; however, none of their literal definitions satisfactorily embraces the wide variation of effects the drugs produce.[8] Nonetheless, these terms are generally used to signify substances that consistently produce changes in thought, perception and/or mood, usually without causing serious disturbances in the autonomic nervous system (when taken at typical doses) or creating such other problems as serious dependence. "Hallucinogen" is the most widely used term of the three; thus, for our purposes it will be the only one employed.

Classes of Hallucinogens[9]

The LSD Family

Known as indolealkylamines, this family bears a similarity to 5-hydroxytryptamine, a transmitter substance that occurs naturally in the brain. Important members include LSD (d-lysergic acid diethylamide), LSA (d-lysergic acid amide, found in the seeds of several varieties of morning glory), psilocybin and DMT (dimethyltryptamine).[10] LSD is a semi-synthetic substance derived from a naturally occurring constituent of ergot, a fungus that grows on certain grains such as rye. LSA, psilocybin and DMT are entirely natural alkaloids. All can be synthesized in a laboratory.

Shortly after ingestion, these drugs can produce a variety of physical symptoms, which include increased heart rate and blood pressure, elevated body temperature, reduced

---

8   "Hallucinogen" literally means hallucination-producing. However, hallucinations are not the main effect of some drugs commonly included in this class; some of these drugs produce hallucinations only at doses substantially higher than the amount typically taken by users. The terms "psychotomimetic" and "psychotogenic" have meant, respectively, mimicking natural forms of psychosis and psychosis-producing; however, there are too many important differences between the states typically produced by these drugs and naturally occurring psychotic states for these names to be generally accurate (although the toxic effects of high doses of some of these drugs can include psychotic effects). The term "psychedelic," coined by the psychiatrist Humphry Osmond, originally meant mind-revealing or mind-manifesting; it has also come to mean that some of these drugs may give rise to states that are allegedly mystical or transcendental.

9   According to structural similarity.

10   Other members of this family, rarely found on the North American illicit drug market, include harmaline, ibogaine, DET (diethyltryptamine) and DPT (dipropyltryptamine).

appetite, nausea, vomiting, abdominal discomfort, exaggerated reflexes, impairment of motor co-ordination and pupillary dilation.[11] At typical doses for each of these drugs (except for DMT), most of these effects tend to be mildly to moderately intense; with DMT, the physical effects tend to be more intense and more rapidly experienced.[12]

The intensity of hallucinogenic effects of the major drugs in this family is related to size of dose; that is, with increasing doses, effects are usually more intense, rather than different in nature. Distortions of any of the senses can occur with any of these drugs, although visual distortions are the most common. At typical doses, users are likely to perceive various phenomena — including a kaleidoscope of visual patterns and objects ("pseudohallucinations") and changes in the size, shape, distance and other characteristics of objects ("pseudoillusions") — which they know are not real. However, even at low doses, such effects can appear quite real to a few users. Distortions of time, space and body image frequently occur, and recognized boundaries between self and the environment may temporarily seem to change and possibly even to disappear. Synesthesias — the melding of two sensory modalities (e.g., music being "seen") — are also common.

In addition, these drugs can markedly affect thought processes and memory. It is not unusual for short-term memory (i.e., of immediately prior events) to be impaired, while distant and forgotten events may be vividly recalled. In fact, recall can be so greatly affected that the person may be unable to discriminate between past and present. Users may also accord heretofore trivial matters or objects new importance and meaning, and they may believe that they are undergoing a profound mystical or religious experience.[13]

The above effects and emotional reactions to them vary greatly among users. The desired reactions are, of course, joy and ecstasy, and many users achieve these states. However, users may also experience transient periods of fearfulness and anxiety during the course of the same hallucinogen-taking episode. Some users, particularly those who have had few or no previous experiences with hallucinogens, encounter

---

11   Many of these symptoms may also be evident at lower intensity later in the same episode.

12   In fact, all of the effects of DMT disappear much more rapidly than those of other members of this family of substances, usually 30 to 60 minutes after ingestion.

13   It is exactly this latter effect that caused psilocybin to be so greatly revered by many pre-Columbian tribes in Mexico and Central America.

only adverse effects on a given occasion. When prolonged periods of highly unpleasant emotions (which can range from persistent anxiety to terror) dominate the episode, the person is said to have had a "bad trip." These effects usually disappear after the drug is metabolized and excreted.[14] Among drugs in this family, DMT most frequently induces agitation and non-psychotic panic states. The major factor contributing to the increased risk with DMT is likely the short time lapse between ingestion of the drug and the peak experience of hallucinogenic effects (usually 10 to 20 minutes); apparently the user needs a gradual psychic adjustment from the drug-free state. A considerably longer period occurs between ingestion and the onset of hallucinogenic effects induced by other members of this family of drugs.

DMT and harmaline are monoamine oxidase inhibitors (i.e., they block the activity of MAO, an enzyme that metabolizes norepinephrine and related compounds). MAO inhibitors (MAOIs) can interact with a variety of drugs and constituents of foods (such as those in red wine and aged cheese) to produce hazardous results.[15]

Mescaline, MDA and MDMA

Mescaline, MDA (3,4-methylenedioxyamphetamine) and MDMA (3,4-methylenedioxymethamphetamine) are the only members of the phenylethylamine group of drugs to have achieved at least moderate popularity among hallucinogen users in North America. (Mescaline is encountered only very rarely in Canada.) Others that have been taken at least occasionally by street drug users since the 1960s include PMA (paramethoxyamphetamine), STP (also known as DOM[16]— 2,5-dimethoxy-4-methylamphetamine), TMA (trimethoxyamphetamine) and MMDA (3-methoxy-4,5-MDA).[17] Mescaline is the only entirely natural alkaloid in this drug family, but it too can be synthesized.

Most phenylethylamines share the psychoactive effects produced by the LSD family

---

[14]   The subject of adverse effects is more generally explored under Abuse of Hallucinogens.

[15]   See chapter on monoamine oxidase inhibitors in Section 4

[16]   The origins of "STP" are unknown. Some claim that the name is an abbreviation for serenity, tranquillity and peace, while others claim that it takes its name from the motor oil additive, because of the drug's potent amphetamine-like effects at higher doses.

[17]   This last substance can be produced from the main psychoactive principle of nutmeg, myristicin.

of hallucinogens.[18] For example, though it is considerably weaker than LSD in doses containing the same number of drug molecules, mescaline produces very similar sensory and psychological effects.

The phenylethylamine structure is common to both these hallucinogens and amphetamines. Drugs such as MDA, MMDA, PMA, STP and TMA share with amphetamine and methamphetamine the basic phenylethylamine chemical structure common to amphetamines, and also share with mescaline a particular type of chemical substitution on the benzene ring portion of their structure. As a result of this combination of chemical features, they are often referred to as "ring-substituted amphetamines." At high doses these drugs can produce amphetamine-like effects such as agitation and marked stimulation of the peripheral nervous system, resulting in both abnormally accelerated heart rate and very high blood pressure. The parallel extends further in that amphetamines may also produce hallucinations at sufficiently high doses.

Because of the simple molecular structure of the phenylethylamines, it has been a simple matter to produce a large number of chemical analogues with a similar range but varying intensity of individual effects. The synthesis of many of these drugs in the 1960s represents the beginning of the "designer drug" phenomenon, that is, the production of unregulated analogues of regulated drugs. This phenomenon has led to a number of drug-abuse crises, the most notable involving the creation and use of the drug PMA. In 1973 and again in 1985 in Ontario, PMA was synthesized in illicit laboratories and sold on the street as MDA. Unfortunately, the slight difference in chemical structure between PMA and MDA had extreme consequences for some users, who were expecting the effects of a typical dose of MDA. PMA's heightened stimulant properties caused hypertensive crisis, seizures and, in some cases, death.

TMA also produces unusual effects as the size of the dose is increased, although these effects are not nearly as hazardous as those produced by PMA. The mescaline-like effects observed at lower doses of TMA tend to be replaced at higher doses by unprovoked anger and aggressive behavior.

---

18   However, at low doses, MDA ordinarily produces a pleasant state of peacefulness and relaxation with few hallucinogenic effects. Moderately high doses produce LSD-like effects. At still higher doses, MDA can produce extreme CNS excitation, occasionally with fatal results.

Like most members of the LSD family, most drugs in the phenylethylamine (mescaline) family are produced only in illicit laboratories for the street user; the small quantities produced legally are intended for research purposes.[19] When produced illegally, these drugs vary in purity and are often adulterated with other substances, which in themselves may cause serious medical problems for the user. Therefore, taking drugs in this category is particularly risky.

Finally, drugs in this group have been traditionally subject to misrepresentation on the street. MDA and mescaline, for example, are seldom available; yet many samples of products supposedly containing one or the other of these drugs come into street-drug analysis centres every year. In the vast majority of cases, the drugs are actually PCP, LSD or the two combined, along with psychoactively inert substances. The popularity over many years of misrepresenting other drugs as mescaline appears to be linked to two factors: the perceived safety of mescaline based on reports of its extensive use by Mexican natives in religious ceremonies, and the perception of mescaline's superiority over LSD and PCP because of its "natural origin."

PCP and Ketamine

These two dissociative anesthetics — phencyclidine (PCP) and ketamine — belong to the arylcycloalkylamine family of drugs. PCP can produce such a wide spectrum of effects that it is difficult for users to predict what they will experience from one drug episode to another, or indeed within a single episode. PCP and ketamine both produce hallucinogenic effects at relatively low dose levels. PCP has been shown to produce stimulant, depressant, analgesic, anesthetic and hallucinogenic effects, depending on the dose level, the user and the situation in which the drug is taken.

The particular combination of effects that a PCP user experiences seems to be somewhat dependent on dose levels. For example, certain effects on the autonomic system at low dose levels can mimic those of stimulants (e.g., increased heart rate and elevated blood pressure), while impairment of muscle co-ordination and respiration mimic the effects of depressants. As the dosage increases, both the stimulant and depressant effects become more severe: a severe rise in blood pressure may occur, as well as seizures, coma and even death.

---

19   However, psilocybin and mescaline can be obtained in some areas from the Psilocybe mushroom and the peyote cactus respectively.

Ketamine may also produce many of the disorienting and paradoxical stimulant/depressant effects of PCP. Even at low to moderate dose levels, both drugs can create delusions and mental confusion progressing to hallucinations and degrees of dissociation bordering on schizophrenic states.

The PCP story began in the 1950s when a pharmaceutical company, Parke Davis, studied it as a general anesthetic. The company was preparing to market PCP for human use when it discovered in clinical trials that possible side effects include seizures during surgery as well as delirium, confusion, visual disorientation and hallucinations as the drug begins to wear off (emergence reaction). A decade later, PCP was easily available to street drug users in San Francisco,[20] and since the 1970s abuse has been widespread throughout North America.

The history of ketamine is less checkered. It is still in use as a general anesthetic despite its dissociative and hallucinogenic side effects. Abuse appears to be on the upswing in the United States, although it does not yet seem to be a significant problem in Canada.

Marijuana and Hashish

The plant *Cannabis sativa* contains THC (delta-9-tetrahydrocannabinol),[21] the most enduringly popular hallucinogen, as its principal psychoactive constituent. Marijuana is prepared from the flowering tops and leafy material of the plant and often contains such natural adulterants as stems and seeds. In North American street samples of marijuana cigarettes, the amount of THC varies widely, sometimes exceeding 10 per cent of the bulk weight. Hashish is a combination of the dried resinous exudate and the compressed flowers obtained from the female plant.[22] The THC content of street samples of hashish ranges up to 15 per cent of the product's weight. (These concentrations change frequently because of frequent shifts in sources.) The thick and much more potent hashish oil is obtained by boiling hashish in an appropriate organic solvent, then filtering out the waste sediment and evaporating solvent from the filtrate; the resulting yield of THC varies widely, from 10 to 70 per cent of the weight of oil. Pure THC is almost never found on the street, although several substances, such as PCP and low-grade cannabis products, are often misrepresented to be pure THC.

---

[20]   It was also reintroduced as an anesthetic and tranquillizer in veterinary medicine.

[21]   THC can also be synthesized in the laboratory, but the process is both expensive and difficult.

[22]   Cannabis is "dioecious" — i.e., there are both male and female plants of this species.

Cannabis use is a phenomenon spanning many cultures and thousands of years. Unlike many of the natural hallucinogens mentioned earlier, cannabis seems to grow in many climates, is very easy to cultivate and retains its psychoactive properties wherever it is grown. Plants can be grown not only outdoors, but also indoors in hydroponic cultivation arrangements, from seeds or by cloning. Effectively restricting its availability is thus almost impossible. Although cannabis is not native to North America, it can be easily grown in most parts of Canada, the United States and Mexico.

At low to moderate doses, cannabis produces relatively mild and transitory physical symptoms, which can include increased heart rate, muscle weakness, mild impairment of co-ordination, slight tremors, reddened eyes, involuntary movement of the eyeballs, slightly increased body temperature, increased appetite, and dry mouth and throat. In this dose range, most users experience euphoria, disinhibition, relaxation and talkativeness; however, drowsiness and sedation often follow the initial stimulation and exhilaration. Hallucinogenic effects are generally dose-related and relatively mild, although the range and intensity of effects varies greatly among users. Typical doses of cannabis (such as a few milligrams of THC in a marijuana cigarette) produce perceptual distortions in some users. In most users higher doses produce LSD- or mescaline-like changes in perception and thought. Vivid visual imagery is much less commonly experienced than it is with most other hallucinogenic drugs, and the main psychoactive effects tend to diminish more rapidly, typically within two hours after smoking.

Cannabis can also cause unpleasant effects in some users, although these seem to occur less frequently and generally with less intensity than with other hallucinogens. In low to moderate doses, users may experience mild to moderate anxiety, most commonly among inexperienced users. More severe consequences occasionally occur at higher doses and less frequently at lower doses; these may include severe anxiety, panic reactions, paranoid thinking and frightening hallucinations.

The Atropinic Family (Solanaceous Alkaloids, Belladonna Alkaloids)

The atropinic drugs — atropine, scopolamine and hyoscyamine — are also collectively designated as solanaceous alkaloids because they are found in many species of Solanaceae (a plant family that includes the potato, nightshade and tobacco, among others). All three of these substances (plus other chemically related alkaloids) are found in the plants *Atropa belladonna*[23] (deadly nightshade), *Datura stramonium* (jimsonweed) and several related species throughout the world.

These drugs have been subject to periodic street abuse in North America, and have long been available in medications. At therapeutic dose levels,[24] scopolamine taken orally is the only member of this family that produces psychoactive effects — such as mild euphoria, sedation and drowsiness — that might be of interest to abusers. At much higher doses,[25] all of these drugs can produce intense central and peripheral nervous system effects, including any of the following:

- **CNS:** visual, auditory and tactile hallucinations; visual illusions; severe disorientation and confusion; memory loss; paranoid thinking; agitation; difficulty articulating and significantly impaired motor co-ordination; dilation of the pupils and seizures.
- **Peripheral nervous system:** rapid and weak pulse, abnormally rapid and ir-regular heart rate and abnormally high blood pressure; headache; fever; dry and burning sensations in the mouth; nausea and vomiting.

The entire episode may last for 24 to 48 hours, compared with six to 12 hours with LSD; psychic effects have been known to last for several days.

Medical Uses

A few hallucinogens are currently used in clinical medicine. Ketamine is employed as an intravenous anesthetic in many surgical procedures when the use of an anesthetic mask is undesirable, as with surgical procedures involving the head and neck, and with children.

The atropinic alkaloids have been used to control smooth-muscle spasms (as anti-spasmodics), hyperirritability of the gastrointestinal tract, excessive salivation and bronchial secretions and, in earlier years, some symptoms of Parkinson's disease. They

---

23 Hence they are also widely referred to as the belladonna alkaloids.

24 1 mg or less.

25 10 mg or more.

have also been used to produce pupillary dilation for certain kinds of eye examination and to combat some types of inflammation of the eye. Scopolamine is used to control motion sickness.[26]

There are, as yet, no widely accepted medical uses for cannabis. However, cannabis, individual cannabinoids and synthetic cannabinoid analogues continue to be studied as potentially useful drugs in the treatment of epilepsy, wide-angle glaucoma, certain types of anorexia, multiple sclerosis and asthma, and for relief of nausea and vomiting caused by cancer chemotherapy.

Several potent hallucinogens, including LSD, MDA and MDMA, were explored in the past as adjuncts to psychotherapy, in the treatment of alcoholism and in a variety of other interventions related to emotional problems. However, such experiments have now been largely discontinued (except for recently approved studies of MDMA and DMT), as there was not enough evidence of the therapeutic value of such potent and potentially disruptive agents to justify their general availability as therapeutic agents.

Effects of Hallucinogen Abuse

Acute Adverse Episodes

Virtually all of the hallucinogens can produce adverse effects. In most cases, these include relatively mild and transient feelings of physical discomfort, anxiety and/or depression. Such symptoms occur routinely, even during otherwise enjoyable hallucinogenic episodes. However, more severe adverse consequences can occasionally occur, sometimes suddenly, even in regular users who have had no prior negative experiences with these drugs. The most common adverse experiences are intense anxiety, panic or paranoid states. The most severe psychic reaction, toxic psychosis, occurs relatively infrequently at typical hallucinogenic doses. Symptoms typically include true hallucinations, delusional thinking, confusion, disorientation, and bizarre and sometimes violent behavior. In most cases, the psychosis clears within a few hours to a few days; however, it may persist in some individuals for several

---

[26]   Over-the-counter scopolamine preparations used in the past in Canada specifically to produce drowsiness and sedation have been replaced by products containing an antihistamine. For motion sickness, scopolamine is currently administered in transdermal patches (which release the drug at a constant rate for absorption into the body through the skin).

months. With many hallucinogens (e.g., the atropinic alkaloids, PCP and MDA) the most important factor contributing to a severely adverse reaction — a "bad trip" — is the size of the dose. Nonetheless, a user may suffer an extremely unpleasant episode on any given occasion, irrespective of the dose size. Little is known about other factors that can precipitate such acutely adverse episodes, why such episodes occur on some occasions and not on others, or why some individuals appear to be more vulnerable to them than others. It seems likely that the user's personality, current emotional state, past hallucinogen experiences and attitudes, as well as the setting in which the hallucinogen is taken are contributing factors; however, none of these variables has been scientifically proven to significantly increase the probability of a severely adverse episode.[27]

Reliable reports of bizarre crimes of violence, homicides, suicides and self-mutilations directly associated with the use of hallucinogens are uncommon, although unsubstantiated rumors are abundant. In fact, given the literally millions of unremarkable hallucinogenic episodes, there appears to be a very low frequency of violent events. In instances when violence has occurred, the hallucinogens most frequently implicated are PCP and, to a lesser extent, LSD. Case histories of dangerously violent behavior indicate that severe paranoia or some other drug-induced psychotic effect was involved and that the individual was typically a regular user of PCP or LSD.

The known incidence of serious hallucinogen-related accidents and accidental deaths also appears to be relatively low. Except for hallucinogen-related traffic crashes (which tend to involve cannabis), PCP and LSD are the hallucinogens most frequently associated with serious and lethal accidents. A number of studies have implicated cannabis as a cause of driving impairment and accidents, both as a primary cause (i.e., by itself) and as a secondary cause (i.e., accentuating the effect of alcohol or other drugs). It has been clearly established that even low doses of cannabis can impair driving performance under a variety of standard conditions. Unfortunately, at this time there is no simple test comparable to the breathalyser or roadside screening devices (used to assess alcohol levels) that can be easily administered to drivers to determine the levels of active cannabinoids in the body.

---

27   No specific user variables have been clearly demonstrated to induce acute toxic psychotic episodes. However, when this disorder persists for long periods of time, the probability is that the individual involved was a latent psychotic or was otherwise severely disturbed prior to the psychosis-inducing drug-related event.

Deaths from acute overdose have been known to occur with some hallucinogens. Fortunately, the two drugs most widely used — cannabis and LSD — are not known to have directly caused any deaths even at extremely high doses; nor have mescaline and psilocybin. Certain other hallucinogens, however, are highly toxic. In fact, atropine, scopolamine and hyoscyamine are so dangerous at very high doses that plants containing high concentrations were specifically used for centuries as poisons in Europe and parts of Asia. PMA has also proven to be highly lethal, and deaths have been associated with MDA and MDMA use. PCP has caused a number of deaths resulting from severe muscular rigidity, very high fever, cardiac irregularity and seizures. Other hallucinogenic substances that are known to have caused deaths from overdose include fly agaric, nutmeg, ibogaine, DOB[28] and MDA.

Flashbacks

The spontaneous, transitory and drug-free recurrence of feelings, perceptions and thoughts that were originally experienced during a hallucinogenic drug episode is relatively common among hallucinogen users. This experience is called a flashback. Various studies have reported flashbacks in up to 25 per cent of users (but most studies report lower rates). Although primarily associated with LSD, flashbacks can occur with other hallucinogens and are frequently produced by cannabis in former LSD users.

Visual flashbacks tend to be the most common, although other sensory flashbacks may occur. For example, recurrence of specific intense feelings; spontaneous recall of forgotten thoughts; distortions of time, body image and reality; or almost any other experience originally occurring during a hallucinogenic "trip" can unexpectedly recur, and the individual's subjective reaction may range from intense pleasure to terror. Usually these experiences are brief, lasting no more than a few seconds to a few minutes; however, on rare occasions they have been known to last for up to several hours. Regular users are more likely to experience flashbacks than those who have used LSD only once or twice. A particular flashback may occur only once or may recur over a period of several months. Recurring visual illusions or prolonged after-images (palinopsia) that persist for months or years after last use of hallucinogens have been recognized as a chronic visual complication of hallucinogen use.

The cause of the flashback phenomenon is not known. While many physiologically based hypotheses have been suggested, none have been scientifically proven. By the

---

28   2,5-dimethoxy-4-bromoamphetamine.

same token, it is not possible to predict when, or in what circumstances flashbacks may occur. Depending on the individual, flashbacks may occur during periods of either stress or relaxation, while under the influence of cannabis or alcohol or in a drug-free state, and while dreaming or awake.

Amotivational Syndrome

The term "amotivational syndrome" designates a collection of characteristics and behaviors reported in some chronic heavy users of hallucinogens, particularly cannabis and LSD. The most commonly reported symptoms are gradually increasing apathy, decreasing interest in both the environment and social contacts, loss of effectiveness, passivity, diminished tolerance for frustration, lack of interest in planning ahead, and a disregard for typical social conventions such as appropriateness of dress and public behavior.

Since some hallucinogen users have been known to exhibit many or all of the above symptoms, and the symptoms tend to clear up if drug use is stopped, a causal relationship between the use of hallucinogens and the syndrome has been postulated. However, this relationship has not been proven. An alternative explanation is that the amotivational syndrome was simply part of a lifestyle adopted by many young people during the 1960s and early 1970s. Conservatively, it may be suggested that in some respects the use of cannabis, LSD and other hallucinogens may serve to foster an amotivational syndrome in certain individuals, while for others the amotivational syndrome as a lifestyle or behavior may foster the use of hallucinogens.

Organic Impairment

Psychological and neurological tests designed to detect organic brain impairment have failed to reveal any consistent and statistically significant differences between small groups of healthy non-users and regular users of LSD. Findings of chromosomal damage in users of LSD and cannabis have been inconsistent; no firm conclusions can be drawn from available evidence.[29] Even in those cases where chromosomal damage has been reported, its significance is not known. Some research studies have found a higher risk of both spontaneous abortion and congenital abnormalities in the

---

[29]   One study compared the rate of chromosomal abnormalities among Mexican Indians who had ritually used peyote for generations with the rate among those who did not use peyote. The authors reported no differences in rate between the two groups. See the chapter on mescaline in Section 3.

offspring when mothers regularly used LSD during pregnancy; however, even these finding must be interpreted with caution, as almost all mothers in these studies also used other drugs during pregnancy.

Nonetheless, it must be kept in mind that almost all of the above findings are preliminary and that well-controlled short-term and longitudinal studies in these areas are few.

Tolerance and Dependence

Overall, it appears that tolerance develops to the psychoactive effects of many hallucinogens, and psychological dependence may develop in some regular users. However, the development of physical dependence is not strongly supported by evidence for most hallucinogens. Specifically, one recent study found that an inability to reduce or control drug use does not appear typical of hallucinogen users. However, there is some evidence of the development of mild physical dependence with long-term cannabis use.

The members of the LSD family of hallucinogens (except for DMT)[30] produce a form of rapidly developing tolerance that is more correctly referred to as tachyphylaxis. With repeated daily administrations over as few as three to four days, users cease experiencing the drug's psychoactive effects, irrespective of the size of the dose. In other words, in contrast to many other drugs of abuse, dose increases cannot be used to maintain the desired original effect (or compensate for acquired tolerance). Original sensitivity is restored only after a period of abstinence lasting several days or more. Cross-tachyphylaxis also operates among drugs within this family;[31] after the user can no longer achieve the effects produced by drug, he or she will also be insensitive to the psychoactive effects of other drugs in this family until after the required period of abstinence.

Physical dependence on any drug in the LSD family is not known to occur, although psychological dependence on LSD has been reported to occur occasionally.

---

[30] A study exploring tolerance to the effects of DMT found considerable variation among subjects in the degree to which they had developed tolerance after daily administration for several days.

[31] Recent evidence indicates that LSD and DMT do not share cross-tachyphylaxis.

Except for mescaline, the members of the phenylethylamine family of hallucinogens have not been thoroughly studied with respect to the development of tolerance and dependence. In the case of mescaline, not only does tachyphylaxis occur, but mescaline also shares cross-tachyphylaxis with some members of the LSD family, including LSD and psilocybin. There is no evidence that physical dependence on mescaline can develop. Tolerance to MDMA has been reported to develop rapidly, and some users systematically increase their dosage over weeks or months of use.

Tolerance to the effects of phencyclidine (PCP) has yet to be clearly demonstrated. However, preliminary investigations of chronic users suggest that, given daily administration, frequent dose increases over several weeks are required to sustain the intensity of effects desired. Physical dependence on PCP has not been observed in humans; however, psychological dependence has been reported in chronic heavy users.

Cannabis smokers, over their first few experiences with the drug, may seem to become more sensitive to its effects; however, they have probably simply learned to smoke more efficiently. In contrast, tolerance develops with regular use, and ever-greater doses are then required to produce the original intensity of pleasurable effects.

In contrast to the evidence relating to other hallucinogens, some research evidence indicates that physical dependence on cannabis develops with chronic high-dose use. Abrupt discontinuation may result in mild withdrawal symptoms including irritability, sleep disturbances, weight loss, inhibition of appetite, sweating and gastrointestinal upsets. Psychological dependence on cannabis may occur in some users.

Tolerance to the effects of the atropinic alkaloids develops to a limited extent in humans; however, these drugs do not appear to produce dependence.

Background Reading

Adlaf, E.M., Ivis, F.J. & Smart, R.G. (1997). *Ontario Student Drug Use Survey 1977-1997*. Toronto: Addiction Research Foundation.

Adlaf, E.M., Ivis, F., Ialomiteanu, A., Walsh, G. & Bondy, S. (1997). *Alcohol, Tobacco and Illicit Drug Use Among Ontario Adults: 1977-1996*. The Ontario Drug Monitor, 1996. Toronto: Addiction Research Foundation, ARF Development Series No. 135.

Chilcoat, H.D. & Schultz, C.G. (1996). Age-specific patterns of hallucinogen use in the U.S. population: An analysis using generalized addiction models. *Drug and Alcohol Dependence, 43 (3)*, 143–153.

Grinspoon, L. & Bakalar, J.B. (1979). *Psychedelic Drugs Reconsidered*. New York: Basic Books.

Miller, L.L. (1990). Visual illusions associated with previous drug abuse. *Journal of Clinical Neuro-Ophthalmology, 10 (2)*, 103–110.

Morgenstern, J., Lagenbucher, J. & Labouvie, E.W. (1994). The generalizability of the dependence syndrome across substances: An examination of some properties of the proposed DSM-IV dependence criteria. *Addiction, 89 (9)*, 1105–1113.

Schultes, R.E. & Hofmann, A. (1980). *The Botany and Chemistry of Hallucinogens* (2nd edition). Springfield, IL: Charles C. Thomas.

Wasson, R.G., Hofmann, A. & Ruck, C.A.P. (1978). *The Road to Eleusis*. New York: Harcourt Brace Jovanovich.

Psychiatric Medications:
Antipsychotics, Antidepressants
and Mood Stabilizers

See the chapters in Section 4 on the following drugs: antipsychotics (typical and atypical), lithium, monoamine oxidase inhibitors (MAOIs), selective serotonin reuptake inhibitors (SSRIs), tricyclic antidepressants and valproic acid and carbamazepine. Section 5 includes brief notes on bupropion, nefazodone, reserpine, trazodone and venlafaxine.

Many psychotropic medications are used to help patients with mental illness. Several of these, for example, CNS stimulants such as methylphenidate and CNS depressants such as the benzodiazepines, are discussed in other chapters. Antipsychotics, antidepressants and mood stabilizers are psychiatric medications that provide therapeutic benefit to many patients but do not fall into the other drug classes discussed in this book. They are generally not considered to be drugs of abuse.

Antipsychotics

In the late 1930s it was reported that antihistamines had a quieting effect on patients suffering from severe psychiatric disorders. Until then it had been necessary to treat these patients with very heavy doses of such sedative/hypnotic drugs as bromides and barbiturates, which often rendered them insensible and unable to carry out all but routine functions. By modifying the chemical formula of the antihistamines, chemists found that they could increase the potency of the calming or tranquillizing activity. Antipsychotic medications were the product of this chemical search; chlorpromazine, the prototype, was synthesized in 1950.

Psychosis is a mental state characterized by disorganized thinking in which an individual is unable to distinguish real from unreal experiences. Psychotic symptoms include delusions and disturbances of perception (e.g., hallucinations). Psychosis may be substance-induced (e.g., cocaine, amphetamines) or may be the result of a mental disorder such as schizophrenia. Early clinical application of chlorpromazine in psychotic patients indicated that it had a broad range of desirable effects: for example, calming of hyperexcited patients; reduction of fearfulness and even of terror associated with hallucinations; and reduction of distressing delusional thinking.

While sedative effects are often readily observed after initial administration of many of the antipsychotics, tolerance to the sedating effects develops gradually. Tolerance to the antipsychotic effects ordinarily does not occur to any appreciable extent. Antipsychotics have little or no abuse potential. Deaths have been known to occur, however, when patients combine them with large doses of alcohol, barbiturates, or other CNS-depressant drugs.

Some scholars point to the introduction of chlorpromazine in the early 1950s as the major breakthrough in the field of psychopharmacology. It has been observed that chlorpromazine had as significant an impact on the major mental illnesses as penicillin had on the major infectious diseases. However, chlorpromazine and its many analogues do not cure mental illness. Their contribution is rather in the management of the symptoms of psychosis, permitting patients to engage in other therapeutic endeavors and to live more productive lives in their community. Prior to the introduction of major tranquillizers, most psychotic patients admitted to mental hospitals became either permanent or long-term residents. Since then, there has been a dramatic decrease in the number of chronic residents of the mental hospitals.

The medications used to treat psychosis and schizophrenia did not change significantly from the 1950s to the late 1980s, when a new generation of drugs including clozapine (e.g., Clozaril®), risperidone (e.g., Risperdal®) and olanzapine (e.g., Zyprexa®) began to appear. Previously available antipsychotics had several limitations. First, they were not always effective. Second, some symptoms such as social withdrawal, restriction in the amount of speech or reduced expression of emotions (known as negative symptoms) did not respond well. Third, these antipsychotics were associated with a variety of adverse effects. The newer antipsychotics have potential advantages in terms of helping previous non-responders and improving negative symptoms. They also have a reduced likelihood of neurological adverse effects (extrapyramidal symptoms, tardive dyskinesia). However, rare, serious side effects restrict the use of clozapine. As experience with these agents continues to grow, more information will be gathered regarding their long-term safety and place in treatment.

Antidepressants

A very slight modification of the original antipsychotics yielded a group of compounds referred to as tricyclic antidepressants. Although the first, imipramine (e.g., Tofranil®), was synthesized in 1948, its mood-altering actions were not discovered until almost a decade later (1957). Shortly thereafter, amitriptyline (e.g., Elavil®), was introduced, and subsequently became the most widely employed drug in this group. There are currently various other antidepressant medications available, such as the monoamine oxidase inhibitors (e.g., Parnate®) and the selective serotonin reuptake inhibitors (e.g., Prozac®).

Antidepressants should not be confused with stimulants, such as amphetamines, caffeine and cocaine, which act at different sites and produce different effects. Antidepressants have been demonstrated to have significant beneficial effects in people suffering from major depression. Depression is characterized as episodes of feeling deep sadness that may not be related to life events and may not go away or may go away but keep returning. Accompanying symptoms can include changes in appetite and in sleep patterns, feelings of guilt, inability to experience pleasure and thoughts of suicide. When depressed patients take antidepressant medications, in most cases there is a gradual but significant improvement in mood — usually observable from three to six weeks after the drug treatment is begun. It is necessary for physicians and pharmacists to alert patients that they may not notice real improvement for a few weeks, because mood elevation is gradual. Without such information patients may stop their medication when they fail to experience obvious improvement after a few days of treatment.

Tolerance to the antidepressant actions does not appear to develop, even after protracted use. In fact, it is not unusual for patients to take a daily maintenance dose for years, since depression can be a chronic episodic illness. Antidepressants are not considered to be drugs of abuse.

Given the prevalence of incapacitating chronic depression in our society, the introduction of antidepressants has been of major significance.

Mood Stabilizers

Bipolar disorder (also known as manic-depressive illness) is a chronic mood disorder characterized by recurring episodes of mania or of mania cycling with depression. A manic episode can be defined as a period of abnormally elevated or irritable mood accompanied by other symptoms such as inflated feelings of self importance, decreased need for sleep, easy distractibility, increased talkativeness and excessive involvement in risky pleasurable activities (e.g., spending sprees, sexual imprudence). The specific goals of treatment are to decrease the frequency, severity and psycho-social consequences of these episodes and to improve functioning between episodes. In 1949, lithium was first noted to have a calming effect in manic patients. However, it was about this same time that lithium chloride caused a number of deaths in patients with heart disease who had been using it as a salt substitute. Therefore, it was not until the 1970s that lithium found its place as a treatment option in psychiatry. Lithium (e.g., Lithane®, Carbolith®, Duralith®) is an effective agent both for treating manic episodes and for preventing manic or depressive episodes, which has led to the terminology "mood stabilizer." Lithium was the mainstay of treatment in these patients for many years, until the discovery of the mood stabilizing properties of the anticonvulsant medications valproic acid (e.g., Epival®) and carbamazepine (e.g., Tegretol®), which provide treatment options for patients who may not have responded to lithium or who could not tolerate its side effects.

Background Reading

Canadian Pharmaceutical Association. (1997). *Compendium of Pharmaceuticals and Specialties* (32nd edition). Ottawa: Canadian Pharmaceutical Association.

Mckim, W.A. (1997). *Drugs and Behavior: An Introduction to Behavioral Pharmacology* (3rd edition). New Jersey: Prentice Hall.

Stahl, S. M. (1996). *Essential Psychopharmacology: Neuroscientific Basis and Practical Applications*. Cambridge: Cambridge University Press.

STIMULANTS

See the chapters in Section 3 on amphetamines, caffeine, cocaine, MDA, MDMA ("ecstasy"), nicotine and volatile solvents. See Section 4 for chapters on diethylpropion, ephedrine, fenfluramine, khat, methylphenidate, phentermine, PMA, PPA, propylhexadrine, strychnine, STP (DOM) and TMA. Section 5 includes brief notes on other stimulants, including betel nut, DOB, lidocaine, mazindol, MDEA, methcathinone, phendimetrazine and phenmetrazine.

The class of drugs known as central nervous system (CNS) stimulants includes a large number of substances that have the common property of increasing activity in the central and autonomic nervous systems. Caffeine and nicotine are the most widely used stimulant drugs in North America. However, because of the relatively low potency in their usual dose forms (coffee, tea and cola drinks and tobacco products respectively) compared with other stimulants, and the very different legislative and regulatory controls to which they are subject, caffeine and nicotine are considered separately in Section 3 of this book. Cocaine and the amphetamines are the most widely abused potent stimulants that are consciously used as drugs to produce feelings of energy and euphoria, and are tightly controlled under drug legislation in North America.

Weaker stimulant drugs include ephedrine, pseudoephedrine and phenylpropanolamine (PPA). Ephedrine *(ma-huang)* is a naturally occurring substance found in various plants that has been used in China for thousands of years. Pseudoephedrine (e.g., Sudafed®) and phenylpropanolamine (e.g., Contac C®, Ornade®) are used for their decongestant properties in non-prescription cold and allergy formulations. Phenylpropanolamine may also be found in over-the-counter diet pills in the United States, but in Canada such preparations are no longer available without a doctor's prescription.

Diethylpropion (e.g., Tenuate®), phentermine (e.g., Fastin®, Ionamin®) and mazindol (e.g., Sanorex®) share some of the pharmacological properties of the amphetamines and thus are used medicinally to control appetite. These drugs generally produce milder CNS stimulation and cardiovascular effects than amphetamines. Methylphenidate (Ritalin®) is a mild CNS stimulant commonly used for treating attention-deficit hyperactivity disorder (ADHD). Pemoline (Cylert®), which is also used less frequently for ADHD, differs structurally from the amphetamines and methylphenidate but has similar pharmacologic activity to other stimulants.

MDA (methylenedioxyamphetamine, "love drug"), MDMA (methylene-dioxymethamphetamine, "ecstasy," "Adam"), MDEA (methylenedioxyethamphetamine, "Eve") and PMA (paramethoxyamphetamine) are designer drugs that are chemically related to the amphetamines and mescaline. These synthetic drugs are used for their euphoric and mood-intensifying effects. Another substance with actions similar to amphetamine is (l)-cathinone, the active ingredient found in the leaves of the khat shrub (*Catha edulis*).

History of Use

Cocaine

Cocaine is a stimulant obtained from the leaves of the South American coca bush, *Erythroxylum (Erythroxylon) coca*. It has been used by Indians in South America for at least the past 1,200 years, according to estimates based on the archeological excavation of graves containing coca leaves and pottery with coca-leaf emblems. In its most primitive use, the coca leaf is chewed. Cocaine, the chief active component (and about one per cent of the weight) of the coca leaf, is absorbed through the mucous membranes of the mouth.

During the pre-Inca era, chewing of coca leaves is believed to have been widespread among Indians in the Andes of Peru, Bolivia and northern Chile. At the height of the Inca era, coca-leaf chewing was forbidden to all but the aristocracy and priesthood, although there is evidence that Inca physicians may have employed cocaine's local-anesthetic properties for trephining (circular perforation and removal of bone tissue from the skull). When the Spanish conquistadors arrived in the early 16th century, however, the practice of coca-leaf chewing had again become widespread. Cocaine use increased endurance, suppressed appetite, and produced a general state of euphoria, all of which were important in allowing Indian workers to perform hard work at high altitudes and to withstand inadequate diet. The Spanish disdained the practice of coca-leaf chewing, and initially attempted to eradicate it. However, they quickly learned that enslaved Indians were both more able and more willing to perform heavy labor if payment was in the form of coca leaves. To this day, many Andean Indians continue to chew coca leaves.

Coca plants were brought to Europe before the end of the 16th century, but attracted little interest until the biochemist Albert Niemann isolated pure cocaine in the early 1860s. Within 20 years of his discovery, cocaine had come into widespread use as a local anesthetic. It was also used, without a scientific basis, as a component of countless patent medicines, confections, lozenges and beverages designed to treat any number of minor and often imagined afflictions.

In the early stages of modern medical use, cocaine was believed to be an effective treatment for morphine addiction. Sigmund Freud strongly advocated such use until a close friend, a fellow physician whom he was treating, became one of the first recorded cases of both cocaine addiction and cocaine-induced psychosis. Robert Louis Stevenson was treated with cocaine for tuberculosis in 1885, at which time he is believed to have sketched the first draft of his classic, *Dr. Jekyll and Mr. Hyde*. Shortly thereafter, the original formulation of Coca-Cola®, which contained cocaine, was introduced in North America where it was marketed not only as a pleasant-tasting beverage but also for relief of fatigue and headaches.

Despite the number of prominent people who praised the effects of cocaine, by the beginning of the 20th century its acceptable uses were drastically curtailed as evidence accumulated on both sides of the Atlantic regarding its very high addiction potential and its ability to induce bizarre behavior at high doses. In 1906, for example, cocaine was replaced by caffeine as a constituent in Coca-Cola. In the United States, regulations were imposed on cocaine importation and distribution under the *Harrison Narcotic Act* of 1914. In Canada, cocaine was one of the first drugs to require a doctor's prescription, beginning in Ontario in 1908.

With increasing legal controls on cocaine and with the growing availability of amphetamines in the 1930s, cocaine quickly disappeared as a significant drug of abuse in North America and Europe. Its medical use for such maladies as depression, alcoholism and gastrointestinal disorders was also increasingly restricted. However, because of its important local-anesthetic properties, it still retains some limited medical use, mainly to induce surface anesthesia on the mucous membranes of the nose and throat. For other purposes, new local anesthetics such as lidocaine and bupivacaine have been synthesized, which lack psychoactive effects.

During the 1970s when the dangers of amphetamines were recognized, cocaine made a substantial comeback. In the late 1970s the drug gained popularity among musicians, sports figures, entertainers, artists and certain groups of intellectuals. At this time the drug was usually administered intra-nasally ("snorted") in a crystalline form.

Heavy users would inject it or inhale a pure form of smokable cocaine base. The latter practice, known as "freebasing," is quite dangerous because of the risk of explosion during the preparation of this form of the drug. In the mid-1980s, "crack" cocaine became available. Crack is a form of smokable freebase cocaine that is less expensive and more easily produced (by a process that does not remove adulterants) and used than the traditional freebase drug. The emergence of crack made cocaine available to younger users and it quickly gained popularity.

Amphetamines

The amphetamines and amphetamine-like drugs are relatively new synthetic compounds. The prototype, amphetamine, is structurally related to the naturally occurring stimulant ephedrine. Amphetamine was first synthesized in 1887, although its medical uses were not recognized until much later. In the 1930s, it was discovered that amphetamines had both vasoconstricting and bronchodilating effects. As a consequence of this last finding, amphetamine was marketed as a non-prescription inhaler for nasal congestion in the early 1930s under the trade name Benzedrine®. Amphetamine was used in its early years as a mixture of two chemical forms: dextroamphetamine and levoamphetamine (i.e., d- and l-amphetamine). When these two components of the original drug were separated and studied individually, it was found that dextroamphetamine (later marketed as Dexedrine®) was a much more potent CNS stimulant than levoamphetamine.

By the 1930s and 1940s the medical importance of this group of drugs was generally acknowledged, and their stimulant and anorexant properties were being used to treat a number of medical conditions such as narcolepsy, hyperactivity in children, depression and obesity.

Early enthusiasm for and endorsements of amphetamines by both medical practitioners and researchers gradually diminished during the late 1940s as evidence mounted that amphetamines were being widely abused. Athletes, professionals and students used Benzedrine inhalers for their endurance-increasing properties. In the United States, the abuse of Benzedrine for its powerful euphoric and stimulant properties was so widespread that in 1949 its manufacturer, Smith, Kline and French, responded to social and legal pressure by replacing it with a new product, Benzedrex®, which contained a weaker stimulant, propylhexedrine. Today, amphetamines and other stimulants are classified as banned substances by the International Olympic Committee.

Certain significant physical and psychological health hazards associated with use and abuse of amphetamines were examined in the medical literature as early as the 1930s. The extremely harmful effects of these drugs, however, were most dramatically brought to light only in the late 1960s after young abusers had discovered that injection greatly enhanced the euphoric effects of amphetamines, particularly methamphetamine ("speed," "crank"). Any lingering doubts regarding the potentially damaging effects of amphetamine abuse were rapidly answered by the introduction of "speed." Its users are characterized both by their numerous serious medical, social, psychiatric and legal problems, and by a lifestyle very similar to that of heroin addicts.

Until the 1970s, the major source of street amphetamines had been supplies illegally diverted from the legitimate pharmaceutical industry. Since then, more stringent controls over production and distribution have resulted in a significant reduction of legally produced amphetamines and a corresponding proliferation of illicit supplies from "basement" laboratories set up mainly to produce "speed." Street-drug analyses indicated a consistent decline in the quality (purity) of available "speed" during the 1970s. The clandestine production of methamphetamine uses a number of potentially toxic chemicals, and serious poisonings have been reported (for example, lead poisoning) from the contaminants remaining in the final product.

Often, less potent stimulant drugs such as caffeine, ephedrine and phenylpropanolamine were sold as amphetamines in tablet shapes and colors designed to mimic proprietary amphetamines. In the United States this led to the "look-alike" business, where these legal drugs were sold by mail order. Now manufacturers no longer attempt to mislead consumers in this way, and these products are promoted as stimulants in their own right. Although generally produced in the United States, these "look-alike" tablets have also been found in Canada.

Since the late 1980s, methamphetamine use has again been reported with the emergence of crystal methamphetamine as a street drug of abuse. Also called "ice," because of its transparent, sheet-like crystals, crystal methamphetamine is a smokable form of methamphetamine that is used in a way similar to "crack" cocaine. Use of ice was first reported in East Asian countries and then spread to Hawaii and some areas in North America.

A decrease has been evident in the medically sanctioned uses of amphetamines, which are now limited to the treatment of only a few disorders. Many of the supposed benefits of amphetamines in their earlier medical uses were later found to be (1) nonexistent (as in the treatment of functional psychosis and opiate dependence); (2) questionable or uncertain (as in the treatment of depression); or (3) only short-term (as in the treatment of obesity).

Pharmacological Effects

Central Nervous System
Most drugs that stimulate the central nervous system can cause heightened feelings of well-being in low to moderate doses. At high enough blood levels many such drugs produce intense euphoria. At some point, usually later in the drug-taking episode, most people will experience mild anxiety, tension, nervousness or even agitation whether or not they experience the desired effects. Stimulants may also increase alertness and mask the signs of fatigue, prolonging the user's ability to perform work that requires endurance or concentration. Other effects include increased talkative-ness, repetitive behavior and movements, diminished appetite, altered sexual behavior, increased body temperature, nausea, tremor and twitching of small muscles. Extreme stimulation may result in seizures, coma and death.

Autonomic Nervous System
Among the more significant effects that many stimulants exert on the body are increased heart rate and blood pressure, constriction of the blood vessels, dilation of the pupils and increased rate of respiration — symptoms that are generally viewed as unfavorable and are often described collectively as the "alarm reaction."

Comparing Cocaine and Amphetamines
From a biochemical perspective, cocaine and the amphetamines have different mechanisms of action. Cocaine increases the concentrations of neurotransmitters (including dopamine, serotonin and norepinephrine) available to transmit nerve impulses by inhibiting their reuptake into neurons. Amphetamines, by contrast, cause the release of neurotransmitters from their storage sites in the neurons, as well as inhibiting their reuptake. Because the overall impact of their mechanisms is the same, however, cocaine and amphetamine use result in similar basic clinical symptoms and behavioral problems. One important difference, however, is that cocaine's effects

dissipate much more rapidly than those of the amphetamines. Cocaine's effects may last less than an hour, compared with several hours for those of methamphetamine and amphetamine. Another significant difference is that amphetamines do not share cocaine's local anesthetic properties.

Stimulant Abuse

Both cocaine and amphetamines have a high potential for abuse. Their attractiveness as drugs of abuse results from the exhilaration, euphoria and increased energy they produce in the user.

Patterns of Use

In high doses and with rapid routes of administration (smoking or injecting intravenously), amphetamines or cocaine produces powerful sensations referred to collectively as a "rush." While many users feel that the rush cannot be adequately described in words, some have compared it to an intense orgasm. Once users experience this type of intense euphoria, their pattern of stimulant use may change from controlled or perhaps daily use to high-dose compulsive bingeing. Compulsive abusers of stimulants are a small proportion of the total number of users.

During a binge, users may readminister cocaine as often as every 10 minutes, causing rapid mood changes. The average length of a binge is about 12 hours, although it could last for days. Because amphetamines have a longer duration of action than cocaine, the time between administrations during a binge is usually longer (up to several hours) and binges often last more than a day.

As the length of binges increases, feelings of anxiety, hyperactivity and irritability are mixed with the euphoria. Paranoid psychosis and feelings of panic can occur. The psychosis resembles acute paranoid schizophrenia in many respects and appears to be related to the level of the drug in the blood and not necessarily to any inherent predisposition or weakness in the user. In other words, given a high enough dose, even psychologically normal individuals may experience a psychotic reaction.

Stimulant psychosis is characterized at first by increases in suspiciousness and paranoid thinking, progressing to full-blown paranoid delusions, typically of persecution.

The user may perceive even close friends and relatives as a danger and may react with unprovoked hostility and (sometimes bizarre) violent behavior. Both suicides and homicides have been committed in a state of stimulant psychosis. Early on, pseudohallucinations occur (i.e., hallucinations the user knows to be unreal), the most common of which are auditory and visual. These are typically followed by true hallucinations (which the user believes to be real). Although auditory and visual hallucinations are more common, users often experience tactile and olfactory hallucinations as well. Tactile hallucinations, such as the feeling that bugs are crawling over one's body or under one's skin, are similar to those experienced by alcoholics undergoing withdrawal. Further, users characteristically engage in seemingly meaningless behavior that is compulsively repeated for extended periods.

Although stimulant psychosis and schizophrenia differ in several respects, the scientific literature largely neglects this fact. The predominant hallucinatory experience in stimulant-induced psychosis is visual, whereas auditory hallucinations occur significantly more frequently in schizophrenics. Furthermore, tactile and olfactory hallucinations that are common to stimulant psychosis are unusual in any of the major schizophrenic disorders. Violent behavior is uncommon among schizophrenics, notwithstanding folklore to the contrary. In contrast, the rate of violence among stimulant-induced psychotics is high. (This led to the street warning "speed kills," which was common in the 1960s and 1970s). Most significant, however, is the fact that after the stimulants have been excreted, the toxic psychosis readily disappears in the vast majority of cases.

High-dose abuse of amphetamine-like and other less potent stimulant drugs has produced psychotic symptoms virtually identical to those produced by cocaine and the amphetamines.

Toxicity

Toxicity from stimulant abuse can result from the acute effects after single or multiple doses or from long-term cumulative effects. These effects are typically not distinguished in the literature.

Sudden death from acute cocaine use may result from arrhythmias (abnormal heart rhythms), status epilepticus (seizures), respiratory arrest or brain hemorrhage. Many medical complications have been associated with cocaine use, including heart disease, lung complications (associated with smoking cocaine), acute renal failure, intestinal disorders, hormonal irregularities, obstetrical complications, changes in sexual function, and diseases of the eyes, mouth and nose.

Amphetamine use may result in cardiovascular complications, brain hemorrhage, seizures, arrhythmias, hyperthermia (dangerously high body temperature) and death. Toxicity may also be due to the contaminants found in clandestinely produced methamphetamine. For example, the presence of lead has resulted in acute lead poisoning.

Indirect complications of stimulant use include infections (e.g., HIV, viral hepatitis and sexually transmitted diseases) through the use of non-sterile needles and syringes and/or unprotected sex, and death associated with homicides, suicides and accidents.

Simultaneous Use of Other Drugs

Amphetamine users also commonly use CNS depressants (e.g., benzodiazepines, opiates or alcohol) or cannabis during the crash phase to help reduce agitation and induce sleep. These drugs are also used, sometimes in combination with stimulants, for their own euphoric properties. "Speedball," for example, refers to the combination of cocaine and heroin.

By the same token, many heroin addicts seek amphetamines and/or cocaine for their euphoric properties, particularly when they can no longer achieve appreciable euphoric effects from their regular dose of heroin. They do, however, continue to use heroin regularly to avoid the discomfort of withdrawal. Neither amphetamines nor cocaine can suppress the withdrawal sickness resulting from abrupt abstinence from heroin and other opioids or from barbiturates or other sedative/hypnotics.

Medical Uses of Stimulants

Obesity

To varying degrees, stimulants that affect the central nervous system have an anorectic effect — that is, they suppress appetite. However, amphetamine, methamphetamine and phenmetrazine are no longer recommended for treating obesity because of their potential for abuse. Newer agents, such as diethylpropion (e.g., Tenuate), phentermine (e.g., Fastin, Ionamin) and mazindol (e.g., Sanorex), have pharmacological properties similar to the amphetamines and are available by prescription as adjunct therapy to promote weight loss. Their place in therapy, however, is still controversial. Although the user may lose weight, the effect of stimulants on weight is transient, since the rate of weight loss plateaus after several months of treatment. In general, anorectic drugs are recommended for those obese patients who are medically at risk due to their excessive weight. These drugs should only be used in conjunction with dietary counselling.

Attention-Deficit Hyperactivity Disorder

Approximately one to four per cent of children experience a nervous disorder known as attention-deficit hyperactivity disorder (ADHD). ADHD is characterized by a short attention span, abnormally high levels of dysfunctional and non-directed activity, impulsiveness, distractibility and low frustration tolerance. Symptoms tend to worsen in group or distracting situations. These children's impaired ability to focus selectively on schoolwork severely limits learning and their excessive activity can also produce marked stress in parent-child relationships. Conflicts with parents and poor academic performance often result in further emotional problems and inordinately low self-esteem.

Stimulants have been found to be effective in improving schoolwork and learning. Dextroamphetamine (e.g., Dexedrine) and methylphenidate (e.g., Ritalin) are the drugs of first choice. When these drugs are not effective, pemoline (e.g., Cylert) and other drugs (antidepressants) are used as alternatives. Other treatment approaches, such as behavioral, educational and psychosocial interventions, are also necessary.

The most common side effects of the use of stimulants to treat ADHD are diminished appetite, upset stomach, headaches and insomnia. Exacerbation of tics may also occur. Some researchers believe that the lower-than-average growth rate of some hyperactive children may be due to inadequate nourishment resulting from anorexia related to the use of stimulants during their formative years. Others claim that long-term treatment with methylphenidate does not result in significant growth impairment.

Until recently it was the practice to discontinue the stimulant therapy when the hyperactive child reached puberty. Not only was there concern about growth suppression, but it was also thought that these children "outgrew" their disorder, and that when this happened, continued treatment would produce a stimulant rather than a calming effect. Now, however, it is recognized that while the affected child may indeed gain some measure of control over the hyperactive behavior, the attention deficits that accompany this disorder often do not recover spontaneously. Consequently, clinicians have tended to maintain drug therapy throughout the school years or even longer in those patients who continue to benefit from it. Patients should spend a period of time off of the medication every year to ensure that it has continued benefit.

Stimulant treatment does not benefit all children with ADHD, and there has been controversy over the appropriateness of this treatment in general. These arguments draw strength from the fact that stimulants have not yet been shown to affect the long-term outcome of ADHD.

Narcolepsy

Stimulants are indicated in the treatment of narcolepsy, a rare but serious sickness characterized by sudden, inappropriate (in terms of time, place or need) and uncontrollable attacks of deep sleep.

Other Uses

Cocaine is now only used very infrequently as a local anesthetic in nose and throat surgery. In Canada, dextroamphetamine is used rarely in the management of the symptoms of parkinsonism. Other stimulants, such as ephedrine, pseudoephedrine and phenylpropanolamine (PPA), are used for their decongestant properties in non-prescription cold and allergy formulations. Caffeine tablets (e.g., Wake-ups®) are available without a prescription, and are promoted for their stimulant properties.

Tolerance and Dependence

When stimulants are specifically and regularly abused for their euphoria- and endurance-producing effects, tolerance develops rapidly. During a binge pattern of non-stop administration, users frequently lose the ability to achieve the desired pleasurable response no matter how much of the drug they take. After several days of abstinence, the sensitivity to stimulants is usually restored.

While stimulants can produce psychological dependence, researchers disagree on whether physical dependence results from regular cocaine use. It has been suggested that long-term abuse of stimulants can lead to sustained neurophysiological changes, especially in the regulation of moods and the experience of pleasure. However, withdrawal from stimulants is primarily a psychological phenomenon. The term "crash" has been used to describe the extreme dysphoria, exhaustion, depression, agitation, anxiety and insomnia that directly follow a binge. As part of the withdrawal, if abstinence is maintained, there may be a period of decreased energy and an inability to experience pleasure (anhedonia), effects opposite to the acute effects of stimulants. Accompanying this may be strong cravings for the stimulant drug.

Tolerance to the appetite-suppressant effects of amphetamines can develop within a few weeks even at therapeutic doses. These properties limit the usefulness of amphetamines in the treatment of obesity. In the treatment of ADHD, tolerance to the desired effects may not develop.

Background Reading

Bray, G.A. (1993). Use and abuse of appetite-suppressant drugs in the treatment of obesity. *Annals of Internal Medicine, 119*, 707–713.

Canadian Centre for Drug Free Sport. (1993). *Drug Free Sport — Banned and Restricted Doping Classes and Methods.* Gloucester, Ontario: Canadian Centre for Drug Free Sport.

Canadian Pediatric Society Mental Health Committee. (1990). Use of methylphenidate for attention-deficit hyperactivity disorder. *Canadian Medical Association Journal, 142 (8)*, 817–818.

Cho, A.K. (1990). Ice: A new dosage form of an old drug. *Science, 249*, 631–634.

Elia, J. (1993). Drug treatment for hyperactive children — Therapeutic guidelines. *Drugs, 46 (5)*, 863–871.

Hall, W.C., Talbert, R.C. & Ereshefsky, L. (1990). Cocaine abuse and its treatment pharmacotherapy. *Pharmacotherapy, 10 (1)*, 47–65.

Kennedy, J. (1985). *Coca Exotica — The Illustrated Story of Cocaine.* Cranbury, NJ: Associated University Presses, Inc.

Lowinson, J.H., Ruiz, P., Millman, R.B. & Langrod, J.G. (Eds.). (1997) *Substance Abuse —
A Comprehensive Textbook.* (3rd edition). Baltimore: Williams & Wilkins.

Miller, M.A. & Kozel, N.J. (1991). *Methamphetamine Abuse: Epidemiologic issues and implications.*
National Institute on Drug Abuse Research Monograph 115. Rahway, NJ: NIDA.

Mitler, M.M., Erman, M. & Hajdukovic, R. (1993). The treatment of excessive somnolence with
stimulant drugs. *Sleep, 16 (3),* 203–206.

Pentel, P. (1984). Toxicity of over-the-counter stimulants. *Journal of the American Medical
Association, 252 (14),* 1898–1903.

Schober, S. & Schade, C. (1991). *The Epidemiology of Cocaine Use and Abuse.* National Institute
on Drug Abuse Research Monograph 110. Rahway, NJ: NIDA.

Silverstone, T. (1992). Appetite suppressants — A review. *Drugs, 43 (6),* 820–836.

Smart, R.G. (1991). Crack cocaine use: A review of prevalence and adverse effects.
American Journal of Drug and Alcohol Abuse, 17 (1), 13–26.

Warner, E.A. (1993). Cocaine abuse. *Annals of Internal Medicine, 119 (3),* 226–235.

3

Some Key Drugs

INTRODUCTION

The descriptions of individual drugs in each chapter in Section 3 are organized under the following headings:[1]

Synopsis

This introduction of each chapter provides a brief overview of the particular drug, including key pharmacological effects, tolerance and dependence, and patterns of use and abuse.

Drug Source

This section indicates whether the drug is produced by the pharmaceutical industry, illicit laboratories or both.

Trade Names

This section provides common commercial names, primarily those used in Canada and, to a lesser extent, in the United States. These listings are generally not exhaustive. A list of trade names used in the book is found in Section 6. Trade names are capitalized while non-proprietary names are not. Complete listings of drug commercial trade names are available in the

---

[1]   For further discussion of the issues addressed under most of these headings, see Section 1: Understanding Drugs, Drug Effects and Drug Use.

Compendium of Pharmaceutical and Specialties (Canada) and the *Physician's Desk Reference* (United States).

Street Names

Common slang names used mainly by non-medical users are listed here.

Combination Products

Examples of two types of combination products are identified here:
1. important legitimate pharmaceutical preparations containing the drug under discussion in combination with one or more other drugs
2. common drug combinations taken by non-medical users and known almost exclusively through street drug abuse.

Medical Uses

Listed here are only those major legitimate uses for which a drug is prescribed or recommended by physicians. In some cases, there may be other less common uses.

Physical Appearance

Generally, only the characteristics of the pure drugs are identified. The form and identifying characteristics of legitimate pharmaceutical products (size, color and so on) are described in standard physicians' references such as the *Compendium of Pharmaceuticals and Specialties* in Canada and the *Physician's Desk Reference* in the United States. The physical appearance of drugs sold on the street is often too deceptive for a description to be reliable.

Dosage

Information about two distinct types of dosage is presented here:
1. the accepted single dose range appropriate for the treatment of certain recognized medical conditions
2. the typical single dose range taken by non-medical users.

It should be noted that the figures provided refer to adults and most situations. Under certain conditions, more or less of the drug may be prescribed and/or taken at any one time.

Routes of Administration

Common methods for taking the drug (e.g., injection, oral) are listed here, including those employed for medical and non-medical use.

Effects of Short-Term Use: Low Doses

Lower doses taken by non-tolerant users are defined in two ways:

1. in the case of the drug that has a common medical use, an amount taken on a specific occasion within the therapeutic dose range
2. in the case of a drug that is used mainly or exclusively in non-medical situations, an amount taken on a specific occasion that is typical (i.e., common) for non-tolerant users.

At such dose levels, most users are unlikely to experience serious toxic effects. Nevertheless, it should be kept in mind that, for a number of drugs, there can be a wide disparity with respect to what constitutes a lower dose.

In describing drug effects, *short-term* (as opposed to *long-term*) means the same as *acute* (as opposed to chronic in the medical sense) and refers to the effects produced as a result of a single drug-taking episode.

Effects refers to the results of the drug's actions and the body's changes in response to a drug. Included in each chapter are those effects that range in incidence between occasionally occurring and frequently occurring. Generally, effects that occur very infrequently are not identified. Effects are divided into several subgroups:

- central nervous system (CNS), behavioral, subjective
- cardiovascular
- respiratory
- gastrointestinal
- other.

Note: In this book, drug effects appear in one subgroup or another according to *the system(s) in which the drug's effects are apparent* rather than the drug's *mechanism of action*. (The latter would refer to the underlying cause of the effects.) Thus, for example, rapid heart rate, a common side effect of many drugs, is consistently listed as a cardiovascular effect even though the underlying causes of drug-induced rapid heart rate can vary.

Effects of Short-Term Use: Moderate Doses

In a few cases, it is useful to separate the effects of moderate doses of a drug from those of lower doses for the sake of clearer understanding. This approach is logical with certain medically used drugs that are prescribed at different dose levels to achieve different ends. Benzodiazepines, for example, are usually prescribed at lower doses to reduce anxiety and at moderate doses to induce sleep.

Effects of Short-Term Use: Higher Doses

Higher doses taken by non-tolerant users are defined in two ways:

1. in the case of a drug that has a common medical use, an amount taken on a specific occasion in excess of the therapeutic dose range for that drug
2. in the case of a drug that is used mainly or exclusively in non-medical situations, an amount taken on a specific occasion that is in excess of that typical for non-tolerant users.

At such dose levels, the probability of experiencing serious toxic effects is substantially greater than with low to moderate doses.

Effects of Long-Term Use

In this context, *long-term* refers to regular continuing (or chronic) use. Effects pertain to the body's persistent reactions to the long-term use of a particular drug.

Lethality

This section describes the propensity of a drug to produce death.

Tolerance and Dependence

Material under this heading describes the propensity of a drug to produce tolerance, as well as physical and psychological dependence, with regular use.

Patterns of Use

Patterns of use include the incidence and prevalence of use, including prescribing practices, where relevant, and non-medical use.

Abuse Potential

This section summarizes the degree to which a given drug is abused, or is likely to be abused, in our society, based on an interaction of its dependence liability, inherent harmfulness and availability.

Amphetamines

CNS Stimulant

Synopsis

The amphetamines are a group of central nervous system (CNS) stimulants. These drugs produce a number of effects including wakefulness, alertness, increased energy, reduced hunger and an overall feeling of well-being.

The original drug in this class, amphetamine, consists of a combination of dextroamphetamine (*d*-amphetamine) and its mirror image, levoamphetamine (*l*-amphetamine).[1] Since dextroamphetamine is more effective as a CNS stimulant, pure dextroamphetamine is more potent than the same weight of the amphetamine mixture. Otherwise, the effects of the two preparations are identical. Throughout this chapter, the term "amphetamines" refers broadly to the amphetamine mixture, pure dextroamphetamine and the close chemical congener, methamphetamine.

Amphetamine was first introduced in the 1930s to combat nasal congestion. These drugs were later found to be effective in treating attention-deficit hyperactivity disorder (ADHD) in children and narcolepsy (uncontrollable sleeping episodes). They were also prescribed to control obesity and disorders involving depression but have been shown to be of limited value in treating these latter problems. Any therapeutic benefits amphetamines may have in treating obesity and depression are short-lived and more than offset by the serious liabilities of chronic use: tolerance to desired effects, physical and psychological dependence, sleep disorders, psychological disturbances and unwanted appetite suppression in those taking them for other reasons.

At high dose levels, these drugs can create a toxic psychosis characterized by paranoid delusions, hallucinations, and, frequently, aggressive or violent behavior.

---

[1]   The combination of equal proportions of dextroamphetamine and levoamphetamine is known as *d,l*-amphetamine or racemic amphetamine

Amphetamines have long been abused for their euphoric and stimulant effects. Truck drivers, students and athletes were among the groups that abused them extensively when they were easily available in Canada because of the drugs' ability to extend considerably the normal periods of wakefulness and endurance. Among street drug users, injectable methamphetamine ("speed") has been used because of its greater potency and more rapid onset of effects.

In North America and elsewhere, abuse of amphetamines has declined from its level in the 1960s. Several factors may have contributed to this decline. Increased awareness of their harmful effects and the limitations of their therapeutic benefits resulted in the severe restriction (through legislation) of the medical use of these agents. The resultant decrease in availability of legitimately produced product was partly offset by illicit production, but the quality of illicit product was much less reliable.

The use of crystal methamphetamine, or "ice," has been reported since the mid-1980s, particularly in Hawaii and other western United States. "Ice" is a smokable form of methamphetamine. Smoking as a route of administration allows a very rapid onset of drug action, comparable to intravenous injection, without the injection-related risks.

In addition to amphetamines, there are "designer drugs" related to the amphetamines, such as MDA (methylenedioxyamphetamine), MDMA (methylenedioxymethamphetamine), STP (methyldimethoxyamphetamine), TMA (trimethoxyamphetamine) and PMA (paramethoxyamphetamine).[2] These agents have hallucinogenic and stimulant properties. (For more information on "designer drugs," see the chapter on hallucinogens in Section 2 and on the individual drugs in Sections 3 and 4.)

Drug Source

Amphetamines are produced through chemical synthesis by the pharmaceutical industry and by illicit laboratories. The drastic reduction in the level of manufacture of legally produced amphetamines since the 1960s led to a sharp reduction in their diversion for illegal distribution. Most street amphetamines are synthesized in "basement" laboratories.

2　　These are sometimes referred to as ring-substituted amphetamines.

Trade Names

- amphetamine[3] — Benzedrine® (no longer marketed)

- dextroamphetamine — Dexedrine® (Canada and the United States)

- methamphetamine — Desoxyn® (USA), Methedrine® (no longer marketed).

Street Names

- amphetamines — bennies, black beauties, copilots, eye-openers, lid poppers, pep pills, uppers, wake-ups

- dextroamphetamine — dexies

- methamphetamine— speed, crystal meth, meth, crank

- smokable methamphetamine — ice, Hawaiian salt, rock candy.

Combination Products

Street combinations include "goofballs" (amphetamines and barbiturates) and "speedballs" (methamphetamine or cocaine and heroin).

Medical Uses

Amphetamines may be used to treat:

- narcolepsy (uncontrolled episodes of sleep)

- attention-deficit hyperactivity disorder (ADHD)

- Parkinson's disease.

---

[3]   *d,l*-amphetamine, the mixture of equal proportions of dextroamphetamine and levoamphetamine.

Physical Appearance

In pure form, amphetamine sulphate and dextroamphetamine sulphate are white, odorless crystalline powders with a bitter taste. They are soluble in water and slightly soluble in alcohol. In pure form, methamphetamine hydrochloride (not legally available in Canada) is a white, odorless, bitter crystalline powder soluble in water and in alcohol.

Illicit preparations, which vary in level of purity, include fine to coarse powders, crystals and "chunks" that are whitish in color, occasionally with traces of grey or pink. They may be supplied loose or in capsules or tablets of various sizes and colors (sometimes imitating commercially produced compounds).

Smokable methamphetamine resembles shaved glass slivers or clear rock salt.

Dosage

Medical

- for narcolepsy: amphetamine or dextroamphetamine in a daily dose range of 5 to 60 mg

- for attention-deficit hyperactivity disorder (ADHD): amphetamine or dextroamphetamine in a daily dose range of 2.5 to 40 mg.

Non-medical

The dosage taken by occasional users may be within the therapeutic range (up to 60 mg per day). However, dependent heavy users are likely to take daily doses several times greater.

It is difficult to assess the doses used by those relying on illegal sources of supply. The gross weight of amphetamines purchased on the street often includes substantial amounts of diluents and impurities. Also, street drug sellers or "pushers" often misrepresent, either knowingly or unknowingly, the substances they are selling. As a result, amphetamines bought on the street may actually be wholly or partly one of the weaker stimulants such as ephedrine or caffeine.

Given the above cautions, a reasonable estimate of daily dose for heavy users is 250 to 1000 mg per day.

Routes of Administration

Most commonly, amphetamines are taken orally, injected or smoked. Less commonly, amphetamines are sniffed or snorted.

Effects of Short-Term Use: Low Doses[4]

The effects of short-term use of low doses of amphetamines include the following:

CNS, *subjective, behavioral*: overstimulation, restlessness, dizziness, insomnia, euphoria, dysphoria, mild confusion, tremor, and, in rare instances, panic and/or psychotic episodes; reduced appetite; dilated pupils; increased talkativeness, alertness and energy, reduction of fatigue and drowsiness, general increase in psychomotor activity, and a heightened sense of well-being; improved performance on fatigue-impaired simple mental tasks.

***Cardiovascular*:** palpitations, increased heart rate (or slowed initially), irregular heartbeat, headache, increased blood pressure.

***Respiratory*:** increased breathing rate and depth.

***Gastrointestinal*:** dryness of the mouth, unpleasant taste, constipation or diarrhea, appetite suppression, abdominal cramps.

***Other*:** increase or decrease in libido, possible temporary impotence.

---

4   Single doses within the therapeutic range, up to 60 mg per day in non-tolerant individuals.

Effects of Short-Term Use: Higher Doses[5]

Intensification of the low-dose effects may occur with higher doses, as well as any of the following effects:

Subjective, behavioral: intense exhilaration and euphoria, rapid flow of ideas, feelings of increased physical strength and mental capacity, talkativeness, excitation, agitation, sometimes panic or irritability. With repeated administrations, the amphetamine user, like the cocaine user, may suffer from a stimulant psychosis consisting of paranoid thinking, confusion and perceptual distortions, including hallucinations. Violent behavior has also been observed. The amphetamine "rush" or "flash," an effect greatly desired by the abuser, is a highly pleasurable sensation experienced almost immediately after intravenous injection and felt to be similar to an intense orgasm or to electric shock.

Neurological: seizures, cerebral hemorrhage, high fever, coma.

Cardiovascular: angina pain, heart attack, abnormal heart rhythm, fainting, high or low blood pressure, and cardiovascular collapse.

The Methamphetamine "Run"

In an attempt to maintain the initial effects of exhilaration and highly enhanced self-confidence, many methamphetamine abusers repeatedly administer the drug several times a day over a period of several days. This is known as an amphetamine "run"— analogous to a cocaine "binge." (People who use injectable methamphetamine in this manner have been called "speeders" or "speed freaks.") During the first day of the run, feelings of euphoria and elevated self-esteem and intense sexual arousal are commonly reported. Thought patterns tend to be rapid and of a decisive nature. Periods of talkativeness may alternate with periods of intense preoccupation with one's thoughts and behavior. Usually by the second day, the euphoria is gradually replaced by increasing agitation. Thoughts can race so rapidly that concentration becomes extremely difficult. Frightening visual images that the user knows to be unreal (pseudohallucinations) often occur under these conditions and cannot be controlled. Although less common, true hallucinations (hallucinations that the user believes to be real) may also occur and may be visual, auditory, tactile or olfactory. Runs usually last three to five days, or longer, and usually end when the drug supply has run out or the user is too exhausted to continue.

---

5   Above the medically recommended level in non-tolerant users, or lower doses in particularly sensitive individuals.

Effects of Long-Term Use

Regular amphetamine use at low or high doses can (directly) produce the following effects: chronic sleeping problems including insomnia, frequent nocturnal awakening and poor-quality sleep; anxiety and tension; appetite suppression, which may result in disorders related to poor nutrition; high blood pressure, and rapid and irregular heartbeat. Regular high-dose use of amphetamines can also (directly) produce suspiciousness and paranoid thinking, severe agitation, repetitious behavior and in some cases a prolonged amphetamine psychosis.

Potentially lethal cardiac complications (heart attack, heart failure) have been associated with chronic use of "ice."

To combat these drug-related effects, chronic abusers often take alcohol, minor tranquillizers, other sedative/hypnotics, cannabis and, when available, opiates. The probability of multiple drug dependence among chronic abusers is therefore quite great.

In addition to the direct effects, serious indirect health risks are associated with chronic amphetamine use. Illicitly produced methamphetamine may be contaminated with other substances (intentionally or due to inadequate processing). For example, lead poisonings have been reported in injectable methamphetamine users. Frequent injection of drugs and needle sharing among users can result in such communicable and serious diseases as viral hepatitis, septicemia, acquired immune deficiency syndrome (AIDS) and bacterial endocarditis. Abscesses, phlebitis and infections may occur at or around the injection sites because of incorrect injection technique, non-sterile needles, or repeated injections at the same spot. Collapsed blood vessels are also possible, and blockage of blood vessels is common among those who inject street preparations, which may contain insoluble particles that can lodge in the small blood vessels of the hands, feet, lungs and brain.

Lethality

The use of amphetamines can cause death. Death has resulted from intravenous injection of as little as 120 mg. However, the lethal dose varies widely among individuals, and non-tolerant persons have been known to survive doses of 400 to 500 mg.

Causes of deaths attributed to amphetamine overdose include rupture of blood vessels in the brain; cardiac failure, hyperthermia (extremely high fever), seizures and coma. Speed (injectable methamphetamine) has a reputation for being particularly dangerous, which is reflected in the popular slogan: "Speed kills."

Like cocaine and other psychoactive drugs, amphetamines may be an indirect cause of death. Numerous violent and sometimes bizarre accidents, homicides and suicides have been documented, where those involved were suffering from amphetamine psychosis at the time of the violent episode. Homicide victims have ranged from close relatives and amphetamine co-users to complete strangers. Both suicide attempts and successful suicides have occurred under heavy intoxication with amphetamines and during or after withdrawal. Some deaths are probably also attributable to disease indirectly resulting from lifestyles associated with amphetamine abuse.

Tolerance and Dependence

Tolerance to many of the significant effects of the amphetamines has been reported to develop when these drugs are used chronically.

Tolerance develops rapidly to the euphoria and other mood-elevating effects of amphetamines, particularly in the case of "speeders." Many users report having increased their daily dose several times over the course of their drug-using career to maintain or increase the pleasurable effects of the drug. During a "run," speeders report that the full effects of the "rush" occur only immediately after the first "hit" (injection) and that the intensity of this effect rapidly diminishes upon successive injections. Significantly, the daily dose ultimately reaches a plateau beyond which no further dose increase can produce the desired effects. Indeed, with uninterrupted use, pleasurable effects can give way to dysphoria, paranoid thinking or even psychosis. Tolerance to the psychosis-producing effects of amphetamines does not develop.

Tolerance has also been reported to develop to the following effects: appetite suppression, dilation of the pupils, slightly increased body temperature (hyperthermia), increased blood pressure and heart rate, increased respiratory rate and increased energy (progressively expressed as agitation and restlessness).

Children do not seem to develop tolerance to the beneficial effects of amphetamine treatment of attention-deficit hyperactivity disorder (ADHD).

Individuals who suffer from narcolepsy (frequent inappropriate and uncontrollable sleeping episodes) usually respond favorably to amphetamines. In such cases, tolerance to the anti-narcoleptic effect does not appear to develop even after years of continued use.

Like cocaine, amphetamines can also produce reverse-tolerance or sensitization to certain effects, such as stereotypy (repetitious, seemingly meaningless behavior). Cross-sensitivity may also occur between cocaine and amphetamines.

When chronic, high-dose use of amphetamines is abruptly discontinued, withdrawal does not include major grossly observable physiological disruptions. Rather, the prominent symptoms are extreme fatigue followed by prolonged but disturbed sleep. Upon awakening, the user typically has a huge appetite. Irritability, lethargy and moderate to very severe emotional depression are also typical. Sleep disturbances and psychotic symptoms may persist after the period of prolonged sleep. Dysphoria and anhedonia (the inability to experience pleasure) may continue for weeks.

Psychological dependence — a persistent craving for the mood-altering effects — can occur. Users may crave the drug effects so intensely that, if the drug is temporarily unavailable, they can experience severe distress or even feelings of panic.

Patterns of Use

Amphetamine use peaked between the 1950s and the early 1970s. Since that time there has been a sharp decline in medical use of these agents. For example, in the United States in 1967 there were 23 million prescriptions for amphetamines for their anorectic effects, compared with only 400,000 amphetamine prescriptions in 1989. This decline in legal use was an important factor in the decline of widespread availability, and therefore use, of amphetamine.

However, in the mid-1980s, increased use of illicit methamphetamine was again being reported. In the United States, the number of methamphetamine drug laboratory seizures increased from 88 in 1981 to 652 in 1989. In the late 1980s, over 80 per cent of all clandestine laboratories seized were involved in manufacturing methamphetamine. Also in the United States, emergency-room visits due to methamphetamine increased by a factor of 1.7 from 1986 to 1989. In Hawaii, the use of "ice," a smokable form of methamphetamine, was considered to be quite high by the late 1980s. Surveys conducted by the Addiction Research Foundation in the early 1990s indicated that approximately one per cent of Ontario students and street youth had tried "ice" in the previous year.

Potential for Abuse

Abuse Liability

Among central nervous system drugs of abuse, the abuse liability of methamphetamine and amphetamine is considered to be extremely high. Both drugs can produce powerful euphoria. (Experienced users claim that the euphoric and stimulant properties of methamphetamine are greater.) Because both drugs are highly water-soluble in their pure salt form, they can be administered in large amounts by injection directly into the bloodstream, resulting in very rapid and intense gratification.

Inherent Harmfulness

It is unclear whether inherent harmfulness is a significant factor in deterring abuse of these drugs. Many experienced abusers, particularly of injectable methamphetamine, frequently engage in repeated use of very high doses. They are generally aware of the heightened risks and are also willing to accept them. However, the overall decline in use of these drugs may have been influenced somewhat by increased awareness of their harmful effects.

Availability

The potential for abuse of the amphetamines is now greatly reduced because of the drastic reduction in their availability since the early 1970s.

Background Reading

Canadian Pharmaceutical Association. (1997). *Compendium of Pharmaceuticals and Specialties* (32nd edition). Ottawa: Canadian Pharmaceutical Association.

Carson, P., Oldroyd, K. & Phadke, K. (1987). Myocardial infarction due to amphetamine. *British Medical Journal, 294,* 1525–1526.

Chandler, D.B. & Norton, R.L. (1990). Lead poisoning associated with intravenous-methamphetamine use — Oregon, 1988. *Journal of the American Medical Association, 263 (6),* 797–798.

Cho, A.K. (1990). Ice: A new dosage form of an old drug. *Science, 249,* 631–634.

Hong, R., Matsuyama, E. & Nur, K. (1991). Cardiomyopathy associated with the smoking of crystal methamphetamine. *Journal of the American Medical Association, 265 (9),* 1152–1154.

King G.R. & Ellinwood, E.H. (1992). Amphetamines and other stimulants.(Chapter 19). In J.H. Lowison, P. Ruiz, R.B. Millman & J.G. Langrod (Eds.), *Substance Abuse — A Comprehensive Textbook* (2nd edition) (pp. 247–270). Baltimore: William & Wilkins.

Miller, M.A. & Kozel, N.J. (1991). *Methamphetamine Abuse: Epidemiologic issues and implications.* National Institute on Drug Abuse Research Monograph 115. Rahway, NJ: NIDA.

Miller, N.S., Millman, R.B. & Gold, M.S. (1989). Amphetamines: Pharmacology, abuse and addiction. *Advances in Alcohol and Substance Abuse, 8 (2),* 53–69.

Smart, R.G., Walsh, G.W., Adlaf, E.M. & Zdanowicz, Y.M. (1992). *Drifting and Doing. Changes in Drug Use Among Toronto Street Youth, 1990-1992.* Toronto: Addiction Research Foundation.

Anabolic Steroids

DRUG CLASS: Anabolic Steroids, Androgens

Synopsis

Anabolic steroids, more precisely defined as androgenic anabolic steroids, include testosterone, the main androgenic hormone (male sex hormone) in males, and all synthetic derivatives of testosterone. These drugs have both anabolic (tissue-building) and androgenic (masculinizing) effects. They are used primarily in veterinary medicine, but they also have medical uses in humans. Anabolic steroids are also used by athletes (e.g., sprinters, weight lifters and football players) in the belief that they will enhance performance, and by body builders to increase muscle bulk and body size. Increasingly, they are used by adolescents to "improve" their appearance. In fact, dissatisfaction with body image — particularly the perception of being too small or not muscular enough — is common in individuals who use anabolic steroids. This disorder has been called "reverse anorexia nervosa." Despite the fact that there is little compelling evidence that anabolic steroids enhance athletic performance, the general public and young athletes in particular are convinced that these drugs can improve both physique and athletic performance.

While it is illegal to sell anabolic steroids in North America (except by a prescription or for veterinary use), possession of these drugs is not illegal. They can often be readily obtained in gyms or other weight-lifting settings.

Anabolic steroids have both acute and chronic side effects, some of which are potentially dangerous to the user. Recent studies have indicated that chronic anabolic steroid use is associated with signs and symptoms of dependence.

Drug Source

Anabolic steroids are regulated under Canada's *Controlled Drugs and Substances Act,* and are legally available for human use only by prescription. It is estimated that 85 to

100 per cent of anabolic steroids used by athletes are obtained through the illegal black market. Mexico is believed to be the largest source of anabolic steroids for non-prescription use in the United States. Many of these compounds are produced in clandestine laboratories, and concerns over safety have been raised, particularly for the injectable preparations. Individuals who sell steroids illegally are likely to be users of steroids themselves, and new users are often recruited at gyms.

Trade Names

The following table indicates representative trade names and therapeutic uses for selected anabolic steroids currently available for human and veterinary use.

Table 1. Non-Proprietary and Representative Trade Names and Therapeutic Applications for Selected Anabolic Steroids

Non-Proprietary Name	Representative Trade Name	Therapeutic Use (Human/Veterinary)
Injectable Anabolic Steroids		
boldenone undecylenate	Equipoise®	veterinary
nandrolone decanoate	Deca-Durabolin®	human/veterinary
nandrolone laurate	Nandrobolin®	veterinary
stanozolol	Winstrol V®	veterinary
testosterone cypionate	Depo-Testosterone®, Cypionate®, Scheinpharm Testone-Cyp®	human
testosterone enanthate	Delatestryl®, PMS-Testosterone Enanthate®	human
testosterone injection	Malogen Aqueous®, Testos 100®, UniTest®, Testosterone Suspension®	human/veterinary
testosterone propionate	Testex®, Malogen® (oil), Anatest®	human/veterinary
Oral Anabolic Steroids (C-17 alkyl derivatives)		
danazol	Cyclomen®, Danocrine®	human
ethylestrenol	Maxibolin®	human
methandrostenolone	Various U.S. manufacturers	human
methyltestosterone	Metandren®	human
oxandrolone	Anavar®	human
oxymetholone	Anadrol®, Anapolon 50®	human
oxymesterone	Oranabol®	human
stanozolol	Winstrol V®, Winstrol®	human/veterinary
testosterone undecanoate	Andriol®	human

Street Names

Steroids, roids, juice. Other street names vary, depending on the agent.

Combination Products

No pharmaceutical combination products are known.

Medical Uses

Human medical uses for anabolic steroids include the treatment of:
- testosterone deficiency in males, including delayed male puberty
- chronic conditions involving tissue wasting (catabolic states)
- certain types of anemia
- certain types of osteoporosis (as one component of treatment)
- certain types of breast cancer (advanced or metastatic)
- hereditary angioneurotic edema (a disorder in which fluid leaks from the blood vessels).

Dosage[1]

Medical
The dose of anabolic steroids varies depending on the agent, route of administration and purpose of use. Androgens are used primarily to treat androgen deficiency in men, in order to develop or maintain secondary sexual characteristics. For this purpose, dose levels are selected to provide the equivalent of 10 mg of testosterone per day. Because orally administered testosterone undergoes extensive metabolism in the liver, intramuscular preparations are widely used. Typically, doses of 25 mg of testosterone propionate are given three times weekly. With some other injectable testosterone derivatives, the drug may be injected every two weeks.

---

[1]   All doses refer to adults.

Non-medical

The primary reason for non-medical use of steroids is their anabolic effects in athletes, body builders and young men seeking to improve their appearance. Doses used by weight lifters and body builders are often 100 times larger than those used medically, while those used by sprinters and endurance athletes may be closer to usual medical recommendations. Non-medical users may take steroids according to one of many dosing regimes, including one of the following:

- *Cycling* refers to periods of steroid use followed by periods of abstinence. These cycles may be short (i.e., six to eight weeks on the drug, followed by six to eight weeks' abstinence) or long (six to eight weeks on the drug and up to 12 months of abstinence).

- *Pyramiding* is a variation of cycling that involves building up to a peak dose and then tapering down.

- *Stacking* involves the use of more than one steroid (up to eight) and combinations of both oral and injectable forms. The technique of progressively increasing the dose and numbers of steroids used before decreasing the doses for a drug-free period is called "stacking the pyramid."

Steroids have also been taken with human growth hormone (HGH) to enhance their anabolic effects.

Routes of Administration

Anabolic steroids are taken orally or by intramuscular injection.

Effects of Use: Low Doses

When androgenic-anabolic steroids are used to treat hormone deficiency, typical sexual characteristics and function are likely to develop (similar to naturally occurring male development in puberty) or be maintained. These effects include deepening of the voice, penis growth, development of body hair and, subsequently, beard growth. These effects are accompanied by large muscle development, increased physical vigor and a feeling of well-being.

Women who use anabolic steroids are at risk of developing masculine features including acne, growth of facial hair and hoarsening or deepening of the voice. Menstrual irregularities may also occur. With long-term use, women may develop male-pattern baldness, growth of excessive body hair, prominent muscles and enlargement of the clitoris.

Effects of Use: High Doses

CNS, behavioral, subjective: Use of anabolic steroids can produce a range of CNS effects including euphoria; anxiety; irritability; aggression (steroid rage); feelings of decreased fatigue and faster recovery from weight-training workouts; insomnia; antidepressant effects or depression, sometimes with suicidal thoughts and/or manic phases; psychosis; delirium; hypomania and mania.

Cardiovascular: The use of high doses of anabolic steroids can contribute to heart attack; enlargement of the heart and abnormalities of the heart muscle leading to cardiac arrest; stroke; blockage of circulation in the legs due to blood clots and blood clots in the lungs; reduction in high density lipoproteins (HDL) and increased blood pressure.

Gastrointestinal: Nausea, vomiting and gastric irritation are associated with high doses of anabolic steroids, especially oral dosing.

Reproductive: Among women, hormone imbalance resulting from use of anabolic steroids can lead to irregular menstrual periods. Among men, steroid use can cause reduction in the size of the testes, decreased sperm production and reduced sperm motility resulting from disruption of the body's production of hormones (including testosterone, follicle-stimulating hormone [FSH] and luteinizing hormone).

Secondary sexual effects: Among women, anabolic steroid use can cause masculinization due to drugs' androgenic effects. These effects include acne, the development of a coarse and deep voice, growth of facial hair, reduction in breast size, male-pattern baldness and clitoral enlargement. Male steroid users may experience feminization due to the metabolism of testosterone into estrogen. Resulting changes can include enlargement and pain in the breasts.

Musculoskeletal: Anabolic steroid use can lead to musculoskeletal problems, such as an increased risk of tendon ruptures and the possibility that adolescents who are still growing will not attain their full height because of premature closure of the long bones.

Liver:[2] Use of high doses of anabolic steroids has been associated with acute elevation of liver enzymes (transaminases), hepatitis, liver enlargement and liver cancer.

Other physical effects: Anabolic steroid use can cause acne and fluid retention.

Indirect effects: Sharing needles and the use of non-sterile equipment can contribute to the transmission of, and increase the user's risk of contracting, bacterial and viral infections, including hepatitis and HIV. Improper injection techniques, repeated injections at the same site or ingredients/impurities in preparations intended for veterinary use may lead to abscesses and blood clots.

Lethality

While steroids have been used in massive doses for their anabolic effects in athletes and body builders, no case reports of lethal overdose are known. Supportive therapy for overdose symptoms is the recommended treatment. Liver toxicity is one potentially serious complication of high doses or long-term use, particularly with the subgroup of anabolic steroids related to methyltestosterone (i.e., the so-called 17 alpha-alkyl subgroup). Because this toxicity may lead to liver cancer, liver functions should be monitored closely.

The potentially lethal side effects that occur with long-term use of anabolic steroids include stroke, liver bleeding and infections (spread by needle use).

Tolerance and Dependence

No evidence suggests that tolerance to anabolic steroids exists. However, it appears that dependence on these drugs can develop. Although anabolic steroid dependence is not included as a substance-related disorder in the American Psychiatric

---

2   These effects have been associated with use of testosterone and related 17 alpha-alkyl steroids.

Association's *Diagnostic and Statistical Manual of Mental Disorders* (DSM-IV), several characteristics of this syndrome are consistent with DSM criteria for dependence:

1. Use continues over a longer period than intended.
2. Unsuccessful attempts are made to stop use.
3. Time spent obtaining, using, and recovering from the effects of steroids interferes with other commitments.
4. Use continues despite psychological problems caused by the hormones.
5. Characteristic withdrawal symptoms occur.
6. The hormones are taken to relieve these withdrawal symptoms.

In one study of 77 anabolic steroid users who completed an assessment based on the DSM-III-R, 14.3 per cent met the criteria for dependence.

The mechanism underlying the development of dependence is unclear. However, the development of psychological dependence may be due to the action of the sex hormones in inducing euphoria and stimulating the reward mechanisms in the brain. It has been suggested that the euphoria from steroids may be caused by the release of naturally occurring opioids.

When use of anabolic steroids is stopped abruptly, the resulting syndrome can simulate opioid withdrawal. In one chronic steroid user, withdrawal was precipitated by the administration of the opioid antagonist naloxone. The symptoms in this case included nausea, headache, dizziness, sweating, "goose-flesh," chills, and increased pulse rate, blood pressure and temperature.

Patterns of Use

Because of their limited medical uses in humans, anabolic steroids are rarely prescribed. Most legal use of these drugs involves veterinary products used to promote muscle development and weight gain in farm animals.

Since many steroid products are designated for veterinary use and are considered unfit for humans, their sale is not regulated in the same way as drugs for human use. Therefore, those abusing the drugs often use veterinary formulations, since such formulations are available, their possession is legal, they are effective in building muscle mass, and they are highly promoted by weight-lifting books and magazines and by other users. While trafficking the drugs for human use is illegal, the penalties imposed tend to be minor.

Anabolic steroids are used extensively by athletes such as football players, power lifters, and track and field competitors who desire more muscular builds. While their use is believed to be extensive among Olympic athletes, the International Olympic Committee bans the use of anabolic steroids, as well as human growth hormone (HGH) and human chorionic gonadotropin (HCG). Athletes who are caught using these agents risk suspension from competition. Many professional sports have also implemented drug testing programs that include anabolic steroid testing.

A disturbing trend in anabolic steroid use has been observed in adolescents. In many of these young people, self-esteem is heavily dependent on body size and shape, and they turn to anabolic steroids to achieve a muscular build. Adolescents are also bombarded with indications that professional and internationally ranked athletes use steroids to improve athletic performance and thereby gain a competitive edge. Finally, the availability and legality of steroids contribute to their use in adolescents. The consequences, both physical and psychological, of long-term use require further investigation.

Potential for Abuse

Dependence Liability
With short-term use, the dependence liability of anabolic steroids appears to be low, perhaps due to a delay in the onset of euphoric effects after administration. However, physical dependence has been demonstrated following extended periods of use, including withdrawal symptoms when these compounds are discontinued abruptly. Tolerance to the effects of these drugs has not been shown.

Inherent Harmfulness
Anabolic steroids are unlikely to cause acute problems with short-term overdose. They are used for short periods by some weight lifters in doses up to 100 times the levels produced by a normal male without evidence of such problems. However, the long-term consequences of steroid use are serious. Psychiatric consequences such as paranoia and a manic-depressive-like disorder can develop. Serious physical side effects are also of concern and include cardiovascular problems, reduction in the size and function of the testes, and sterility. Masculinizing effects in female users are not reversible.

Availability

Anabolic steroids are readily available in local gyms and are often supplied by other gym patrons. They may be diverted from veterinary sources, smuggled in from other countries or produced by local manufacturers.

Background Reading

Appleby, M., Fisher, M. & Martin, M. (1994). Myocardial infarction, hyperkalemia and ventricular tachycardia in a young male body-builder. *International Journal of Cardiology, 44 (2)*, 171-174.

Bahrke, M.S., Wright, J.E., Strauss, R.S. & Catlin, D.H. (1992). Psychological moods and subjectively perceived behavioral and somatic changes accompanying anabolic-androgenic steroid use. *American Journal of Sports Medicine, 20 (6)*, 717-724.

Brower, K.J. (1992). Anabolic steroids: Addictive, psychiatric and medical consequences. *American Journal of Addiction, 1* , 100-114.

Brower, N.J., Blow, F.C., Young, J.P. & Hill, E.M. (1991). Symptoms and correlates of anabolic-androgenic steroid dependence. *British Journal of Addiction, 86*, 759-768.

Canadian Centre for Drug Free Sport. (1993). *Drug Free Sport: Banned and Restricted Doping Classes and Methods.* Gloucester, Canada: Canadian Centre for Drug Free Sport.

Dickerman, R.D., Schaller, F., Prather, I. & McConathy, W.J. (1995). Sudden cardiac death in a 20-year-old bodybuilder using anabolic steroids. *Cardiology, 86 (2)*, 172-173.

Friedl, K. (1990). Reappraisal of the Health Risks Associated with High Doses of Oral and Injectable Androgenic Steroids. Rockville MD: National Institute on Drug Abuse, *NIDA Research Monograph No., 102.*

Galloway, G.P. (1997). Androgenic Steroids. In J.H. Lowinson, P. Ruiz, R.B. Millman & J.G. Langrod (Eds.), *Substance Abuse: A Comprehensive Textbook* (3rd edition). Baltimore: Williams and Wilkins.

Kennedy, M.C. & Lawrence, C. (1993). Anabolic steroid abuse and cardiac death. *Medical Journal of Australia, 158 (5)*, 346-348.

Moss, H.B., Panzak, G.L. & Tarter, R.E. (1993). Sexual functioning of male anabolic steroid abusers. *Archives of Sexual Behavior, 22(1)*, 1-12.

Pope, H.G. Jr. & Katz, D.L. (1994). Psychiatric and medical effects of anabolic-androgenic steroid use. *Archives of General Psychiatry, 51*, 375-382.

Williamson, P.J. & Young, A.H. (1992). Psychiatric effects of androgenic and anabolic-androgenic steroid abuse in men: A brief view of the literature. *Journal of Pharmacology, 6*, 20-26.

Antihistamines

DRUG CLASS: Histamine Antagonist

Synopsis

Antihistamines are a chemically heterogeneous class of drugs (e.g., diphenhydramine, chlorpheniramine) that can block the effects of histamine, a naturally occurring substance found in tissue throughout the body. Histamine is released from the cells when the body experiences a hypersensitivity reaction (i.e., an allergic reaction), when cells are injured, or in reaction to a variety of drugs and poisons. Histamine, by binding to H_1 receptors, causes flushing, itching and other unpleasant symptoms associated with allergic reactions. The term "antihistamine" traditionally refers to agents that block H_1 receptors.

Drugs that block the stomach acid-producing actions of histamine at H_2 receptors (e.g., cimetidine, ranitidine, famotidine and nizatidine) are also available. However, the pharmacology of these H_2 receptor antagonists is very different from that of antihistamines, and these drugs lack the abuse potential of H_1 receptor antagonists. Therefore they are not included in this chapter.

In addition to their H_1 receptor antagonist effects, many antihistamines also have sedative and anticholinergic effects (see the chapter on anticholinergic agents in Section 4). Some antihistamines that produce drowsiness and sedation as side effects are used in a number of over-the-counter (i.e., non-prescription) products marketed worldwide to promote sleep and relaxation. In Canada, diphenhydramine and doxylamine are sold in over-the-counter products intended for these purposes. Antihistamine products are only mildly effective when compared with the sedative/hypnotic prescription drugs used for the same purposes.

Newer ("non-drowsy") antihistamines, such as terfenadine (Seldane®), astemizole (Hismanal®) and loratadine (Claritin®), which have a different pharmacology from the antihistamines described in this chapter, have also become available. Although they also block H_1 receptors, they generally do not have sedative or anticholinergic properties, and do not share the abuse potential of the older antihistamines.

Many people underestimate the potentially toxic effects of antihistamines on young children, and fail to store the drugs safely out of reach. Several children have been accidentally and seriously poisoned, and some have died as a result. Large quantities of antihistamines can also be hazardous to adults, particularly when they are taken with other central nervous system (CNS) depressants.

As is the case with other anticholinergic agents, higher doses of antihistamines may have hallucinogenic, mood-elevating and stimulant effects (see the chapters on anticholinergic agents and dimenhydrinate in Section 4). Some antihistamines enhance the pleasurable effects of alcohol and other CNS-depressant drugs of abuse. For these reasons, and because they are easily available, antihistamines have a moderate abuse potential.

Drug Source

Antihistamines are produced through chemical synthesis by the pharmaceutical industry.

Trade Names

Trade names of some of the commonly used products include:

- brompheniramine — Dimetane®

- chlorpheniramine — Chlor-Tripolon®

- cyproheptadine — Periactin®

- diphenhydramine — Benadryl®, Nytol®, Sominex®, Sleep-Eze®

- doxylamine — Unisom®

- tripelennamine — Pyribenzamine®.

Street Names

None in common use.

Combination Products

Antihistamines are ingredients in many prescription and over-the-counter cough-suppressant medications, analgesics, cold and decongestant preparations, and anti-allergic and antispasmodic products.

Street drug combinations include "blue velvet" (paregoric and tripelennamine) and "Ts and Blues" (pentazocine and tripelennamine).

Medical Uses

- Antihistamines are effective in combating the symptoms associated with certain types of allergic reactions, such as hay fever and acute skin rashes.

- Several antihistamines can produce drowsiness and sedation, and some are marketed specifically for those properties. Diphenhydramine and doxylamine preparations for the treatment of transient insomnia are available over the counter in most Canadian pharmacies. These agents are generally thought to be less effective than prescription sedative-hypnotics but are nonetheless commonly used for this purpose. Their effectiveness in chronic insomnia has not been evaluated, and concerns have been raised over their safety, especially in the elderly, because of their anticholinergic side effects.

- Antihistamines are commonly found in cough and cold preparations in combination with decongestants and analgesics. Their effectiveness for this purpose has been debated. However, they may help relieve some cold symptoms in adults. Their benefit in children is less clear.

- Some antihistamines (e.g., diphenhydramine) have anticholinergic properties and may be used to treat parkinsonian symptoms and other antipsychotic-induced side effects.

Physical Appearance

Most antihistamines occur in pure form as white, odorless crystalline powders that have a bitter taste. They vary considerably with respect to their solubility in water and alcohol.

Dosage[1]

Medical

Dosage for the treatment of a particular disorder varies, depending on the antihistamine chosen or prescribed and the severity of the condition. The following are examples of typical therapeutic doses of commonly used products:

- for combating the symptoms of hay fever and similar allergic conditions — 50 mg of tripelennamine up to four times per day

- for inducing sleep — 25 to 50 mg of diphenhydramine at bedtime.

Non-medical

There have been reports of diphenhydramine abusers ingesting up to 2500 mg of the drug per day.

Routes of Administration

Most antihistamines are administered orally by tablet or capsule or in solution (as in syrup formulations). Injection may be used in emergency treatment of severe allergic reactions. Diphenhydramine is also contained in creams and other (topical) products for use on the skin and in eye drops. The street drug combinations noted above are usually injected intravenously.

---

[1]   All doses refer to adults.

Histamine and Antihistamines

Histamine is a naturally occurring substance found in almost all body tissue. Its concentration is particularly high in the cells of the skin tissue, the lungs and the intestinal mucosa. The release of histamine can be brought about under several conditions, including hypersensitivity (allergic) reactions, cell injury and the presence of a range of drugs and poisons (e.g., bee venom). When histamine is released, it is thought to interact with certain cells in the body (histamine receptors) to cause a number of effects. Some key actions include:

- stimulation of the smooth muscles
- vasodilation in capillary beds, particularly on the surface of the face and upper body (the so-called "blushing area"), which causes flushing, a rise in skin temperature and a drop in blood pressure
- increased heart rate
- stimulation of nerve endings on the body surface, which results in itching and pain
- lung and eye secretions
- pronounced gastric secretions.

Antihistamines are substances that act to block histamine (H_1) receptors. Drugs that effectively block only the H_2 histamine receptors that stimulate excessive gastric secretions (e.g., cimetidine, ranitidine, famotidine and nizatidine) are referred to not as antihistamines but as H_2 receptor antagonists. Antihistamines tend to diminish significantly (i.e., to antagonize) the effects of histamine on the body.

Effects of Short-Term Use: Low Doses[2]

The short-term effects produced by many antihistamines include the following, although the occurrence and intensity of these effects may vary from one substance in this class to another.

CNS, *behavioral, subjective:* drowsiness, dizziness, mild impairment of concentration and co-ordination, lassitude, sedation or sometimes insomnia, excitation and nervousness (more commonly in children than in adults), mild euphoria, blurred vision, ringing in the ears and tremors.

Cardiovascular: palpitations, headache and elevated or reduced blood pressure.

---

[2]   Single doses within the therapeutic range taken orally by non-tolerant users.

Respiratory: dryness of the nasal, throat and other respiratory passages.

Gastrointestinal: dryness of the mouth, gastric discomfort, loss of appetite, relief from nausea or increased nausea and vomiting, constipation or diarrhea.

Other: urinary retention or frequency, heaviness and weakness in the hands, muscle pain and tightness in the chest.

Effects of Short-Term Use: Higher Doses[3]

Intensification of the low-dose effects of antihistamines may occur with higher doses. Sleep is the most probable result, following a period of drowsiness, lethargy and sedation. When antihistamines are taken with alcohol or other CNS-depressant drugs, their effects tend to be intensified.

The effects of very high doses (i.e., overdose) on children can be extremely severe. Symptoms include flushing, fixed and dilated pupils, agitation, lack of muscle co-ordination, hallucinations, very high fever and convulsions. These symptoms may be followed by coma, profound cardiovascular and respiratory depression, and sometimes death.

The effects of very high but non-lethal overdose on adults can include confusion; toxic psychosis characterized by hallucinations, delusions and disorientation; tremors; muscle twitching; irregular heartbeat; abnormally high blood pressure and, rarely, convulsions.

Effects of Long-Term Use

When antihistamines are used regularly at therapeutic dose levels, adverse effects are generally mild, tend to be similar to short-term low-dose effects and often disappear over time. Regular topical application of certain antihistamines can cause allergic skin rashes.

Little is known about the effects of chronic high-dose abuse.

---

[3]   Single doses in excess of the therapeutic range taken orally by non-tolerant users, or lower doses in particularly sensitive individuals.

Lethality

As is the case with ASA, parents often underestimate the danger of antihistamines to very small children. Failure to store the drugs out of children's reach has led to accidental poisonings. An overdose of diphenhydramine in the range of 20 to 40 mg/kg body weight can be lethal.

The margin of safety for adults is considerably greater than that for children. Nonetheless, deaths of adults have resulted from severe overdose of antihistamines. In general, toxicity can occur after ingestion of three to five times the usual daily dose. Lethal overdoses of antihistamines in adults have produced coma followed by a period of hyperexcitability, often including delirium and convulsions. The terminal phase is characterized by severe CNS depression, and death results from respiratory arrest and/or cardiovascular collapse. Antihistamines have been used in intentional overdoses.

Tolerance and Dependence

Tolerance to some of the anticholinergic effects (e.g., dry mouth, urinary hesitancy) and physical withdrawal from antihistamines has been described, similar to those associated with other agents with anticholinergic properties. Tolerance to the subjective effects (e.g., euphoria, elevated mood) is suggested by the increasing doses administered by antihistamine abusers reported in the literature. The therapeutic benefit of antihistamines used chronically for sleep has not been evaluated.

When an antihistamine is regularly used for its psychoactive effects, users may become psychologically dependent. They develop a craving for the psychological effects and a sense of urgency with respect to maintaining an adequate supply of the drug. Diphenhydramine dependence, according to DSM-IV criteria for substance use disorders, has been reported.

Patterns of Use

Products containing antihistamines are so commonly used for such a variety of purposes that at least one antihistamine product is likely to be found in the medicine cabinet of most North American homes. Antihistamines, either alone or in combination preparations, are easily available both over the counter and by prescription. In many instances, the identical antihistamine is marketed for several different purposes. In Canada, for example, diphenhydramine is found in cough and cold preparations, anti-allergic preparations and sleep-promoting preparations. It can also be used for relief from the symptoms of motion sickness.

Since antihistamines may be used for their anticholinergic properties to treat and prevent extrapyramidal symptoms associated with antipsychotic medications, they are among the agents that patients with mental health problems may abuse (see the chapter on anticholinergic agents in Section 4).

Antihistamines alone are rarely taken by street drug abusers. However, it is not unusual for these drugs to be consumed with other CNS depressants such as alcohol or the opioid pentazocine, because some antihistamines seem to enhance the desired effects of the latter drugs.

Potential for Abuse

Although antihistamines may produce euphoria or feelings of well-being in some individuals, the side effects experienced at the higher doses needed to achieve these effects likely limit their widespread abuse. However, their abuse potential is moderate because of their easy availability to those seeking their psychoactive effects.

Background Reading

de Nesnera, A.P. (1996). Diphenhydramine dependence: A need for awareness. *Journal of Clinical Psychiatry, 57 (3)*, 136–137.

Feldman, M.D. & Behar, M. (1986). A case of massive diphenhydramine abuse and withdrawal from use of the drug. *Journal of the American Medical Association, 255*, 3119–3120.

Glickman, L. (1986). Diphenhydramine abuse and withdrawal. *Journal of the American Medical Association, 256*, 1894.

Krenzelok, E.P., Anderson, G.M. & Mirick, M. (1982). Massive diphenhydramine overdose resulting in death. *Annals of Emergency Medicine, 11*, 212–213.

Lasagna, L. (1995). Over-the-counter hypnotics and chronic insomnia in the elderly. *Journal of Clinical Psychopharmacology, 15 (6)*, 383–386.

Showalter, C.V. (1980). Ts and Blues: Abuse of pentazocine and tripelennamine. *Journal of the American Medical Association, 144*, 1224–1225.

Smith, M.B.H. & Feldman, W. (1993). Over-the-counter cold medications. A critical review of clinical trials between 1950 and 1991. *Journal of the American Medical Association, 269*, 2258–2263.

Wells, B.G., Marken, P.A., Rickman, L.A., Brown, C.S., Hamann, G. & Grimmig, J. (1989). Characterizing anticholinergic abuse in community mental health. *Journal of Clinical Psychopharmacology, 9 (6)*, 431–435.

Barbiturates

DRUG CLASS: Sedative/Hypnotic

Synopsis

Barbiturates are potent central nervous system (CNS) depressants. At low doses, these drugs generally induce a state of relaxation and tranquillity, and can mildly impair cognitive and motor functions. At moderate doses, they can both induce sleep and increase the amount of uninterrupted sleep time. However, prior to the onset of sleep or on occasions when sleep does not result, cognitive and motor functions can be moderately impaired and many users experience a state of pleasurable intoxication. At even higher doses, barbiturates induce anesthesia — a state of unconsciousness wherein even such powerful stimuli as severe pain are not experienced. At these levels, a more severe condition of impairment and intoxication (similar to that induced by large amounts of alcohol) typically precedes unconsciousness. As the size of the dose increases, barbiturates also cause ever-greater depression of the respiratory control centres of the brain. This last action constitutes the major toxic effect of barbiturates and many overdose deaths have resulted from respiratory arrest.

Only a few barbiturates remain in clinical use, which physicians prescribe for a variety of purposes. The choice of a drug for a specific clinical purpose is partly based on its duration of action: the ultrashort-acting barbiturates are used only for inducing anesthesia; the short- and intermediate-acting agents are used for sedation and sleep induction; and the long-acting agents are used to control epileptic seizures, for prolonged sedation and occasionally to induce sleep.

In addition to their therapeutic uses, barbiturates have been subject to widespread abuse for their pleasurably intoxicating effects. Because tolerance to the desired effects can develop very rapidly with regular use, higher daily doses become necessary to maintain these effects. However, taking progressively higher doses of barbiturates to compensate for acquired tolerance can lead to life-threatening complications. On one hand, there is the risk of death from overdose. On the other hand, when chronic and regular high-dose abuse has resulted in profound physical dependence, abrupt withdrawal can present symptoms so severe that they may cause death. For this reason, barbiturates are considered to be among the most dangerous of the widely abused drugs.

Because of the risks associated with barbiturate abuse, and because new and safer drugs such as benzodiazepines are now available, barbiturates are less frequently prescribed than they were in the past.

Drug Source

Barbiturates are produced through chemical synthesis by the pharmaceutical industry.

Trade Names

Examples of the non-proprietary names of some commonly used barbiturates, along with some example trade names, include:

- amobarbital — Amytal®

- butabarbital — Butisol Sodium®

- methohexital — Brietal®

- pentobarbital — Nembutal Sodium®, Barbilixer®, Barbita® (USA), Solofton® (USA)

- phenobarbital — Luminal® (USA)

- secobarbital — Seconal Sodium®

- thiopental — Pentothal®.

Street Names

There are literally dozens of street names for barbiturates. Some of the more common street names applied to all barbiturates include "barbs," "downers" and "goofballs."

Many individual barbiturates are named for the colors of well-known trade-named products. Examples of such names include "blues" or "blue heavens" (Amytal), "yellow jackets" (Nembutal), "red birds" or "red devils" (Seconal), and "rainbows" or "reds and blues" (Tuinal®).

Combination Products

- Cafergot-PB® (pentobarbital, belladonna, caffeine, ergotamine tartrate)

- Donnatal® (phenobarbital, atropine, hyoscyamine, scopolamine)

- Fiorinal® (butalbital, ASA, and caffeine)

- Fiorinal C® (butalbital, codeine, ASA, and caffeine).

- Phenaphen® with Codeine (phenobarbital, ASA, codeine)

- Tuinal® (amobarbital and secobarbital)

Medical Uses

Traditionally, barbiturates were classified as ultrashort-, short-, intermediate- and long-acting, depending on their duration of action.

- Ultrashort-acting barbiturates, such as thiopental (half-life: eight to 10 hours) and methohexital (half-life: three to five hours), are used as intravenous anesthetic agents. They may be the exclusive anesthetic used in brief surgical procedures, or may be used in longer procedures to induce anesthesia prior to the use of another anesthetic.

- Short- and intermediate-acting barbiturates, such as secobarbital (half-life: 15 to 40 hours), amobarbital (half-life: 10 to 40 hours) and butabarbital (half-life: 35 to 50 hours), are used mainly for daytime sedation and for induction of sleep. They are also used for pre-anesthetic sedation. Butalbital (half-life: 35 to 88 hours) is available in analgesic products.

- Long-acting agents, such as phenobarbital (half-life: 80 to 120 hours), are used to prevent or mitigate epileptic seizures. Phenobarbital is also available in combination products with antispasmodics or anti-migraine agents.

Physical Appearance

In salt form,[1] barbiturates are generally white, odorless powders that are bitter and water soluble.

Dosage[2]

Medical

- daytime sedation: amobarbital 50 to 300 mg daily in divided doses, butabarbital 15 to 30 mg three or four times a day, pentobarbital 20 mg three or four times a day, secobarbital 30 to 50 mg three or four times a day

- induction of sleep: amobarbital 60 to 200 mg, butabarbital 50 to 100 mg, pentobarbital 100 mg, secobarbital 100 mg at bedtime

- prevention or mitigation of epileptic seizures: phenobarbital 60 to 250 mg per day.

Non-medical

Non-medical users often take barbiturates initially at doses within the therapeutic range. As tolerance develops, users may progressively increase their daily dose to many times their original intake. While abusers have been known to take 500 mg to 4000 mg daily, it is important to emphasize that these extremely high doses could be lethal even for tolerant abusers.

Routes of Administration

For medical use, barbiturates are administered orally by tablet or capsule or in liquid solution, rectally by suppository, or subcutaneously, intramuscularly or intravenously by injection. Administration by injection is restricted almost exclusively to medical settings, and must be undertaken with great care because of the potentially life-

---

1   Barbiturates have the chemical properties of weak acids and form salts by reaction with bases. The salt forms are more soluble in water, so that they may be administered in a smaller volume of solution than the corresponding acid form of the drug. However the acid and salt forms of a given drug share the same pharmacological properties.

2   All doses refer to adults.

threatening effects. Injection is sometimes used to control seizures in emergency situations. Some street drug users, such as heroin addicts, inject barbiturates in order to obtain a "rush" effect, despite the risks.

Effects of Short-Term Use: Low Doses[3]

CNS, behavioral, subjective: tranquillity; relaxation; mild euphoria; reduced interest in external environment; dizziness; lethargy; drowsiness (in some cases sufficient to induce sleep); mild impairment of motor co-ordination, particularly of fine dexterity functions; mild impairment of thought processes and of short-term memory; increased reaction time; occasionally, mild release of inhibition and mood swings; paradoxical excitement in some users; exacerbation of pre-existing pain.

Gastrointestinal: occasionally nausea, vomiting, diarrhea and constipation.

Effects of Short-Term Use: Moderate Doses[4]

The low-dose CNS-depressant effects of barbiturates are intensified at moderate doses. These and other symptoms include:

CNS, behavioral, subjective: Moderate doses result in sleep. However, many symptoms occur prior to this or when sleep does not result. These include a brief period of heightened activity; a pleasurable state of intoxication and euphoria in some, although others may experience hostility, depression and/or anxiety; over-sedation and confusion; greater impairment of fine and gross motor functions, as well as of memory and thought processes; moderate release of inhibitions; and mood swings. Other effects, similar to those produced by moderate amounts of alcohol, include slurred speech, disturbed vision, possibly impaired judgment, increased libido, and "hangover" after the barbiturate effects wear off.

---

3   The therapeutically recommended dose taken orally by non-tolerant users to induce sedation, e.g., 50 mg or less.

4   The therapeutically recommended dose taken orally by non-tolerant users to induce sleep, e.g., 100 to 200 mg, or less in particularly sensitive individuals.

Cardiovascular: slight drop in blood pressure.

Respiratory: slight respiratory depression.

Effects of Short-Term Use: Higher Doses[5]

CNS, behavioral, subjective: Progressively higher doses cause ever-greater CNS depression. Onset of sleep is highly probable, and may progress to deeper levels of unconsciousness. Prior to the onset of sleep, symptoms are very similar to those exhibited by someone highly intoxicated by alcohol: exaggerated levels of activity may occur for a brief period; emotions are often intense and their expression is likely to be unpredictable and extreme; and thinking and other cognitive functions may be severely impaired, as may motor and perceptual functions.

Cardiovascular: progressive decline in blood pressure.

Respiratory: progressive respiratory depression.

Very high doses (i.e., severe overdose) characteristically produce slow, shallow and irregular breathing, lack of responsiveness of superficial reflexes, low body temperature, very low blood pressure, weak pulse and coma. Death may result from respiratory arrest.

Effects of Long-Term Use

Protracted high-dose abuse tends to produce effects similar to those resulting from short-term use, not unlike a state of chronic inebriation. Effects may include impaired memory, judgment and thinking; hostility, depression or mood swings. The effects of barbiturates on liver function include speeding up the metabolism of certain vitamins and steroids. Rarely, rickets and osteomalacia, a disorder that causes the deterioration of bone, have been reported after long-term use.

---

5   Single doses higher than those indicated for induction of sleep, taken orally by non-tolerant users, or lower doses in particularly sensitive individuals.

Lethality

In keeping with the trend toward decreased numbers of prescriptions for barbiturates, a marked decline has occurred in the incidence of deaths and of hospital emergency admissions related to barbiturates.

The principal toxic effect of barbiturates is respiratory depression. Although mild tolerance may develop to this effect, it develops much less rapidly than does tolerance to the desired level of pleasurable effects or to the level necessary to produce sleep. Therefore, the margin of safety between a lethal dose and a pleasure-producing dose decreases as the daily dose increases.

Generally, the lethal dose range is one to three grams (1,000 to 3,000 mg) for the shorter-acting barbiturates (e.g., secobarbital, pentobarbital), with the longer-acting barbiturates (e.g., phenobarbital) tending to be fatal at higher doses (5 grams). When taken with other CNS depressants, such as alcohol or other sedative/hypnotics, the lethal dose of barbiturates can be substantially smaller.

In contrast to opioid poisoning, for which antagonists are capable of reversing overdose effects, there are no known antagonists for barbiturates.

In addition to deaths from barbiturate overdose, deaths in heavily dependent users have occurred as a result of withdrawal. This withdrawal syndrome is discussed below.

Tolerance and Dependence

Tolerance

The many barbiturates have such different pharmacokinetic characteristics that it is difficult to generalize about the development of tolerance to them. Furthermore, there is a wide variation among users in the rate at which tolerance develops to the same drug. Tolerance can develop very rapidly to the sleep-induction and mood effects of barbiturates, often within weeks of consecutive nightly administrations. With regular use, tolerance to both impaired motor co-ordination and slowed reaction time appears to develop at least partially. Tolerance to the anti-convulsant property of phenobarbital develops much more slowly.

There is a high degree of cross-tolerance among barbiturates and also between barbiturates and most other sedative/hypnotic drugs; that is, a desired effect will not result if the user who is tolerant to one of these drugs ingests another at a dose level that would otherwise be sufficient to produce this desired effect.

Tolerance rapidly diminishes following a short period of abstinence (a few weeks) from both barbiturates and other sedative/hypnotic drugs, and normal sensitivity is then restored.

Psychological Dependence

Psychological dependence on barbiturates can result after regular use, irrespective of the size of the dose taken. In this case, users crave the psychological effects of the drug even though they may not use it every day. The drug takes on exaggerated importance to users, and anxiety or even feelings of panic may ensue if they are temporarily unable to obtain an adequate supply. In fact, users will adamantly resist any attempt by others to curtail their use of barbiturates, even when the drugs no longer produce any significant psychoactive effects. The craving may in fact persist long after drug use is terminated.

Physical Dependence/Withdrawal

Withdrawal syndrome typically follows abrupt abstinence after chronic consumption of even low doses of barbiturates. In such cases, the only symptom of this syndrome may be sleep disturbances. A more severe withdrawal sickness tends to follow abrupt abstinence after chronic and regular consumption of higher doses (e.g., over 400 mg daily) of the short- or intermediate-acting barbiturates. Early symptoms appear within 12 to 24 hours after the last administration and may include tremors, anxiety, weakness and insomnia, as well as a rapid drop in blood pressure when the user attempts to stand, severe weakness, and hyperactive blink reflex and deep reflexes. The intensity of the syndrome peaks 24 to 72 hours after the last administration, and symptoms likely to occur at this time include tonic-clonic seizures (ranging from a single seizure to uninterrupted seizure activity), delirium, visual hallucinations and a very high body temperature. Death can occur during this period of peak intensity. Provided the person survives, the symptoms gradually decline in intensity and disappear after several days.

As there is a high degree of cross-dependence among barbiturates and also between barbiturates and other sedative/hypnotics (including alcohol), many of these drugs, if taken in sufficient quantities, can partially or fully postpone the withdrawal syndrome induced by abstinence from any of the others. Gradual withdrawal under medical supervision usually involves administration of the long-acting barbiturate phenobarbital. Under these conditions, severe withdrawal symptoms are unlikely to be experienced.

Patterns of Use

Recently, there has been a notable decline in the prescribing of barbiturates. Three important factors have contributed to this trend:

- awareness of the highly addictive properties of barbiturates
- the substantial number of barbiturate-implicated deaths from suicide, accidental overdose and severe withdrawal
- the availability of safe and effective alternatives (e.g., the benzodiazepines).

The butalbital-containing products (e.g., Fiorinal C®) remain among the most frequently prescribed agents in Canada, ranking 154th of the top 200 prescription products in 1996.

Heroin-dependent individuals may use barbiturates. Sometimes these individuals combine barbiturates with street heroin and intravenously inject the combination to obtain a pleasurable "high" — a hazardous practice, as both drugs depress respiratory control centres in the brain. Some methamphetamine ("speed") abusers inject a combination of barbiturates and methamphetamine. They claim that the euphoria produced by the combination is greater than that produced by either drug taken alone. Stimulant abusers also take barbiturates to combat the often severe agitation resulting from repeated administrations of methamphetamine or cocaine over the several days of a "run," as well as to relieve the sleep problems often associated with chronic stimulant abuse.

Potential for Abuse

Abuse Liability
The abuse liability of the shorter-acting barbiturates is substantially greater than that of the longer-acting ones because the desired effects of the former are experienced more rapidly and intensely. The pleasurable effects of the shorter-acting barbiturates are very similar to those produced by alcohol, and their abuse liability is at least as great.

Inherent Harmfulness
Few other widely encountered drugs of abuse present the extreme hazards associated with excessive use of barbiturates. Both abuse of and withdrawal from barbiturates have frequently resulted in death.

Availability
Although the medical use of barbiturates has declined substantially, these drugs continue to be used, and they remain available to the abuser through both licit and illicit sources.

Background Reading

American Society of Health-Service Pharmacists. (1991). *American Hospital Formulary Service (AHFS) Drug Information*. Bethesda, MD: American Society of Health-Service Pharmacists.

Canadian Pharmaceutical Association. (1997). *Compendium of Pharmaceuticals and Specialties* (32nd edition). Ottawa: Canadian Pharmaceutical Association.

Hardman, J.G., Limbird, L.E., Molinoff, P.B., Rudden, R.W. & Gilman, A.G. (Eds.), (1996). *Goodman and Gilman's The Pharmacological Basis of Therapeutics*. (9th edition). New York/Toronto: McGraw-Hill Health Professions Division.

IMS. (1996). The top 200 drugs of 1996. *Pharmacy Practice, 12 (12)*, 67–79.

McKim, W.A. (1997). *Drugs and Behavior. An Introduction to Behavioral Pharmacology*. (3rd edition). New Jersey: Prentice-Hall, Inc.

Robinson, G.M., Sellers, E.M. & Janacek, E. (1981). Barbiturate and hypnosedative withdrawal by a multiple oral phenobarbital loading dose technique. *Clinical Pharmacology and Therapeutics, 30 (1)*, 71–76.

Benzodiazepines

DRUG CLASS: Anxiolytic, Sedative/Hypnotic

Synopsis

Benzodiazepines are the most widely prescribed psychoactive drugs in the world. They are effective in the management of a wide range of anxiety and tension states and in the management of insomnia. At low to moderate doses, taken orally, they are highly effective in relieving mild to moderate anxiety. At higher therapeutic doses, they can control more severe states of emotional distress.

Benzodiazepines have significant advantages over older agents prescribed essentially for the same purposes, such as meprobamate and the barbiturates. In addition to their fewer and milder side effects, they have the following desirable features: (1) they possess a much wider margin of safety than the older agents when taken in overdose quantities, (2) they have a lower abuse liability, and (3) when physical dependence occurs after long-term use, the withdrawal syndrome that results from abstinence tends to be far less severe than is the case with barbiturate or meprobamate withdrawal.

While most prescribed use of benzodiazepines is appropriate, these drugs have the potential to be abused and severe dependence may occur. Diazepam, and perhaps alprazolam and lorazepam, may have greater abuse potential than other drugs in this class and are attractive to street drug abusers. Abusers often take benzodiazepines in large quantities in combination with other central nervous system (CNS) depressants such as alcohol in order to achieve a pleasurable "high." This practice is dangerous, as all of the benzodiazepines can intensify the toxic effects of other CNS depressants.

Drug Source

Benzodiazepines are produced through chemical synthesis by the pharmaceutical industry.

Trade Names

Non-proprietary names and examples of the corresponding trade names for benzodiazepines include:

- alprazolam — Xanax®

- bromazepam — Lectopam®

- chlordiazepoxide — Librium®

- clobazam — Frisium®

- clonazepam — Retrovil®

- clorazepate — Tranxene®

- diazepam — Valium®, Vivol®

- flurazepam — Dalmane®

- lorazepam — Ativan®

- midazolam — Versed®

- nitrazepam — Mogadon®

- oxazepam — Serax®

- temazepam — Restoril®

- triazolam — Halcion®.

Street Names

Tranks, downers, Vs (Valium®).

Combination Products

Librax® (chlordiazepoxide and clidinium bromide) is used to treat gastrointestinal disorders.

Medical Uses

Medical uses of benzodiazepines include:

- management of a broad spectrum of mild to severe anxiety states, including panic disorders

- management of insomnia

- inducing of sedation and amnesia for diagnostic and surgical procedures

- symptomatic relief from acute agitation, tremor and impending delirium tremens associated with alcohol withdrawal

- controlling seizures

- skeletal muscle (e.g., back, neck) relaxation.

Physical Appearance

Most benzodiazepines occur as crystalline powders that vary considerably in their solubility in water and alcohol.

Dosage

Medical

Typical medical dosages of benzodiazepines are indicated in the following table.

Drug	Typical Oral Daily Adult Dose[i]	Elimination Half-life[ii]	Active Metabolites (Elimination Half-life)	Marketed Uses
Short to Intermediate Elimination Half-life				
alprazolam	0.5 - 1.5 mg	6 - 20 hours		anxiety; panic disorder
bromazepam	6 - 30 mg	8 - 19 hours		anxiety
clobazam	5 - 15 mg	10 - 30 hours	Desmethylclobazam (36 - 46 hours)	seizures
clonazepam	1.5 - 10 mg	18 - 50 hours		seizures
lorazepam	2 - 3 mg	12 - 15 hours		anxiety; status epilepticus
midazolam	(injection only)	3 - 4 hours	Hydroxymethylmidazolam (3-4 hours)	surgical or diagnostic procedures; sedation and anesthesia
nitrazepam	5 - 10 mg	16 - 48 hours		insomnia; myoclonic seizures
oxazepam	30 - 120 mg	5 - 15 hours		anxiety
temazepam	15 - 30 mg	8 - 10 hours		insomnia
triazolam	0.125 - 0.25 mg	1.5 - 5.5 hours		insomnia
Long Elimination Half-life (parent drug and active metabolites)				
chlordiaze-poxide	10 - 40 mg	5 - 30 hours	Desmethylchlordiazepoxide (18 hours) Demoxepam (14 - 95 hours) Desmethyldiazepam (30 - 100 hours) Oxazepam (5 - 15 hours)	anxiety
clorazepate	15 - 60 mg		Desmethyldiazepam (30 - 100 hours) Oxazepam (5 - 15 hours)	anxiety
diazepam	4 - 40 mg	20 - 70 hours	Desmethyldiazepam (30- 100 hours) Oxazepam (5 - 15 hours)	anxiety; alcohol withdrawal; muscle **spasms**
flurazepam	15 - 30 mg	2 - 3 hours	Desalkylflurazepam (47 - 100 hours) Hydroxyethylflurazepam (2-4 hours)	insomnia

i Doses may vary depending on the reason for use.

ii Elimination half-life is the time required for half of the amount of drug in the body to be eliminated or converted to another substance.

Non-medical

The user may initially take daily doses within the therapeutic range. Dependent users may develop tolerance and take higher doses to maintain the original intensity of desired effects. Severely dependent users may take 100 to 200 mg diazepam equivalents daily, although higher doses have been reported.

Routes of Administration

Benzodiazepines are most commonly taken orally in tablet or capsule form. Chlordiazepoxide, lorazepam and diazepam are also available for intravenous administration. Lorazepam is effective when administered intramuscularly but chlordiazepoxide and diazepam are too slowly absorbed via this route. Lorazepam is also available as a tablet that is dissolved under the tongue (sublingually). Midazolam is only administered intravenously.

Rates of Absorption and Duration of Effects

A similar spectrum of pharmacological effects is produced by all of the drugs in this class when they are taken orally. However, various members of the class are absorbed into the bloodstream at different rates, and the rate determines how rapidly the drug effects are experienced. For example, diazepam is readily absorbed into the system and its plasma concentration peaks within approximately one hour. This rapid absorption may be the main reason why some users of diazepam experience euphoria or a pleasant "high," and it may account for this drug's popularity among street users, who often take large quantities at a time.

Duration of effects is determined to a significant extent by two key pharmacological factors: (1) the elimination half-life of the particular drug and (2) the elimination half-lives of any of the psychoactive metabolites of the parent drug (i.e., those chemical products created by the metabolism of the parent drug). Triazolam, for example, generally has a short elimination half-life in the body and it is not transformed into any psychoactive metabolites. Therefore, a single dose of triazolam has one of the shortest durations of action of all the oral benzodiazepines, and the drug does not appreciably accumulate in the body with repeated use. By contrast, a single dose of diazepam has one of the longest durations of action in the body, while the elimination half-life of one of its principal psychoactive metabolites, desmethyldiazepam, is longer than that of the parent drug itself. Because both diazepam and desmethyldiazepam are eliminated so slowly, repeated use of diazepam may cause accumulations of both the parent drug and the metabolite in the body. It is important to note that there is substantial individual variation among users with regard to elimination half-life of each drug and its metabolite(s).

Another important factor influencing the duration of a drug's effect is its distribution throughout the body. Diazepam, for example, has a fairly rapid peak effect (approximately one hour) because it reaches the brain very quickly and then is redistributed throughout other fatty areas in the body.

Effects of Short-Term Use: Low to Moderate Doses[1]

CNS, behavioral, subjective: The principal desired effects are relief from anxiety and tension, relaxation and calmness. When benzodiazepines are used to induce sleep, morning and daytime drowsiness and other "hangover" symptoms have been reported (most commonly with flurazepam). Other effects may include mild to moderate impairment of motor co-ordination, drowsiness, lethargy, fatigue, mild impairment of thinking and memory functions, confusion, sometimes emotional depression, blurred vision, double vision, vertigo, slurred speech, tremors, stuttering and euphoria. On rare occasions, benzodiazepines may cause hyperexcited states, hallucinations and disorientation.

Cardiovascular: Therapeutic doses of these drugs rarely affect cardiovascular functions.

Respiratory: Respiratory depression may follow rapid intravenous injection.

Gastrointestinal: nausea, constipation, dry mouth, abdominal discomfort and loss of appetite; less commonly, vomiting and diarrhea.

Other: urinary retention, changes in libido and allergic reactions.

Benzodiazepines and Driving

All benzodiazepines can impair the user's psychomotor co-ordination. This impairment, which varies with the size of the dose, can interfere with driving performance and increase the risk of traffic crashes. While both laboratory driving-simulation studies and open-road driving tests have indicated a link between benzodiazepine use and an increased risk of accidents, there is conflicting evidence of this

---

1   Refers to single doses within the therapeutic range taken orally by non-tolerant users.

relationship. These studies are very difficult to conduct because driving effects are influenced by many factors, including the specific drugs used, their duration of action and the duration of drug use. Additionally, the effect of anxiety disorders on driving performance has not been fully evaluated. In general, there is evidence that the risk of problems with driving is increased in those taking higher doses of benzodiazepines, in those taking longer-acting benzodiazepines, among elderly benzodiazepine users and during the first few weeks of benzodiazepine use.

Effects of Short-Term Use: Higher Doses[2]

The most frequently encountered effects of higher doses of benzodiazepines are drowsiness, over-sedation and sleep. Prior to the onset of sleep, or when sleep does not occur, the clinical picture may resemble the intoxicated state produced by alcohol or barbiturates. Symptoms may include blurred vision, impairment of motor co-ordination, confusion, slurred speech, slowed reflexes, impaired thought and memory (particularly short-term memory), paradoxical excitement, mood swings, and hostile and erratic behavior. Some users of benzodiazepines report euphoria.

These symptoms become more intense as the size of the dose increases. At very high doses (i.e., overdose), deep sleep may progress to stupor or coma. Significant cardio-vascular and respiratory depression tends to occur only at extremely high doses. These hazardous symptoms, however, may occur at lower doses when benzodiazepines are taken with other CNS depressants such as alcohol or barbiturates.

Effects of Long-Term Use

The slowly eliminated benzodiazepines accumulate gradually in the body and do not reach peak concentrations until several days after the start of daily therapy. Therefore, side effects of over-sedation or daytime drowsiness may be delayed in appearance. The effects of chronic abuse (i.e., taking daily doses in excess of the therapeutic maximum) can vary considerably among individual users. Clinical observations suggest that some tolerant abusers take excessively large doses without significant evidence of intoxication. However, other abusers experience symptoms similar to those caused by chronic

---

2   Refers to single doses in excess of the therapeutic range taken orally by non-tolerant users, or lower doses in particularly sensitive individuals.

sedative/hypnotic intoxication, and any or all of the following may occur: impaired thinking, memory and judgment; disorientation; confusion; slurred speech; lack of muscle co-ordination and muscle weakness.

Lethality

Benzodiazepines are among the most commonly implicated substances in drug overdose situations, accidental or otherwise. Fortunately, these drugs have a very wide margin of safety when taken alone, and deaths resulting from overdose of any of them, without involvement of alcohol or some other drug, are very rare. Enormous overdoses of benzodiazepines are generally necessary to cause dangerous levels of respiratory and cardiovascular depression. Very rapid intravenous injection of benzodiazepines also sometimes causes hazardous depression of respiratory and/or cardiovascular function. However, the risk of lethal consequences can be increased significantly when the benzodiazepine overdose is combined with large doses of alcohol, barbiturates or other CNS depressants. Such toxic combinations have resulted in a number of deaths, by both accident and suicide.

Tolerance and Dependence

Tolerance

Tolerance develops to the effects of benzodiazepines, especially to effects such as sedation and impairment of co-ordination. Tolerance to the anxiolytic effects appears to be less common. The development of tolerance does not necessarily imply abuse or dependence, nor actual increase in dose. Many patients taking benzodiazepines over an extended period claim continued efficacy for their psychiatric condition at a constant dose. For those using benzodiazepines for non-therapeutic purposes, tolerance may develop to the desired effects (i.e., euphoria) and result in dosage increases to achieve the same effect.

A high degree of cross-tolerance occurs among benzodiazepines and other sedative/hypnotic drugs such as barbiturates and alcohol. That is, once the user is tolerant to a specific effect produced by a given benzodiazepine, he or she will also be tolerant to the same effect produced by an equivalent dose of any of these other drugs.

Physical Dependence/Withdrawal

It is generally acknowledged that for the millions of patients who take benzodiazepines for relatively short periods (i.e., a few weeks to a few months), the risk of physical dependence is very low. However, for those who have been using benzodiazepines chronically, sudden discontinuation may produce withdrawal symptoms. The severity of the withdrawal depends on the specific benzodiazepine used, the dose and duration of use, and the abruptness of the discontinuation. The most severe symptoms are likely to occur after abrupt discontinuation of high doses of a short- to intermediate-acting benzodiazepine. These symptoms include agitation, paranoia, seizures and delirium. These extreme symptoms, however, are much less commonly encountered than in cases of barbiturate withdrawal. For many years it was debated whether physical dependence developed following the use of therapeutic doses of benzodiazepines, but Busto and colleagues (1986) found unequivocal evidence that a mild but distinct withdrawal syndrome occurs after discontinuation of long-term therapeutic use of benzodiazepines. The 10 most common symptoms were anxiety, headache, insomnia, tension, sweating, difficulty concentrating, tremor, sensory disturbance, fear and fatigue. Gradually tapering down the benzodiazepine dose helps to reduce the number and severity of withdrawal symptoms.

Three types of benzodiazepine discontinuation syndrome have been described. However, it may be difficult to determine which is (are) occurring in a particular individual, since more than one may occur simultaneously. The effects of discontinuing benzodiazepines can include:

- *Recurrence,* which refers to the reappearance of the original symptoms for which the benzodiazepine was being taken. Usually onset is more gradual and symptoms persist over time.

- *Rebound,* which refers to the return of symptoms that existed before treatment but occur in a more intense form following discontinuation. These symptoms have a rapid onset and are temporary.

- *Withdrawal,* which refers to symptoms that did not exist before treatment but occur following discontinuation of the drug. These symptoms vary in intensity and typically last two to four weeks or even longer after drug discontinuation.

Psychological Dependence

Psychological dependence on benzodiazepines may develop in some users. Dependent users may experience a persistent craving for the psychological effects of the drug and feel a compulsion to continue taking the drug even when it no longer produces any significant psychoactive effects. The drug takes on magnified importance in the daily life of the psychologically dependent user, and anxiety or even feelings of panic may occur if it is temporarily unavailable.

Patterns of Use

Benzodiazepines are among the most widely used drugs in the world. Approximately 10 per cent of Canadians report using a benzodiazepine at least once per year, with one in 10 of these individuals continuing use for more than a year. In the United States, 1.5 billion prescriptions for benzodiazepines were filled between 1965 and 1985. There has been an overall decline in the use of long-acting benzodiazepines in recent years, with the trend shifting toward use of intermediate-acting benzodiazepines, such as lorazepam and alprazolam. The principal consumers are women and middle-aged and elderly patients. In general, concerns about extensive over-prescribing and patient misuse of benzodiazepines have not been supported by research evidence. Most prescribing of benzodiazepines appears appropriate and most individuals take the drugs as prescribed. Of those individuals who take benzodiazepines for extended periods for therapeutic reasons, it appears that dose escalation is not common. Patients may change their pattern of use when required for symptom control and they frequently try to stop their drug use.

Abuse and dependence on benzodiazepines for recreational purposes do occur. Severe benzodiazepine dependence generally occurs in those individuals who are dependent on or who abuse other substances. There is evidence that certain benzodiazepines, primarily diazepam and perhaps alprazolam and lorazepam, are preferred for recreational uses. In the context of polydrug abuse, benzodiazepines may be taken to produce euphoria or to enhance the euphoria from other drugs such as opioids (including methadone) or alcohol. A high percentage, 30 to 76 per cent, of alcohol abusers use benzodiazepines. Cocaine abusers may use benzodiazepines to help ease the "crash." Although more women use benzodiazepines for medical reasons, an equal proportion of men and women abuse or are dependent on benzodiazepines.

Potential for Abuse

Abuse Liability

Benzodiazepines have a relatively low abuse liability. In general, benzodiazepines have weaker reinforcing properties than do other sedative/hypnotics, including alcohol, opioids and stimulants. Diazepam and perhaps alprazolam and lorazepam may be more reinforcing than other benzodiazepines.

Inherent Harmfulness

The margin of safety with benzodiazepines is quite high. They may cause psychomotor impairment and sedation, but are generally safe even in overdose, except if combined with other CNS depressants.

Availability

Benzodiazepines are widely available. In Canada and the United States, a physician's prescription is required for their legal purchase by consumers. Their availability contributes to concerns of overuse and misuse.

Background Reading

American Psychiatric Association. (1990). *Benzodiazepine Dependence, Toxicity and Abuse. A Task Force Report of the American Psychiatric Association*. Washington: APA.

"Benzodiazepine/Driving" Collaborative Group. (1993). Are benzodiazepines a risk factor for road accidents? *Drug and Alcohol Dependence , 33 (1)*, 19–22.

Busto, U.E., Sellers, E.M., Naranjo, C.A., Cappell, H., Sanchez-Craig, M. & Sykora, K. (1986). Withdrawal reaction after long-term therapeutic use of benzodiazepines. *New England Journal of Medicine, 315*, 854–859.

Busto, U.E., Romach, M.K. & Sellers, E.M. (1996). Multiple drug use and psychiatric comorbidity in patients admitted to the hospital with severe benzodiazepine dependence. *Journal of Clinical Psychopharmacology, 16 (1)*, 15–57.

Hemmelgarn, B., Suissa, S., Huang, A., Boivin, J.F. & Pinard, G. (1997). Benzodiazepine use and the risk of motor vehicle crash in the elderly. *Journal of the American Medical Association, 278 (1)*, 27–31.

Ray, W.A. (1992). Psychotropic drugs and injuries among the elderly: A review. *Journal of Clinical Psychopharmacology, 12*, 386–396.

Shader, R.I. & Greenblatt, D.J. (1993). Use of benzodiazepines in anxiety disorders. *New England Journal of Medicine, 328(19)*, 1398–1405.

van Laar, M.W., Volkerts, E.R. & van Willigenburg, A.P.P. (1992). Therapeutic effects and effects on actual driving performance of chronically administered buspirone and diazepam in anxious outpatients. *Journal of Clinical Psychopharmacology, 12*, 86–95.

Buprenorphine

DRUG CLASS: Partial Opioid Agonist

Synopsis

Buprenorphine possesses a unique combination of partial opioid agonist and antagonist properties. It is a partial agonist at μ (mu) opioid receptors and an antagonist at κ (kappa) opioid receptors. It is highly fat-soluble and dissociates very slowly from its receptors. As a result, its duration of action is longer than that of many other opioids.

Buprenorphine is used to treat moderate to severe pain, being 25 to 50 times more potent as an analgesic than morphine. It has also been shown to be useful in treating opioid dependence. Buprenorphine produces morphine-like subjective effects, has a long duration of action similar to methadone, produces only limited withdrawal symptoms and blocks opioid-induced euphoria. Although buprenorphine has low oral potency, owing to extensive first-pass metabolism, it is effective parenterally and sublingually. The sublingual route is preferred when buprenorphine is being used to treat opioid dependence. It may be possible to start buprenorphine treatment immediately after methadone or illicit opioid use without precipitating withdrawal symptoms. As a partial opioid agonist, the maximum effect of buprenorphine is less than that of a full agonist. However, the clinical significance of this difference varies from system to system. For example, within the therapeutic dose range there is a ceiling for buprenorphine's respiratory-depressive effect, while its analgesic effect remains dependent on the size of the dose. Thus, when compared with full opioid agonists such as methadone, buprenorphine may be safer with respect to respiratory depression and sedation.

Drug Source

Buprenorphine hydrochloride is a semi-synthetic opioid derived from thebaine and manufactured by the pharmaceutical industry.

Trade Names

Trade names for buprenorphine include:

- Subutex® (France) — sublingual tablets

- Buprenex® Injection (United States)

- Temgesic® (United Kingdom) — injection and sublingual tablets.

Buprenorphine hydrochloride was not available in Canada in 1997.

Street Names

Not applicable.

Combination Products

Bu-Nx® tablets (New Zealand) contain 0.2 mg of buprenorphine and 0.17 mg of naloxone. A similar combination product (Suboxone®) may become available in the United States. Naloxone is poorly absorbed when the tablet is placed under the tongue, but is included to deter intravenous misuse of buprenorphine in tablet form.

Medical Uses

Medical applications of buprenorphine include:

- use as an injectable analgesic for moderate to severe pain — 0.4 mg of buprenorphine is approximately equivalent to 10 mg of morphine given intramuscularly

- use as an adjunct to anesthesia — buprenorphine antagonizes the respiratory depression produced by anesthetic doses of fentanyl, without completely preventing opioid pain relief.

Other possible therapeutic applications that are under clinical investigation include:

- use for detoxification and maintenance treatment of opioid-dependent patients

- use in treatment for cocaine dependence, although studies show conflicting results to date. Buprenorphine may also be an effective treatment for concurrent dependence on intravenous cocaine and opioids.

- use as an antidepressant and for treatment-unresponsive schizophrenia.

Physical Appearance

Buprenorphine hydrochloride in pure form is a white, crystalline powder.

Dosage[1]

Buprenorphine is effective both parenterally and sublingually (sl), but is poorly absorbed from the gastrointestinal tract. In the United States, buprenorphine has been administered sublingually in the form of (buffered) water-and-ethanol solutions as well as in sublingual tablets in clinical trails. In Japan, buprenorphine is also available in a suppository form.

Medical
- for analgesia:

  - 0.3 to 0.6 mg[2] every six to eight hours by the intramuscular or intravenous route

  - 0.4 to 0.8 mg sublingually

  - has been used epidurally.

---

[1]   All doses refer to adults.

[2]   Approximately 0.4 mg of buprenorphine is equivalent to 10 mg morphine given intramuscularly as an analgesic.

- for the treatment of opioid dependence:

  - a range of 2 to 32 mg per day, administered sublingually, has been used, although the manufacturer recommends a daily limit of 16 mg. Once-daily sublingual dosing is preferred, though less-than-daily dosing may be possible in some patients.

  - 2 mg sublingually may be approximately equivalent to 30 mg of methadone orally, although other dosage equivalencies have also been suggested.

Non-medical

There have been reports of users dissolving and injecting both sublingual buprenorphine tablets and buprenorphine-naloxone combination tables.

Routes of Administration

Compared with the subcutaneous route of administration, buprenorphine is two-thirds as potent when administered sublingually and only one-fifteenth as potent when administered orally. The low potency of orally administered buprenorphine is due to extensive metabolism to inactive metabolites in the liver. For the treatment of opioid dependence, the sublingual route is preferred since it avoids the needle-related cues associated with injectable drugs. However, in order to avoid illicit diversion, opioid-dependent individuals receiving buprenorphine doses should be observed for a longer time after administration of the sublingual dose than after dosing with an oral medication, e.g., methadone solution. One study of a sublingual solution of buprenorphine in ethanol found that, compared with intravenous injection, only 30 per cent of the administered dose is available in the body, even when the solution was held in the mouth for more than three minutes.

For analgesia, intramuscular, slow intravenous and sublingual routes are used.

Abuse may also take the form of crushing and snorting buprenorphine tablets.

Effects of Short-Term Use: Low Doses

CNS, behavioral, subjective: At doses of up to 1 mg subcutaneously or 0.8 mg intramuscularly, buprenorphine has a potent analgesic effect, and may be longer in duration than that of morphine. Some of the subjective effects are slower in onset and longer-lasting than those of morphine. Opioid-dependent patients have reported "liking" buprenorphine and reported opioid-like effects following its administration. Drowsiness, dizziness and headache are among the more common side effects.

Cardiovascular: hypotension.

Respiratory: Respiratory depression, which may not increase proportionately with dose, may be slower in onset and last longer than that produced by morphine.

Gastrointestinal: nausea and vomiting.

Other: sweating, pupillary constriction.

Effects of Short-Term Use: Higher Doses

CNS, behavioral, subjective: At doses greater than 1 mg subcutaneously or 0.8 mg intramuscularly, the opioid agonist activity of buprenorphine decreases and the opioid antagonistic activity predominates. Intravenous abusers of buprenorphine report no "rush" after injection but experience euphoria for hours.

Two milligrams of buprenorphine administered sublingually has been shown to be as effective as 30 mg of oral methadone in preventing withdrawal symptoms during short-term detoxification from heroin, but less effective in blocking the subjective effects of opioids.

Four to 8 mg of buprenorphine given daily sublingually reduces or blocks the euphoria produced by morphine and other opioids. At doses of 8 mg sublingually, buprenorphine suppresses heroin use as well as or better than 60 mg of oral methadone and significantly better than 20 mg of oral methadone over 17 weeks. In a study of volunteers with a history of substance abuse, 8 mg doses did not interfere with the ability to work by causing sedation or intoxication.

Respiratory: Although respiratory despression is possible with buprenorphine, it does not produce lethal respiratory depression even at 10 times the analgesic dose and does not increase respiratory depression in combination with other opioids. Its effectiveness in antagonizing the respiratory depression produced by fentanyl anesthesia is approximately equal to that of naloxone.

Gastrointestinal: nausea, constipation.

Other: urinary hesitancy.

Effects of Long-Term Use

Buprenorphine produces morphine-like subjective behavioral and physiological effects with chronic administration.

Lethality

Buprenorphine does not appear to be strongly linked to death by overdose. In reviewing the treatment of 1,900 opioid-dependent individuals with buprenorphine, Segal and Schuster (1995) reported only four deaths, none of which were attributable to buprenorphine. However, abuse of sublingual tablets by injection carries with it the behavioral risks of shared needles and syringes and consequently the possibility of hepatitis, HIV and bacterial infections.

Increases in the dose of buprenorphine do not necessarily produce proportional increases in respiratory depression, as there appears to be a ceiling on the drug's respiratory depressant effect. If respiratory depression occurs, it is relatively slow in onset and of long duration. The effects of buprenorphine are not readily reversed by naloxone, and higher doses of antagonist may be required.

Tolerance and Dependence

Tolerance and withdrawal symptoms do not appear to be major features of buprenorphine use. However, tolerance to the side effects of sedation and drowsiness can be expected to develop. Further, buprenorphine is thought to produce a low level of physical dependence and may produce psychological dependence. Typical opioid withdrawal symptoms have been described with buprenorphine abstinence; abrupt termination of buprenorphine may produce mild to moderate withdrawal effects within three to five days; these symptoms last from eight to 10 days. The limited withdrawal may make buprenorphine appropriate for opioid detoxification treatments, allow less-than-daily dosing in buprenorphine maintenance regimens, and facilitate the rapid induction of naltrexone maintenance following the discontinuation of buprenorphine. Buprenorphine binds slowly to and dissociates slowly from the receptor site. The drug is eliminated slowly from the central nervous system. This may explain why withdrawal symptoms are less intense and more delayed than those associated with morphine.

Patterns of Use

At present, buprenorphine is not available in Canada. In the United States, the injectable dosage form is used primarily to manage post-operative pain. Buprenorphine, usually as a sublingual solution or tablet, is being evaluated in opioid detoxification and maintenance programs.

Potential for Abuse

Buprenorphine appears to have a lower potential for producing dependence than morphine, but it has been abused. Patients have reported "liking" buprenorphine. Its ability to produce euphoric effects yet limited withdrawal are factors that may render it liable to abuse.

Intravenous misuse of buprenorphine 0.2 mg sublingual tablets has been reported. Although the combination tablet containing buprenorphine and naloxone may have less misuse potential, it has also been intravenously abused. Crushed tablets have been snorted for greater effect than is achieved by the sublingual route.

Background Reading

Blaine, J.D. (Ed.), *Buprenorphine: An Alternative Treatment for Opioid Dependence*. Rockville, MD: NIDA Research Monograph 121.

Cowan, A. & Lewis, J.W. (Eds.) (1995). *Buprenorphine: Combating Drug Abuse with a Unique Opioid*. New York: Wiley-Liss.

Gastfriend, D.R., Mendelson, J.H., Mello N.K., Teoh, S.K. & Reif, S. (1993). Buprenorphine pharmacotherapy for concurrent heroin and cocaine dependence. *American Journal on Addictions*, 2 (4), 269–278.

Greenstein, R.A., Fudala, P.J. & O'Brien, C.P. (1992). Alternative pharmacotherapies for opiate addiction. In J.H. Lowinson, P. Ruiz, R.B. Millman & J.G. Langrod (Eds.), *Substance Abuse — A Comprehensive Textbook* (2nd edition). Baltimore: William and Wilkins.

Jaffe, J.H., Epstein, S. & Ciraulo, D.A. (1991). Opioids. In D.A. Ciraulo & R.I. Shader (Eds.), *Clinical Manual of Chemical Dependence*. Washington: American Psychiatric Press Incorporated.

Kosten, T.R., Morgan, C. & Kleber, H. (1991). Treatment of heroin addicts using buprenorphine. *American Journal of Drug and Alcohol Abuse*, *17(2)*, 119–129.

Kosten, T.R., Schottenfeld, R., Ziedonis, D. & Falconi, J. (1993). Buprenorphine versus methadone maintenance for opioid dependence. *Journal of Nervous and Mental Disease*, *181 (6)*, 358–364.

McEvoy, G.K. (Ed.) (1993). *American Hospital Formulary Service (AHFS) Drug Information*. Bethesda, MD: American Society of Hospital Pharmacists.

Segal, D.L. & Schuster, C.R. (1995). Buprenorphine: What interests the National Institute on Drug Abuse? In A. Cowan & J.W. Lewis (Eds.), *Buprenorphine: Combating Drug Abuse with A Unique Opioid*. New York: Wiley-Liss.

Caffeine

DRUG CLASS: CNS Stimulant

Synopsis

Caffeine is the most widely and regularly consumed psychoactive substance in the world. When taken in moderate amounts — such as that contained in one to three cups of coffee — caffeine can produce elevated mood, increased alertness and a slight increase in heart rate and blood pressure. If taken before bedtime, it can interfere with sleep. Although low to moderate daily doses of caffeine do not appear to produce harmful effects in otherwise healthy adults, higher doses (more than three to four cups of coffee) can result in insomnia, nervousness, irritability, tremor, headache, and rapid and irregular heartbeat. Children, especially newborns, may be particularly sensitive to caffeine's adverse effects. Stopping or decreasing caffeine consumption can produce withdrawal symptoms.

Drug Source

Caffeine is derived from any of a number of plants including:

- the fruit of *Coffea arabica* and related species (coffee)
- the leaves of *Thea sinensis* (tea)
- the seeds of *Theobroma cacao* (cocoa, chocolate)
- the nuts (cotyledons) of *Cola acuminata* and *Cola nitida*
- the dried leaves of *Ilex paraguariensis* (yerba maté) and other plants of the holly species
- the seeds of *Paullinia cupana* or *sorbilis* (guarana).

Trade Names

Some examples of non-prescription caffeine products available in Canada are Stay Awake®, Stay Alert®, Wake-Up® and Alert®.

Examples of oral products available in the United States include No Doz® and Vivarin®.

Street Names

None in common use.

Combination Products

Various beverages — including some soft drinks (soda pop), tea and coffee — and chocolate contain caffeine.

Examples of combination drug products that contain caffeine include:

- ASA or ASA combined with codeine— e.g., Anacin®, Midol®, 222®, 292®
- acetaminophen; or acetaminophen with codeine — e.g., Excedrin®; Tylenol with Codeine® Nos. 1, 2 and 3
- ergotamine — e.g., Cafergot®, Ergodryl®.

Caffeine may also be found as an ingredient in street stimulant preparations, often in combination with ephedrine and/or phenylpropanolamine (see the chapter on ephedrine in Section 4). These preparations may be manufactured to look like and be marketed as more potent stimulants such as amphetamines. The Food and Drug Administration (FDA) in the United States has banned the combination of caffeine with other sympathomimetic (adrenaline-like) drugs.

Medical Uses

Caffeine has the following medical uses:

- in combination products, to treat pain including migraine and other types of headaches. Although it has no intrinsic analgesic activity, it has been argued that caffeine augments the analgesic action of other medications (e.g., ASA, acetaminophen, codeine, ergotamine) and/or antagonizes the CNS depressant effect of codeine. Its clinical benefit in such combinations has been questioned.

- as a mild stimulant to aid in staying awake

- by injection to treat apnea and other types of respiratory failure among newborns.

Physical Appearance

In its pure form, caffeine occurs as an odorless, silky white powder, usually matted together, or as a white crystalline powder.

Dosage[1]

Medical

The amount of caffeine in headache medications ranges from 15 to 100 mg per dose. In non-prescription products the dose ranges from 100 to 200 mg in Canada, and up to 250 mg in the United States.

Non-medical

A cup of coffee contains about 100 mg of caffeine, while decaffeinated coffee contains about 2 to 6 mg per cup. A cup of tea contains approximately 50 mg of caffeine, as do soft drinks with caffeine. A cup of cocoa may contain 5 to 50 mg of caffeine and a chocolate bar 3 to 35 mg. However, the caffeine content of foods and beverages varies widely. With coffee or tea, the methods of preparation, the amount used and the origin of plant (e.g., Colombia, Java, etc.) account for considerable variations.

---

1   All doses refer to adults.

Routes of Administration

For medical use, caffeine is usually given orally in tablets or capsules. When taken orally in medicines or beverages, caffeine is rapidly absorbed and reaches maximum concentration in the blood within 30 to 60 minutes. Caffeine has also been administered by injection to neonates to treat respiratory difficulties.

Effects of Short-Term Use: Low Doses[2]

The effects of short-term use of low doses of caffeine can produce the following effects.

CNS, behavioral, subjective: Caffeine can produce mild mood elevation and reduce drowsiness and fatigue. There is contradictory evidence regarding caffeine's effect on performance and the expectations of the individual may play an important role. Caffeine has been reported to produce a more clear and rapid flow of thought and increased capacity for sustained intellectual effort. When taken by abstainers or sensitive individuals, however, caffeine can produce nervousness and may cause a jittery feeling. When caffeine is consumed shortly before bedtime, symptoms including difficulty in falling asleep, more frequent awakenings and altered sleep patterns may result.

Cardiovascular: constriction of cerebral blood vessels; increased peripheral blood flow, except in the brain; stimulation of the cardiac muscle, which may result in slightly increased blood pressure and small increases in heart rate. A decrease in heart rate has also been reported.

Respiratory: mild stimulation of respiration, and relaxation of bronchial smooth muscle.

Gastrointestinal: Gastric secretion (and irritation) is stimulated by both caffeine and other components of coffee.

---

[2]   Not more than 250 mg, or the equivalent of approximately one to two cups of medium-strength coffee.

Other: stimulation of voluntary skeletal muscle, with increased force of contraction and a reduction in muscle fatigue; increase in basal metabolic rate; increase in urine flow and interference in glucose and fat metabolism with possible alterations in blood glucose and plasma lipid levels.

Among patients with panic disorders caffeine is associated with increased symptoms of anxiety. These individuals may be particularly sensitive to the effects of caffeine and may benefit from avoiding its use.

Despite popular belief, caffeine is not an antidote to alcohol intoxication. The common practice of drinking coffee after drinking alcohol does not help an individual to "sober up." Rather, it is often described as "turning a sleepy drunk into a wide-awake drunk."

Effects of Short-Term Use: Higher Doses[3]

Intensification of caffeine's low-dose effects may occur at higher doses, as well as any of the following effects:

CNS, *behavioral, subjective:* irritability, restlessness, nervousness, insomnia, rambling flow of thoughts and speech, and psychomotor agitation (agitated movement of voluntary muscles).

Cardiovascular: rapid and irregular heartbeat.

Other: increased capacity for muscular work.

Note: The International Olympic Committee has banned large amounts of caffeine by athletes. In Canadian sports competitions, a urine sample is considered to test positive for caffeine if its concentration exceeds 12 mcg/mL. This concentration normally results from consuming the equivalent of several cups of strong coffee, although in some individuals lower levels of consumption may produce positive test results.

---

[3]   Single doses of several hundred milligrams or more, or lower doses in particularly sensitive individuals.

At very high doses (1,000 mg or higher), caffeine may produce insomnia, restlessness and excitement, which may progress to mild delirium; vomiting and seizures; muscle tension; highly abnormal heart rates and rhythms, and rapid respiration.

Effects of Long-Term Use

Daily use in low to moderate doses in most healthy adults does not appear to produce any harmful effects. Substantial daily doses — and in some individuals even as little as 250 mg per day — can lead to adverse consequences including restlessness, nervousness, excitement, insomnia, flushed face, increased urination, gastrointestinal disturbances, muscle twitching, rambling flow of thought or speech, abnormally rapid and irregular heartbeat, and periods of inexhaustibility and agitation. These clinical features have been described as "caffeinism," and appear very similar to the features associated with general anxiety disorder, especially sleep disturbances and mood changes.

Other long-term health consequences of heavy caffeine use are less well established than the behavioral effects. One of the difficulties inherent in studying the relationship between caffeine and chronic disease is that heavy caffeine users also tend to smoke more tobacco and drink more alcohol than do light users. It is not surprising, therefore, to find a relatively high prevalence of cardiovascular disease and cancer among people who regularly consume large quantities of caffeine. There appears to be no link between caffeine use of up to 600 mg per day and the risk of cardiovascular disease, although some clinicians have disagreed with this view. While previous studies linked caffeine consumption with cancer, particularly of the pancreas and urinary tract, these studies were found to have flaws in their methodology and such links have not been satisfactorily established. It has been suggested that lifelong use of coffee or other forms of caffeine may be associated with loss of bone density in women.

Caffeine and Pregnancy

At very high doses, caffeine appears to increase the likelihood of birth defects in mammals. In 1980, the FDA removed caffeine from the list of compounds generally regarded as safe during pregnancy. Consumption of caffeine in higher doses (above 300 mg/day) may be associated with spontaneous abortions and delivery of infants with lower birthweights. Since the safe level of caffeine consumption has not been determined, it appears prudent for women to minimize or eliminate caffeine intake during pregnancy. It is also important to note that pregnant women have a reduced capacity to metabolize caffeine, as do infants, who may be exposed to caffeine because of its ability to passes into breast milk.

Lethality

Death resulting from severe overdose of caffeine is very rare. The lethal dose in humans appears to be 5 to 10 grams, although toxic symptoms may appear with lower doses. In particular, pregnant women and children (especially newborn infants) may experience toxicity at relatively low doses. Early symptoms of toxicity include insomnia, restlessness and excitement, which may progress to mild delirium. Vomiting and seizures are prominent; muscles become tense and tremulous; and a rapid and irregular heartbeat appears, along with rapid breathing.

Tolerance and Dependence

Tolerance

There is evidence that tolerance develops with repeated use of caffeine. However, the ritualistic behavior surrounding drinking a cup of coffee with breakfast appears to have a strong psychological influence and even if tolerance does occur, the drinker's expectations of mild stimulation appear to outweigh it. For many regular users, a single cup of coffee can retain its value as a "pick-me-up" without a need to increase the amount to produce the same effects.

Dependence

Abruptly stopping regular consumption of caffeine-containing beverages can result in a withdrawal syndrome with symptoms including headaches, drowsiness, fatigue, and decreased activity and alertness. Caffeine withdrawal could be an important but often overlooked cause of headaches, even in moderate coffee drinkers. Many regular caffeine users develop some of these symptoms upon cessation and the likelihood of symptoms increases with amount consumed. Symptoms begin within 12 to 24 hours after last use, peak at 20 to 48 hours, and last about seven days. These symptoms can be relieved by taking caffeine, which, in turn, serves to reinforce regular consumption. Gradually reducing caffeine intake may be preferable to stopping abruptly.

Patterns of Use

Caffeine is the most widely used psychoactive substance in the world. In North America, 82 to 92 per cent of adults regularly consume caffeine. Worldwide per-capita caffeine consumption (including that of children) is estimated to be 70 mg per day, or approximately equivalent to one cup of coffee. Average intake for Americans is about 200 mg/day and is twice that of Sweden and the United Kingdom. High caffeine consumption is especially common among psychiatric patients — 22 per cent of psychiatric patients consume more than 750 mg/day as compared with nine per cent of the general population. Heavy caffeine use has also been associated with alcohol and drug abusers. Consumers of high doses of caffeine report greater use of sedative-hypnotic and anti-anxiety agents than do low- or moderate-level users. Recovered alcoholics and heavy smokers also report high levels of caffeine consumption.

Potential for Abuse

Abuse Liability
The abuse liability of caffeine is considered to be moderately low. Caffeine does have reinforcing properties in some individuals, but not as reliably as do other stimulants such as cocaine or amphetamine. Since caffeine products are consumed orally, there is a lag time before the substance reaches the brain, which decreases caffeine's potential for abuse.

Inherent Harmfulness
Low to moderate daily doses of caffeine are well tolerated by most adults, although for some even one or two cups of coffee a day can produce adverse effects. At higher doses (e.g., six to eight cups of coffee per day), a number of unpleasant effects, such as irritability, tremors, insomnia, and rapid and irregular heartbeat, may occur. These effects may tend to restrict regular high-dose use.

Availability
The ready availability and high degree of social acceptability of caffeine-containing beverages and foods tend to increase caffeine's abuse potential.

Background Reading

Briggs, G.G., Freeman, R.K. & Yaffe S.J. (Eds.) (1990). *Drugs in Pregnancy and Lactation, A Reference Guide to Fetal and Neonatal Risk*, (3rd edition). Baltimore: Williams and Wilkins.

Canadian Centre for Drug Free Sport. (1993). *Drug Free Sport*. Gloucester, ON: Canadian Centre for Drug Free Sport.

Charney, D.S., Heninger, G.R. & Jatlow, P.I. (1985). Increased anxiogenic effects of caffeine in panic disorders. *Archives of General Psychiatry, 42*, 233–243.

Eskenazi, B. (1993). Caffeine during pregnancy: Grounds for concern? *Journal of the American Medical Association, 270 (24)*, 2973–2974.

Infante-Rivard, C., Fernandez, A., Gauthier, R., David, M. & Rivard, G. (1993). Fetal loss associated with caffeine intake before and during pregnancy. *Journal of the American Medical Association, 270 (24)*, 2940–2943.

Lowinson, J.H., Ruiz, P., Millman, R.B. & Langrod, J.G. (Eds.) (1997). *Substance Abuse: A Comprehensive Textbook*, (3rd edition). Baltimore: Williams and Wilkins.

Mills, J.L., Holmes, L.B., Aarons, J.H., Simpson, J.L., Brown, Z.A., Jovanovic-Petersen, L.G., Conley, M.R., Graubard, B.I., Knopp, R.H. & Metzger, B.E. (1993). Moderate caffeine use and the risk of spontaneous abortion and intrauterine growth retardation. *Journal of the American Medical Association, 269 (5)*, 593–597.

Myers, M.G. & Basinski, A. (1992). Coffee and coronary heart disease. *Archives of Internal Medicine, 152*, 1767–1772.

Shapiro, S. (1991). Coffee, caffeine and cardiovascular disease. *New England Journal of Medicine, 324 (14)*, 991.

Silverman, K., Evans, S.M., Strain, E.C. & Griffiths, R.R. (1992). Withdrawal syndrome after the double-blind cessation of caffeine consumption. *New England Journal of Medicine, 327 (16)*, 1109–1114.

Strain, E.C., Mumford, G.K., Silverman, K. & Griffiths, R.R. (1994). Caffeine dependence syndrome — Evidence from histories and experimental evaluations. *Journal of the American Medical Association, 272 (13)*, 1043–1048.

van Dusseldorp, M. & Katan, M.B. (1990). Headache caused by caffeine withdrawal among moderate coffee drinkers switched from ordinary to decaffeinated coffee: A 12 week double blind trial. *British Medical Journal, 300*, 1558–1559.

Cannabis
(Marijuana, Hashish, Hashish Oil)

DRUG CLASS: Hallucinogen

Synopsis

Marijuana,[1] hashish and hashish oil are obtained from the plant *Cannabis sativa*, a tough annual that grows in both tropical and temperate climates. The principal psychoactive constituent of this plant is tetrahydrocannabinol (THC),[2] a hallucinogenic substance that is much less potent than an equal weight of LSD. The concentration of THC in marijuana can range from as little as one per cent to 10 per cent or more (by weight) of the dried leaf products, while the concentrations in resin preparations (hashish and hashish oil) can range up to 20 and 70 per cent respectively. While actual concentrations in products sold on the street in North America are usually lower and vary widely according to source of supply, very potent material from cloned and hydroponically grown plants has become increasingly common.

When taken at low to moderate doses, cannabis usually induces a general feeling of well-being, relaxation and emotional disinhibition. A wide spectrum of perceptual and sensory distortions may be experienced, although at these dose levels the effects are not nearly as intense as those associated with LSD. Mild cognitive and motor impairment typically occurs during cannabis-taking episodes. Other common physiological effects involve the cardiovascular system and include increased heart rate and a small drop in blood pressure.

At the very high dose levels normally associated with the use of hashish oil, the effects of cannabis can be more similar to those of LSD in nature and intensity, and

---

1   An alternative spelling is marihuana.

2   Tetrahydrocannabinol exists in *Cannabis sativa* in several chemical forms. The main psychoactive constituent is delta-9-tetrahydrocannabinol (also called delta-1-tetrahydrocannabinol). "Delta-9" and "delta-1" are often replaced by the symbols Δ^9 and Δ^1 respectively.

the probability of adverse psychological reactions increases. True hallucinations can occur and may be accompanied by disorganized thought, paranoia and panic. Fortunately, such severe reactions are infrequent — because the effects of smoked cannabis are rapidly experienced, most users are able to stop their intake before adverse effects become too serious. In contrast, those who swallow the drug are more likely to experience an adverse reaction, both because they have much less control over the size of the dose and because the rate of absorption into blood is highly variable.

Tolerance develops to the desired psychoactive effects of cannabis with regular use, and regular use may also cause psychological and mild physical dependence. Abrupt abstinence after protracted and regular high-dose use can result in a withdrawal syndrome, the symptoms of which include sleep disturbances, anxiety, restlessness, sweating, loss of appetite and upset stomach.

The effects of chronic daily or almost-daily use have recently become the subject of extensive research. Many findings are preliminary (and sometimes contradictory). However, there is growing evidence that chronic heavy cannabis smoking is particularly harmful to the body's respiratory system.

Although survey evidence in North America indicates that cannabis is the most widely used illegal psychoactive drug (with the exception of alcohol and tobacco used by minors), most evidence suggests that the majority of North Americans have never used cannabis, and that most of those who have used it have done so infrequently and experimentally.

Recent advances in understanding of cannabinoid pharmacology have set the stage for development of potent synthetic cannabinoid-like drugs with more selective actions.

Drug Source

Cannabis sativa, the botanical name for the Indian hemp plant[3], is an annual from which marijuana, hashish and hashish oil are prepared. More than 60 constituents,

---

[3]   Hemp plants containing virtually no psychoactive principles are grown commercially in many countries for their fibre content.

known as cannabinoids, occur naturally only in this plant. The principal psychoactive cannabinoid is delta-9-tetrahydrocannabinol, often referred to as Δ^9-THC.[4] *Cannabis sativa* readily grows in both tropical and temperate zones, and numerous cultivated and naturally occurring strains (varying in hallucinogenic potency) are found throughout the world.[5] Frequently, cannabis is bought and sold on the street under a name associated with the alleged (but often incorrect) geographical origin of the particular preparation, e.g., Colombian, Acapulco Gold, Jamaican, Mexican and Panamanian.

Trade Names

There is no generally accepted medical use for crude cannabis, although it has been used as a folk remedy in some parts of the world. When used in research, cannabis preparations and individual cannabinoids are usually referred to by a botanical or chemical name respectively. However, THC is marketed under the name dronabinol (Marinol®) to treat nausea and vomiting caused by cancer chemotherapy. The related synthetic compound nabilone (Cesamet®) is available for the same purpose.

Street Names

Few psychoactive drugs have as many street names as does marijuana. The name "marijuana" likely derives from the Mexican slang for any cheap tobacco. Among the drug's more common English colloquial names are Acapulco Gold, ace, bhang, Colombian, ganja, grass, hemp, Indian, Jamaican, jive (sticks), joint, Mary Jane, Mexican, Maui wowie, Panama Red, Panama Gold, pot, reefer, ragweed (low-grade marijuana), sativa, sinse, tea, Thai sticks, weed. "Roach" refers to the remainder of a marijuana cigarette, or "joint," after most of the drug has been smoked. A "roach clip" (which may be an ornamental commercial product or simply a bobby pin) holds the small remainder until virtually all has been consumed.

---

4   In some earlier literature, this cannabinoid is named as delta-1-tetrahydrocannabinol.

5   *Cannabis sativa* is a species of plant generally considered to exist in several varieties; therefore, reference is often made to *Cannabis sativa var. indica* and *Cannabis sativa var. ruderalis* as particular varieties within the *Cannabis sativa* species. However, the view is held by some botanists that these "varieties" are actually cannabis species different from *Cannabis sativa* — i.e., that *Cannabis sativa*, *Cannabis indica* and *Cannabis ruderalis* are three different species of cannabis.

The derivation of the name hashish may be from the Arabic for "dry grass" or, more colorfully, from Hasan-ibn-al-Sabbah, the founder of the 11th-century Assassins. According to legend, the Assassins carried out ritual murders after achieving hashish intoxication.[6] The only widely used street name is "hash," although many geographically local terms exist.

The viscous, highly potent oil of cannabis resin is most frequently referred to as "hash oil" or "honey oil." Oil derived from leaf material is called "weed oil."

Drug Combinations

- cannabis and PCP, referred to as "supergrass" or "killer weed"

- cannabis and opium, referred to as "O.J." (i.e., opium joint)

- cannabis and heroin, referred to as "atom bomb" or "A-bomb"

- cannabis added to a cigar, referred to as a "blunt."

Medical Uses

While there are, as yet, no widely accepted medical uses for cannabis, its use in the treatment of a range of ailments has been the subject of a growing debate in the 1990s. In 1996, voters in two U.S. states passed referenda that would allow physicians to recommend or prescribe marijuana use for severely ill patients, while in 1997, Canada's prohibition on the medical use of cannabis was subjected to challenges in the courts. Marijuana, THC and structurally similar synthetic chemicals are currently under study in the treatment of epilepsy,[7] wide-angle glaucoma, anorexia nervosa, multiple sclerosis and asthma; for relief of nausea and vomiting produced by cancer chemotherapy; and to combat anorexia among patients with advanced cancer and AIDS (see the note on nabilone in Section 5).

---

6   It is now thought that the Assassins were provided with hashish, women, etc., and then told that the continuing provision of their pleasures was contingent upon their performing the murders.

7   In 1997, an Ontario court dismissed charges relating to possession and cultivation of cannabis because the individual charged was using the cannabis preparations as part of the drug treatment for epilepsy, which was not adequately controlled by conventional drug therapies.

Recent breakthrough advances in understanding cannabinoids' pharmacology at the molecular level have set the stage for a much better understanding of the effects of marijuana and hashish and the development of synthetic cannabinoid agonist and antagonist drugs. Recently, researchers have identified two cannabinoid receptors, CB_1 and CB_2, which are distributed predominantly in the central nervous system and immune system respectively. These receptors are believed to be the molecular sites of action of some of the active constituents of marijuana and hashish. Further research identified two substances[8] in the CNS and other tissues, that bind to cannabinoid receptors and act as agonists. These substances are known as CB endogenous ligands. Another chemical has been synthesized that appears to act as an antagonist at CB_1 receptors.[9] Together these findings provide a platform for development of highly potent synthetic drugs designed to have specific types of cannabinoid effects or to antagonize cannabinoid effects.

Physical Appearance

The plant *Cannabis sativa* can grow to heights of five metres (16 ft.), although most strains grown in North America are considerably shorter. The plant has both a male and a female form (i.e., it is dioecious). Both sexes have large leaves (consisting of five to 11 leaflets with serrated margins) that are deep green on the upper side and light green on the lower. The female plant secretes an abundant sticky resin that covers the flowering tops and upper leaves.

Marijuana is prepared from the dried flowering tops and leaves of the harvested plant. The THC concentration in the resulting marijuana depends on the growing conditions, the genetic characteristics of the plant and the proportions of flowering parts, upper leaves, lower leaves, stems and seeds present in the marijuana preparation.[10] Marijuana may range in color from greyish-green to greenish-brown, depending on where it was grown. Its texture can vary from a dry powder to a dry leafy material to

---

8   The endogenous ligands are known as anandamide (arachidonyl ethanolamide) and 2-AG (i.e., sn-2- arachidonylglycerol).

9   This substance is known by the code name SR141716A.

10   For a given plant, the THC concentration is usually greatest in the bracts (the small leaves at the base of the flowers), and decreases from the flowering tops to upper leaves to small stems to large stems to seeds to roots. However, hydroponic growth of cloned material from high potency plants is increasingly common in North America, and can yield marijuana with a THC content of 10 per cent or more.

a finely divided tea-like product. Occasionally, materials such as tea or tobacco are added to dilute the marijuana before it is offered for sale on the street.

Hashish consists of dried cannabis resin and compressed flowers, and ranges in color from light ochre brown to almost black. It is usually available on the street in the form of hard chunks or cubes. The concentration of THC in hashish sold in North America can be as high as 15 to 20 per cent.

The viscous, highly potent oil of cannabis is obtained by extracting the cannabinoids, including THC, from hashish (or, less often, marijuana) with an organic solvent, concentrating the filtered extract, and in some cases subjecting it to further puri-fication. The color may range from green or pale yellow, through brown, to almost black. The concentration of the THC in "hash oil" is generally 10 to 20 per cent, although samples as high as 70 per cent have been confiscated. Oil extracted from marijuana is usually less potent than "hash oil."

Dosage

Medical

In experimental studies in which THC is administered orally in capsules, single doses have ranged up to 20 mg. The THC derivative, delta-9-tetrahydrocannabinol hemisuccinate has been administered rectally in suppository formulation at doses of up to 5 mg in studies of THC's effectiveness in relieving spasticity and rigidity.

Non-medical

A 500-mg "joint" of marijuana typically contains about 9 to 10 mg of THC. While some street purchases from unreliable sources may contain less, joints rolled from the more potent varieties (e.g., Californian sinsemilla)[11] may contain 20 to 30 mg or more.

---

11   If the female plant is kept unfertilized (i.e., by preventing pollen from the male plant from reaching the female plant), it will flower more abundantly and thereby produce more resin. Marijuana so cultivated is called sinsemilla (literally, "without seeds") and usually contains four to six per cent THC.

A very small amount of cannabis (e.g., containing 2 to 3 mg of THC) can produce a brief pleasurable high for the occasional user, and a single typical joint may be sufficient for two or three non-tolerant smokers. A heavy regular smoker may consume five or more joints per day.

Routes of Administration

Almost all possible routes of administration have been used, but by far the most common method is smoking (inhaling) a hand-rolled joint resembling a cigarette (usually with the ends twisted or folded). Smokers inhale deeply, and then hold their breath for several seconds in order to ensure maximum absorption of the THC by the lungs. Experienced smokers can absorb about a quarter of the THC contained in a joint. Both marijuana and hashish are also frequently smoked through a pipe, and various types of pipes are available for this purpose (some of which are quite exotic in appearance). Hash oil is used sparingly because of its extremely high psychoactive potency — often a single drop is applied to a joint, a cigarette or another smokable substance. Very heavy users, however, may use as much as a gram of this potent product per day.

Crude aqueous extracts of cannabis have on occasion been injected intravenously. However, because THC is virtually insoluble in water, little or no drug is actually present in these extracts. Moreover, the injection of tiny undissolved particles (in addition to water-soluble non-cannabinoid plant components) has caused very unpleasant side effects, including severe pain and inflammation at the site of injection and a variety of toxic systemic effects.

Cannabis, particularly hashish, may be cooked or baked in foods and eaten. In clinical research, THC is usually prepared in gelatin capsules and administered orally. The oral dose must be three to five times greater than the smoked dose to produce the equivalent intensity of effect. Preliminary results indicate that THC is much less effectively absorbed when administered orally than when administered rectally in the form of its hemisuccinate.

Effects of Short-Term Use: Low to Moderate Doses[12]

Short-term use of low to moderate doses of cannabis can produce the following effects:

CNS, *behavioral, subjective:*

- Early effects include disinhibition and talkativeness. Many users also experience relaxation and drowsiness. By contrast, many other hallucinogens, such as LSD, initially induce a state of excitation.

- The user usually experiences a general feeling of well-being, which can be manifested as exhilaration and euphoria.

- Distortions of the perception of time, body image and distance frequently occur. Users may also experience increased auditory and visual acuity and thus may perceive ordinary objects as taking on magnified importance.

- The senses of touch, smell and taste, as well as body awareness and perception are often enhanced.

- Spontaneous laughter commonly occurs.

- There may be mild impairment of short-term memory and concentration as well as mild confusion and disorientation.

- Attention span may be reduced and the user's ability to process information may be impaired.

- Balance and stability when standing can be impaired, and the user tends to experience decreased muscle strength and hand steadiness; slight tremor may also occur.

- Ability to perform complex motor tasks (e.g., in simulated driving tests) can be impaired.

- Some users experience such adverse reactions as fearfulness and anxiety, as well as mild paranoia. However, at relatively low dose levels, abusive or violent behavior associated with cannabis use is rare.

- Cannabis use may also trigger flashbacks in individuals who have experienced prior hallucinogen use.

---

12   Doses of 5 mg of THC or less (equivalent of one low- to medium-potency marijuana "joint") smoked by non-tolerant users.

Cardiovascular: increased heart rate, increased peripheral blood flow, rapid fall in blood pressure and faintness when standing up after being in a lying position, reddening of the eyes.

Respiratory: irritation of the mucous membranes lining the respiratory system, bronchodilation.

Gastrointestinal: increased appetite, dryness of the mouth and throat.

Other: changes in sex drive, slight changes in body temperature. Headache and "hangover" may occur when effects begin to wear off.

The intoxication produced by a single typical joint lasts about 45 minutes. However, where several "typical" joints are smoked at hourly intervals the result is a continuous "high," which persists for approximately 2.5 hours after the last smoking. Smoking much weaker joints (containing approximately 3 mg of THC) shortens both the duration of high from a single joint (to approximately 20 minutes) and the duration of effect after the last smoking (to approximately one hour). However, some behavioral effects may persist for three to five hours. If cannabis is taken orally (swallowed), the effects may last for up to 24 hours. Many of the mental and behavioral effects of cannabis are at least additive with those of alcohol, and combined use of alcohol and cannabis is common.

Effects of Short-Term Use: Higher Doses[13]

Intensification of cannabis's low-dose effects may occur with higher doses, as well as any of the following effects:

CNS, behavioral, subjective: Synesthesias, the melding of one sensory modality with another (such as music being "seen") may occur. Pseudohallucinations — hallucinations that the user knows are unreal — occasionally occur. The probability of adverse psychological consequences tends to increase as the size of the dose increases. Judgment is impaired; reaction time is slowed; performance in simple motor

---

13   Doses of 10 to 20 mg of THC or more smoked by non-tolerant users, or lower doses in particularly sensitive individuals.

tasks is impaired. There may be confusion of past, present and future. True hallucinations may occur, as well as delusions and feelings of depersonalization (i.e., the belief that one is "unreal"). Thoughts are increasingly confused and disorganized; pronounced paranoia, agitation and panicky feelings may replace early euphoria; sometimes the user fears that the drug-induced state will never end. These adverse reactions are more likely to occur if the drug is swallowed rather than smoked, as the user has much less precise control over the size of the dose.

Heavy marijuana use has been shown to result in greater impairment in attention and some learning functions than does light use, even after a day of abstinence from the drug.

At very high doses, some users experience an acute toxic psychosis characterized by hallucinations, paranoid delusions, disorientation, intense feelings of depersonalization, severe agitation and loss of insight. The use of cannabis may also unmask latent schizophrenia, a condition that may be experienced indefinitely.

Cannabis and Driving

The effects of cannabis on driving performance have been studied by testing intoxicated subjects either in driving simulators or in cars driven on test tracks or city streets. On the basis of these experiments, it can be concluded that the drug interferes with many brain processes considered to be essential for safe driving (motor co-ordination, tracking, perception and vigilance), and that actual performance on the road is impaired. Although the degree of disruption is related to dose, as little as one joint can cause noticeable impairment in sensitive individuals. The simultaneous use of alcohol and cannabis intensifies the adverse effects of each drug on driving performance.

Earlier field studies did not permit any conclusion as to the degree of risk posed by a driver who had been smoking cannabis. In several studies, THC or its metabolites were found in the body fluids of 10 to 20 per cent of fatally injured drivers and pedestrians.[14] However, in some of these studies THC itself was found only in the urine, so that it could not be concluded that the individual had been under the influence of THC at the time of death. In addition, most of the drivers with positive blood tests for

---

14   THC is extensively metabolized in the body. Although at least one of the resulting metabolites (11-hydroxy-tetrahydrocannabinol) has psychoactive properties, most of the THC metabolites have negligible psychoactive potency. Further, these metabolites continue to be formed and excreted in urine in very small quantities for long periods (often weeks) after use of a single dose of cannabis. Therefore detection of THC metabolites in urine is an indicator that THC was used at some time in the past, but does not indicate intoxication at the time the urine was collected.

THC also had alcohol present in concentrations that could produce impairment by themselves. However, more recent studies using improved analytical techniques have shown, both in fatally injured drivers and in uninjured drivers arrested for impaired driving, that 10 to 15 per cent tested positive for cannabinoids, and many of these had no alcohol or other drug present in their systems.

Effects of Long-Term Use

Psychological Effects

The occasional low-dose use of cannabis does not appear to produce harmful psychological effects in healthy adults. Even more regular low-dose use (i.e., smoking a single marijuana cigarette or less one or two times a week) probably does not significantly affect normal psychological functioning in healthy adults, although mild psychological dependence may develop. The risk of more pronounced psychological dependence is particularly high among users with emotional problems who turn to cannabis to relieve psychological stress. They may come to depend inappropriately on cannabis instead of learning drug-free means of coping with stress.

Very regular high-dose use of cannabis may be associated with significant psychological adjustment problems in some users. The degree and type of maladjustment is the subject of disagreement among researchers. One pattern of behavior, often referred to as the "amotivational syndrome," has been reported to be manifested in some chronic heavy users of cannabis and/or LSD. One of the early descriptions of this syndrome is contained in the following passage:

> personality changes that seem to grow subtly over long periods of time: diminished drive, lessened ambition, decreased motivation, apathy, shortened attention span, distractibility, poor judgment, impaired communication skills, loss of effectiveness, introversion, magical thinking, derealization and depersonalization, diminished capacity to carry out complex plans or prepare realistically for the future, a peculiar fragmentation in the flow of thought, habit deterioration and progressive loss of insight (West, 1970).

Some of the described symptoms of amotivational syndrome are quite similar to some of the attributes of lifestyle adopted by many young people in the 1960s and early 1970s, especially among the "hippies" and other marginalized members of society. It was therefore not clear whether these symptoms were caused by the lifestyle, by heavy marijuana use that was frequently part of that lifestyle, or by a combination of both.

However, it has been a common experience among psychiatrists dealing with adolescent patients that these symptoms usually clear up fairly quickly when the drug use ends and detoxification progresses. Consequently, many psychiatrists now believe that the amotivational syndrome is simply a manifestation of chronic intoxication.

Among the symptoms that occur fairly frequently in chronic heavy users of cannabis, the most important are impairments of short-term memory, concentration and abstract thinking. Placebo-controlled studies have shown that a single marijuana cigarette can cause a significant increase in the number of memory lapses and intrusions of extraneous material during recall tests. Since the half-life of THC in the plasma is very long, these effects are likely to become intensified and prolonged during chronic heavy use. These symptoms tend to disappear after a few weeks of abstinence, although persistent dysfunction has been described in a few instances after abstinence has been established. The question of whether permanent brain tissue damage in humans arises from chronic heavy use of cannabis has not yet been settled, although some animal studies have shown the possibility of irreversible impairment of learning and memory associated with structural changes in the brain.

Other Adverse Effects

The respiratory system appears to be particularly affected by chronic heavy cannabis smoking. Bronchitis, asthma, sore throat and chronic irritation of and damage to the sensitive mucous membranes lining the respiratory tract are conditions generally acknowledged to have a much higher incidence among heavy smokers of cannabis than among occasional users and non-users. Recent well-designed clinical studies have shown impaired gas exchange, increased signs of airway obstruction and chronic inflammatory changes in lung tissue in the lungs of heavy users. These symptoms are additive with the effects of tobacco smoking. The available evidence also suggests that regularly smoking marijuana may increase the smoker's risk of developing cancer of the respiratory tract.

These problems should not be surprising: an individual cannabis "joint," when smoked, yields substantially more tar than a cigarette made with strong tobacco, and the tar from cannabis smoke possesses a higher concentration of certain cancer-producing agents (e.g., benzo[a]pyrene) than that from tobacco smoke.[15] A greater

---

15   Tar is the residue of tiny particles produced by the combustion of cannabis or tobacco.

percentage (by weight) of the available benzo[a]pyrene in smoked cannabis is probably retained by the lungs than is the case with smoked tobacco, as the cannabis smoker generally inhales more deeply and typically holds cannabis smoke in the lungs for much longer periods with each inhalation. The prolonged holding of cannabis smoke in the lungs ensures maximum absorption of its desired psychoactive constituents but this practice may increase the risk of lung cancer for heavy regular smokers of cannabis, particularly if they are also heavy cigarette smokers.

Other Areas of Investigation

- The long-term effects of chronic cannabis smoking on cardiovascular functions do not appear to be significant in users without a history of heart disease or other cardiovascular disorder.

- The findings on the long-term effects of cannabis use on sexual functioning in human males are not uniform. However, most current evidence suggests that although there are disruptions in hormone balance and a decrease in sperm count in adult users, there is little or no substantial effect on fertility. There has been practically no research on the effects of long-term cannabis use on human female sexual function, although there are concerns about possible disruptions in menstrual cycles. Adolescents, who experience rapid maturation of their reproductive systems, may be particularly vulnerable to cannabis-induced effects. Concerns also remain about an increased risk of congenital abnormalities or developmental delays in children whose mothers have consumed cannabis during pregnancy. However, researchers find it difficult to separate out the effects of cannabis use during pregnancy from the effects of other drugs, diet and poor levels of prenatal care.

- There is some evidence that chronic heavy use of cannabis may adversely affect certain components of the body's immune system. This issue has attracted increasing attention since CB_2 receptors were found primarily in the immune system. However, findings are not uniform, and epidemiological studies in this area are necessary before any firm conclusions can be drawn.

Lethality

In North America, there have been no reports of deaths directly attributable to cannabis overdose in humans. However, a number of deaths are likely to have resulted indirectly from cannabis use. Cannabis has almost certainly contributed to fatal car accidents, for example, since it has adverse effects on such important driving skills as judgment, perceptual/ motor co-ordination, ability to concentrate and depth perception.

Tolerance and Dependence

Tolerance

Cannabis users can become increasingly sensitive to the drug over their first few smoking experiences. In such cases, the user experiences the psychoactive effects more readily and with smaller amounts of the drug on the second and subsequent occasions than on the first occasion. This pattern is accounted for largely by an increase in smoking efficiency (and hence an increase in effective dose). Other factors, such as the development of a more relaxed "set" (i.e., more favorable expectations and attitudes), and greater awareness of the body's responses to the drug may also play a role.

However, in research experiments involving frequent and longer-term regular administration of high daily doses of cannabis, users become less sensitive over time to the desired effects. Clinical observations of chronic heavy cannabis users also suggest that tolerance develops. Therefore, if very regular high-dose smokers wish to maintain the desired intensity of initial psychoactive effects, they must increase their daily dose or abstain for at least several days to restore their original sensitivity.

After very regular high-dose use, tolerance develops to several other effects of cannabis: rapid heart rate, other adverse cardiovascular effects, impairment of performance on psychomotor tasks, and other forms of cognitive impairment. Daily low-dose use of cannabis in some users may not result in any appreciable tolerance to the desired effects, although tolerance to impairment of psychomotor functioning does occur, with a resultant improvement in task performance. The acceleration of heart rate is also somewhat reduced with chronic daily low-dose use.

There is no evidence that cross-tolerance develops between cannabis and other hallucinogens.[16]

Psychological Dependence and Physical Dependence/Withdrawal

With regular use, psychological dependence on cannabis can develop. Users may acquire a persistent craving for its psychoactive effects, and the drug consequently takes on a central role in their lives. If cannabis is temporarily unavailable, anxiety related to the drug supply, or even feelings of panic, may result.

Physical dependence on cannabis may develop in those who use high doses daily and abrupt termination of use can produce a mild withdrawal syndrome, with symptoms including sleep disturbance, irritability, loss of appetite and consequent weight loss, nervousness, anxiety, sweating and upset stomach. Sometimes chills, increased body temperature and tremors occur. The withdrawal syndrome usually lasts for less than a week, although the sleep disturbances may persist for a longer period.

Patterns of Use

Repeated surveys of the prevalence of cannabis use among populations of high school students revealed a significant increase during the late 1960s and the entire 1970s. By 1979, 54 per cent of Grade 12 students polled in a U.S. nationwide survey reported having used cannabis at least once within the previous year, and almost 11 per cent of them were "daily"[17] users. The situation in Canada and in other western countries appeared to be comparable. For example, in a similar survey conducted in 1979 in Ontario, almost 50 per cent of students aged 16 and older reported using cannabis within the previous year, although prevalence of use in the younger age groups was considerably lower.

In the early 1980s, cannabis use began to stabilize and subsequently to decline among the high school population. By 1983, 42 per cent of U.S. high school seniors reported use within the previous year, and 5.5 per cent reported daily use. In Ontario, about 40 per cent of those aged 16 and over had smoked cannabis within the previous

---

16   Cross-tolerance does develop among LSD, mescaline and psilocybin.

17   Defined as 20 or more occasions of use within the previous 30 days.

12 months. During this period, cannabis remained the third most popular psycho-active drug (after alcohol and tobacco), and use was still significantly higher among males than females.

More recent surveys have provided evidence that the decline in adolescent drug use in the 1980s has been followed by a resurgence in the 1990s. Use by Ontario students in Grades 7 through 13[18] increased from 1989 to 1995. However, a recent study found that the level of use remained unchanged from 1995 to 1997, when 24.9 per cent of the survey sample reported use of cannabis in the preceding year.

The use of cannabis among adults is also highly sex- and age-dependent. Over the past 20 years, approximately eight to 11 per cent of Canadian adults acknowledged some use of cannabis during the 12 months prior to the survey. In a 1997 Ontario survey, 8.7 per cent of adults reported cannabis use within the past year. Use is consistently higher among men than women, and higher in 18- to 29-year-olds than in other age groups.

A key factor in the much higher rate of occasional use of cannabis among students as compared to adults is that the large majority of youthful users are experimenters who try cannabis on only a few occasions and then stop. It is possible that after having satisfied their curiosity they lose interest, or that after having bowed to peer-group pressure to try it, they are then relieved of further pressure to use it. The most recent Ontario adult study supports the experimentation hypothesis: while 26.8 per cent of respondents had used cannabis at some time in their lives, only 8.7 per cent of these same people had used it within the past 12 months. However, a previously identified trend was confirmed: the number of "past-year" adult users of cannabis aged 30 to 49 years has increased from 15.4 per cent of this age group in 1977 to 46.5 per cent in 1997. This trend indicates that many cannabis users who began their use as adolescents in the 1970s and 1980s are continuing it into middle age.

---

[18]   In Ontario schools, the traditional Grade 13 has been replaced by an Ontario Academic credit (OAC) year. The term Grade 13 has nevertheless been retained in the Ontario survey and thus in this text to facilitate comparison with previous surveys.

Potential for Abuse

Dependence Liability

The euphoria ("high") produced by cannabis is generally not as intense as that produced by drugs with a high dependence liability, such as cocaine or heroin. In fact, many users claim they take cannabis because of the mellow and relaxed state it tends to create. These pleasurable effects do not appear to be great enough to induce dependence in most users. A small minority, however, appear to experience significant problems when trying to give up use of the drug. It would be best, therefore, to categorize the dependence liability of this drug as mild to moderate.

Inherent Harmfulness

It is generally acknowledged that occasional use of cannabis is not ordinarily harmful to healthy adults. For those who heavily and regularly abuse it, the quick gratification obtained from cannabis smoking apparently greatly outweighs any concern they may have over possible long-term harmful consequences.

Availability

Most cannabis users, including young people, are normally able to obtain the drug through illicit means without great difficulty. Furthermore, compared with many other illicit drugs, cannabis is relatively inexpensive. Both factors contribute to the widespread abuse of cannabis in North America.

Background Reading

Adams, I.B. & Martin, B.R. (1996). Cannabis: pharmacology and toxicology in animals and humans. *Addiction, 91 (11)*, 1585–1614.

Adlaf, E.M., Ivis, F.J. & Smart, R.G. (1997). *Ontario Student Drug Use Survey 1977-1997*. Toronto: Addiction Research Foundation.

Adlaf, E.M., Ivis, F., Ialomiteanu, A., Walsh, G. & Bondy, S. (1997). *Alcohol, Tobacco and Illicit Drug Use Among Ontario Adults: 1977-1996. The Ontario Drug Monitor, 1996*. Toronto: Addiction Research Foundation. ARF Document Series No. 135.

Corrigal, W., Hall, W., Kalant, H. & Smart, R.G. (Eds.). (1998). *The Health Effects of Cannabis.* Toronto: Addiction Research Foundation and World Health Organization (forthcoming).

Hall, W., Solowij, N. and Leeka, J. (1994). *The Health and Psychological Consequences of Cannabis Use.* Sydney: Australian National Task Force on Cannabis, National Drug Strategy Monograph No. 25. [See also Hall et. al. (1996) "Comments on Hall et. al.'s Australian National Drug Strategy Monograph No. 25." Addiction, 91(6), 759-775.]

Institute of Medicine. (1982). *Marijuana and Health.* Washington: National Academy Press.

Matsuda, L.A. (1997). Molecular aspects of cannabinoid receptors. *Critical Reviews in Neurobiology, 11 (2-3),* 143–166.

Pope, H.G. Jr. & Yurgelun-Todd, D. (1996). The residual effects of heavy marijuana use in college students. *Journal of the American Medical Association, 275 (7),* 521–527.

West, L.J. (1970). On the marihuana problem. In D. Efron (Ed.), *Psychotomimetic Drugs.* New York: Raven Press.

World Health Organization. (1997). *Cannabis: A Health Perspective and Research Agenda.* Geneva: World Health Organization, Division of Mental Health and Prevention of Substance Abuse.

Cocaine

DRUG CLASS: CNS Stimulant, Local Anesthetic

Synopsis

Cocaine is a powerful central nervous system (CNS) stimulant that increases alertness, reduces appetite and the need for sleep, and produces intense feelings of euphoria. It is prepared from the leaf of the coca bush, found primarily in Peru and Bolivia. Originally isolated in Europe in the 1860s, pure cocaine was introduced as a tonic in patent medicines to treat a spectrum of maladies. Later it was found to be useful as a local anesthetic for eye, ear and throat surgery. Today, cocaine has been largely replaced by synthetic local anesthetics such as lidocaine, but it continues to have limited use in certain surgical procedures.

Because of its very potent euphoric and energy-increasing properties, cocaine was widely abused in the latter part of the 19th century, and early this century legislation was introduced to restrict its use. For many years thereafter, levels of illicit use remained low. Since the 1970s, however, the number of illicit cocaine users in North America has increased, as has the number of users experiencing problems with the substance. One factor contributing to this increase has been the widespread availability since the 1980s of "crack cocaine," an extremely potent freebase form of the drug.

Drug Source

Cocaine is prepared from the leaves of the *Erythroxylon* (or *Erythroxylum*) *coca* bush of Peru and Bolivia. A crude extract called coca paste is made from the leaves and sold on the street in South America. Coca paste is usually smoked. Several additional purification steps yield the hydrochloride salt of cocaine, which is smuggled into and sold illicitly in North America and elsewhere.

Trade Names

Not applicable.

Street Names

- Cocaine hydrochloride — C, coke, flake, snow, stardust.

- Cocaine base — crack, rock, freebase.

Combination Products

Cocaine plus heroin is called "dynamite" or "speedball." Crack impregnated with heroin is called "moonrock." Crack dipped in PCP is called "space cadet" or "tragic magic."

Medical Uses

In the past, cocaine was used as a local anesthetic for eye, nose and throat surgery. Today it is used only rarely for topical anesthesia of the upper respiratory tract.

Physical Appearance

In its pure form, cocaine hydrochloride is an odorless, white crystalline powder with a bitter, numbing taste. It is very soluble in water and soluble in alcohol.

Street cocaine is often adulterated with such related (but non-psychoactive) substances as lidocaine or benzocaine, both of which, when sniffed, produce a numbing effect in the nasal passages similar to that produced by cocaine. Other adulterants may mimic the taste or appearance of cocaine, and still others (e.g., caffeine) produce mild stimulating effects.

In addition to its salt (hydrochloride) form, cocaine is widely used in two forms as a base: freebase cocaine and crack cocaine. These forms of the drug have different physical properties from the traditional cocaine hydrochloride. For example, they are more volatile than the hydrochloride salt, and can therefore be "smoked" (i.e., vaporized and inhaled) to produce an extremely rapid and intense drug experience. These two forms of cocaine base are produced from cocaine hydrochloride using somewhat different methods.

Freebase cocaine is produced by making a solution of cocaine hydrochloride more alkaline (i.e., increasing its pH), and then extracting the cocaine base from the mixture using an organic solvent that is usually highly flammable. This process yields a very pure solution of cocaine base, without many of the adulterants commonly present in cocaine hydrochloride products. Before the cocaine can be smoked, however, the organic solvent must be evaporated. This is often done using an open flame, which presents a very high risk of fire and injury because of the flammability of the solvent. A user is said to be "freebasing" when using this form of cocaine, and many freebasers have been seriously burned in the course of preparing their drug.

The process for producing crack cocaine, which became popular in the mid-1980s, is more simple. This process does not include a solvent extraction step, and thus does not remove adulterants present in the original cocaine hydrochloride, but also reduces the risk of accidental fire. Crack cocaine is produced by treating the cocaine starting material with an alkaline solution, drying the resulting material, and selling it in the form of small lumps, which are then smoked. Crack derives its name from the cracking or popping sound it makes when it is heated, usually in a pipe.

Dosage[1]

Medical
Solutions used clinically for surface anesthesia vary in concentration from 10 mg/mL (one per cent) to 100 mg/mL (10 per cent).

---

[1]   All doses refer to adults.

Non-medical

A common pattern among users in social settings involves sniffing ("snorting") 20 to 30 mg of cocaine hydrochloride powder into each nostril. The powder is usually finely chopped with a razor blade, arranged into thin strips (or "lines") about 0.3 cm wide and 2.5 cm long, and sniffed through a thin tube. Intravenous doses of cocaine hydrochloride may range from 25 mg to over 200 mg. Smokers of freebase cocaine may use 250 to 1000 mg. Crack is often sold in rocks, each weighing 100 to 150 mg.

Routes of Administration

Cocaine hydrochloride is often "snorted" into the nose, where it is rapidly absorbed across the mucous membranes of the upper respiratory tract. It is also sometimes applied to other mucous membranes, including those of the mouth, vagina and rectum. Since it is readily water soluble, this form of the drug may also be injected intravenously.

Cocaine freebase is not water soluble, but is much more volatile than the hydro-chloride salt. Therefore, it is most commonly vaporized and inhaled into the lungs, where it is rapidly absorbed across the membranes of the alveoli (air sacs). Cocaine freebase, including crack, can be smoked in pipes or in cigarettes, mixed with tobacco or marijuana.

Effects of Short-Term Use: Low Doses[2]

The effects of the short-term use of low doses of cocaine include the following.

CNS, behavioral, subjective: dilation of the pupils; exaggerated reflexes; euphoria and a sense of well-being; postponement of physical and mental fatigue; reduced appetite and need for sleep; increased talkativeness or quiet contemplation and rapture; elevated self-confidence and feelings of mastery over the environment; increased speed of performance on fairly simple physical and intellectual tasks (but the ability to perform more complex functions is not enhanced). Performance may be

---

2   Single doses up to approximately 20 mg.

impaired because of the overestimation of one's abilities. The euphoric phase is often followed by a period of dysphoria characterized by agitation and anxiety.

Cardiovascular: constriction of the blood vessels, increase in heart rate after initial slowing, and increased blood pressure.

Respiratory: increased respiratory rate.

Gastrointestinal: dry mouth.

Effects of Short-Term Use: Higher Doses[3]

Intensification of cocaine's low-dose effects may occur at higher doses, as well as any of the following effects.

Behavioral, subjective: intense euphoria followed by a state of severe agitation. Users may experience anxiety, rapid flight of ideas, feelings of grandiosity, paranoid thinking, and often bouts of repeated, seemingly meaningless behavior (stereotypy). With repeated use, the cocaine user may suffer from a paranoid psychosis.

Neurological: tremor and muscle twitches, seizures, headache, hemorrhagic stroke and cerebral infarction.

Cardiovascular: high blood pressure, headache, pallor, rapid weak pulse and heart attack.

Gastrointestinal: nausea and vomiting.

Respiratory: Hazardous dose levels may cause rapid, irregular and shallow breathing; pulmonary edema (fluid accumulation in the lungs) and other lung damage including hemorrhage (coughing up blood), lung tissue diseases and hypersensitivity lung reactions. Lung trauma may also result from the high pressures sometimes used to force cocaine into the lungs rapidly or from the cocaine-anesthetized airways allowing inhalation of foreign objects and very hot vapors.

---

3   Doses of several hundred milligrams or more, or lower doses in particularly sensitive individuals.

Renal: acute renal failure, secondary to the deterioration of muscle tissue.

Other: elevated body temperature and cold sweat.

The Cocaine "Binge"

Heavy cocaine users may take the drug repetitively over several hours or days. Such "binges" are in many respects similar to the amphetamine "run," but the cocaine binge usually involves more frequent use and covers a shorter period of time. Users may experience toxic psychosis, which in most cases disappears when the drug is metabolized. However, these symptoms may persist if the user continues to take the drug. The user may attempt to end the binge by administering a depressant drug such as alcohol, a benzodiazepine or barbiturate, methaqualone or heroin. The binge is followed by the "crash," a period characterized by intense depression, lethargy and hunger. These symptoms tend to be most intense in the heaviest users (intravenous users and smokers of freebase). Users will often try to treat the "crash" symptoms by taking more cocaine.

Effects of Long-Term Use

The chronic cocaine user tends to administer the drug in high-dose "binges" interrupted by "crashes." The heavy user will appear nervous, agitated and excitable. Dramatic mood swings may occur, depending on how recently the drug has been taken. Users may experience symptoms of a toxic psychosis, including paranoid thinking. They may also become hypersensitive to sensory stimuli, sometimes to the point of visual and auditory hallucinations or sensations of insects crawling under the skin. Some evidence suggests that once a user has experienced psychotic symptoms, these effects are likely to recur with future use, even at lower doses.

Sleep disorders (insomnia followed by exhaustion), eating disorders (appetite suppression alternating with intense hunger) and sexual dysfunction (often impotence) are common among heavy users. Neurological effects can include cerebral atrophy (wasting of the brain) and impairment of neuropsychological functioning. Cardiovascular symptoms include high blood pressure and irregular heartbeat.

Other complications depend partly on the characteristic effects of the drug and partly on how it is taken. If the drug is sniffed, constriction of the blood vessels in the lining of the nose may lead to local tissue damage and perforation of the nasal septum. The long-term effects of cocaine smoking on pulmonary (lung) function have not been determined. Users who inject cocaine or other drugs with non-sterile needles or syringes risk such harmful effects as abscesses at the site of injection and infectious diseases such as viral hepatitis and AIDS.

Heavy users of cocaine often experience considerable social problems to which cocaine may contribute in several ways. Users may be so preoccupied with purchasing, preparing, using and recovering from use of cocaine that other important areas of their lives are neglected. Drug-induced irritability also contributes to interpersonal problems, and job performance tends to suffer. In addition, the large amount of money spent on the drug frequently leads to financial difficulties and occasionally to serious legal problems. The user waking up from a "binge" may have intense cocaine-related depression. Not surprisingly, users frequently have thoughts of suicide during this period and often see taking more cocaine as the only way out of the situation.

Cocaine and Pregnancy

The prevalence of cocaine use among pregnant women is unknown. However, since many cocaine users are between the ages of 20 and 30, which are prime childbearing years, use by pregnant women may be relatively common. Cocaine rapidly crosses the placenta and has the same pharmacological effects on the fetus as on the mother. These include constricting blood vessels, which increases fetal blood pressure and heart rate and can decrease vital oxygen delivery to developing tissues. Also important is the potential impact of cocaine's effect on neurotransmitters on the fetus's developing central nervous system. The potential harms from cocaine exposure during pregnancy include spontaneous abortion, *abruptio placentae,* premature birth, decreased weight and head circumference at birth, blocked blood vessels in the brain around the time of birth, various malformations. Newborns exposed to cocaine *in utero* may also experience abnormal sleep patterns, poor feeding and irritability for the first few days after birth. The longer-term neurological and behavioral effects experienced by these "cocaine babies" are still unclear. This is primarily due to the difficulties in conducting adequate research, since many factors may influence the central nervous system development of these children. These factors include prenatal exposure to other substances in addition to the cocaine (e.g., alcohol, tobacco) and poor prenatal care. However, there is evidence that prenatal cocaine exposure may be associated with neurotoxicity that results in long-term effects.

Lethality

The use of cocaine can cause death. The lethal dose of cocaine is quite variable and depends on many factors, including individual tolerance, the route of administration and the presence of other drugs and underlying medical conditions. Generally, higher blood levels of cocaine are obtained with intravenous injection or inhalation but serious complications have also occurred after snorting. Sometimes smugglers have swallowed large amounts of cocaine wrapped in condoms so as to avoid detection while passing through customs (a practice called "body-packing"). The cocaine released into the gastrointestinal tract from a burst condom is rapidly absorbed and can be fatal.

Sudden death from cocaine use is usually the result of cardiac arrhythmias (heart rhythm abnormalities), status epilepticus (continuous seizures), intracranial hemorrhage (bleeding in the brain), hyperthermia or respiratory arrest. In these cases of cocaine overdose, death may occur so quickly that there is no time to obtain medical assistance.

Like the amphetamines and many other psychoactive drugs, cocaine is often indirectly associated with suicides, homicides and fatal accidents.

Tolerance and Dependence

Users can develop tolerance to the euphoric effects of cocaine over the course of months or years of use, or even within a few days during a binge. Users often increase their daily intake — amounts of several grams per day have been reported — presumably to intensify and prolong the effects produced by the drug. On the other hand, with repeated use, an increased sensitivity to cocaine's adverse effects, including anxiety, depression, suicidal thinking, seizures and psychosis, has been reported.

Regular cocaine users who suddenly abstain can experience symptoms that appear to be qualitatively similar to those that occur following abstinence from other CNS stimulants. Exhaustion, depression, extended but restless sleep with increased REM (rapid eye movement activity) and hunger upon waking are common after abrupt termination of use. The severity of the symptoms partly depends on the length of the "binge," the amount of the drug used and the route of administration. Intravenous users and freebasers tend to suffer from the most intense post-abstinence symptoms because of the higher blood drug levels obtained through these methods of administration.

Regular cocaine users can experience intense psychological dependence in the form of a persistent craving for the drug's mood-altering effects. The strength of this dependence is illustrated by users who continue to take the substance despite seemingly overwhelming physical, psychological and social consequences. It should be noted that even though an effect is psychological it can still have a physical basis, in this case in the user's neurophysiological adaptations to regular cocaine use.

Despite the intensity of these abstinence symptoms, there is no medical need to withdraw users from the drug gradually.

Potential for Abuse

Abuse Liability
The abuse liability of cocaine is among the highest of all the drugs of abuse because of two key factors. First, the euphoria produced by cocaine is powerful when high blood levels are achieved. Second, this euphoria can occur rapidly and be tremendously intense, particularly when users inject cocaine hydrochloride intravenously or smoke freebase cocaine or crack.

Inherent Harmfulness
It is unclear whether cocaine's inherent harmfulness restricts its potential for abuse. Many regular users of cocaine are aware of the risks, but are willing to accept them. Users often continue to take the substance even after experiencing significant physical and psychological problems, including seizures, respiratory arrest and psychosis. However, evidence also suggests that concerns about the risk of addiction and other harmful effects may act as a deterrent to heavy use among those who have tried cocaine. It has been estimated that only five to 10 per cent of those who have ever tried cocaine eventually use it on a more intensive basis.

Availability

Cocaine is illegally exported from South America to North American and European markets. Law enforcement agencies vigorously pursue smugglers, and courts generally impose stiff penalties on those convicted of trafficking (or even of possessing cocaine for personal use). For these reasons, as well as the cost of production, the price of cocaine hydrochloride is relatively high. However, since the mid-1980s, the availability of relatively inexpensive freebase cocaine in the form of crack has increased the accessibility of cocaine to many more potential (especially younger) users. In 1995, 2.4 per cent of Ontario students reported using cocaine in the past year (up from 1.5 per cent in 1993), while 1.7 per cent of the students reported past-year crack use.

Background Reading

Adlaf, E.M., Ivis, F.J., Smart, R.G. & Walsh, G.W. (1995). *The Ontario Student Drug Use Survey, 1977-1995*. Toronto: Addiction Research Foundation.

Chasnoff, I.J. (1992). Cocaine, pregnancy and the growing child. *Current Problems in Pediatrics, (August)*, 302-321.

Erickson, P.G, Adlaf, E.M., Smart, R.G. & Murray, G.F. (1994). *The Steel Drug: Cocaine and Crack in Perspective* (2nd edition). New York: Lexington Books.

Gingras, J.L., Weese-Mayer, D.E., Hume, R.F. & O'Donnell, K.J. (1992). Cocaine and development: Mechanisms of fetal toxicity and neonatal consequences of prenatal cocaine exposure. *Early Human Development, 31*, 1–24.

Graham, K. & Koren, G. (1991). Characteristics of pregnant women exposed to cocaine in Toronto between 1985 and 1990. *Canadian Medical Association Journal, 144 (5)*, 563-568.

Hall, W.C., Talbert, R.L. & Ereshefsky, L. (1990). Cocaine abuse and its treatment. *Pharmacotherapy. 10 (1)*, 47-55.

Laposata, E.A & Mayo, G.L. (1993). A review of pulmonary pathology and mechanisms associated with inhalation of freebase cocaine ("crack"). *The American Journal of Forensic Medicine and Pathology, 14 (1)*,1–9.

Lathers, C.M., Tyau, L.S.Y., Spino, M.M. & Agarwal, I. (1988). Cocaine-induced seizures, arrythmias and sudden death. *Journal of Clinical Pharmacology, 28*, 584-593.

Rieder, M.J. (1994). How much fire under the smoke? The effects of exposure to cocaine on the fetus. *Canadian Medical Association Journal, 151 (11)*, 1567–1569.

Volpe, J.J. (1992). Effect of cocaine use on the fetus. *The New England Journal of Medicine, 327 (6)*, 399–407.

Warner, E.A. (1993). Cocaine abuse. *Annals of Internal Medicine, 119*, 226–235.

Codeine

DRUG CLASS: Opioid

Synopsis

Codeine is a naturally occurring substance produced by the opium poppy, *Papaver somniferum*. Codeine has mild euphoric and analgesic effects and is used clinically in managing mild to moderate pain and controlling cough. Tolerance to the main effects of codeine tends to develop gradually, while physical dependence occurs infrequently. However, a withdrawal syndrome can occur after chronic high-dose abuse (i.e., daily doses in excess of the therapeutic range), with symptoms that are similar to, but less intense than, those occurring during withdrawal from morphine.

Because of the mildness of its desired effects and its potentially dangerous side effects (e.g., seizures) at high doses, codeine is rarely the drug of choice for experienced abusers of opioids. Some products containing codeine can be purchased over the counter in Canadian pharmacies. These products contain a low dose of codeine in combination with at least two other medicinal ingredients. Although such products present a very low risk of dependence when used at recommended dose levels, heavy long-term users may develop dependence.

Drug Source

Codeine is isolated from crude opium, the resinous preparation derived from the opium poppy, *Papaver somniferum*.

Examples of Trade Names

Codeine Contin®.

Street Names

Schoolboy.

Combination Products

- 222®, 282®, 292® (ASA, caffeine citrate and codeine phosphate)

- Tylenol with Codeine No. 1®, No. 2®, No. 3® (acetaminophen, caffeine and codeine phosphate)

- Tylenol with Codeine No. 4® (acetaminophen and codeine phosphate)

- Fiorinal-C 1/4®, C 1/2® (ASA, butalbital, caffeine and codeine phosphate)

- Benylin Codeine® 3.3 mg-D-E (OTC) Syrup (codeine phosphate, guaifenesin and pseudoephedrine hydrochloride)

- Sinutab with Codeine® (acetaminophen, chlorpheniramine maleate, codeine and pseudoephedrine hydrochloride)

- elixir of terpin hydrate with codeine.

Tylenol with Codeine No. 1® and 222® are examples of codeine-containing analgesics that can be sold over the counter (OTC) in Canadian pharmacies without a prescription. Such products must contain two or more non-opioid medicinal ingredients together with no more than 8 mg codeine per dosage unit. Benylin Codeine® 3.3 mg-D-E is a codeine-containing cough suppressant that is similarly available over the counter in pharmacies. To qualify for OTC sale, cough syrups must include at least two non-opioid drugs and no more than 3.8 mg codeine per 5 mL.

Medical Uses

Medical uses of codeine include:

- suppression of cough reflex

- relief of mild to moderate pain.

Physical Appearance

Codeine phosphate is an odorless, white crystalline powder freely soluble in water and slightly soluble in alcohol.

Dosage[1]

Medical

The typical dosage of codeine for suppression of cough ranges from 5 to 10 mg taken orally every three to four hours.

For relief of mild to moderate pain (not adequately relieved by non-opioid analgesics such as ASA) dosages can be as high as 60 mg, taken orally or by injection every three to four hours.

Non-medical

While daily doses of up to 1,800 mg have been reported, codeine abusers ordinarily administer substantially less of the drug because of the potentially serious side effects that may occur at very high doses.

Routes of Administration

Orally or by subcutaneous or intramuscular injection.[2]

Effects of Short-Term Use: Low Doses[3]

Effects of the short-term use of codeine at low doses include the following.

---

[1]　　All doses refer to adults.

[2]　　Intravenous injection is rare, as it can produce severe flushing of the skin, puffy face, and occasionally a severe drop in blood pressure.

[3]　　Single doses within the therapeutic range administered orally to non-tolerant persons, to a maximum of 200 to 250 mg per day in divided doses.

*CNS, **behavioral, subjective:*** suppression of the sensation of and emotional response to mild to moderate pain,[4] suppression of cough reflex, dizziness, lightheadedness, drowsiness, mild euphoria or mild anxiety, mild clouding of mental functions, slight pupillary constriction.

Gastrointestinal: nausea, vomiting, constipation.

Other: itching sensation on the skin.

Codeine and Driving

Because of codeine's ready availability and widespread use in Canada, its possibly deleterious effects on driving performance are important. In one Finnish research study, the performance of professional drivers was tested on a simulated driving task 30 minutes after administration of codeine (50 mg), diazepam (10 mg) or alcohol (0.5 grams per kilogram of body weight). Those who drove under the codeine condition had more "collisions" than drivers in the alcohol or diazepam groups, and many more than drivers in the drug-free control group. Furthermore, the codeine group "drove off the road" more often than the alcohol, diazepam and drug-free groups. Although not all of the drivers were noticeably affected by codeine, such findings suggest that patients prescribed codeine should be cautioned about the increased risks associated with driving.

Effects of Short-Term Use: Higher Doses[5]

Intensification of low-dose effects may occur with the administration of higher doses, while the duration of effects increases with size of the dose. In addition, higher doses of codeine can lead to:

- increasing agitation in some users, and euphoria or sedation in others
- increasing impairment of the ability to concentrate
- gradual decreases in blood pressure, and in some cases, rapid and irregular heart beat
- progressively slower and more shallow breathing.

---

4   When administered by intramuscular injection, codeine 120 mg is approximately equivalent to morphine 10 mg. A principal advantage of codeine, however, is that it retains a high degree of effectiveness when administered orally, whereas morphine does not.

5   Single doses in excess of the therapeutic range administered orally to non-tolerant persons, or lower doses in particularly sensitive individuals.

At very high doses (i.e., overdose), codeine can cause tremors, seizures, delirium, coma, filling of the lungs with fluids, shallow and markedly reduced rate of breathing, low blood pressure, abnormally rapid heart rate, and pinpoint pupils.

Effects of Long-Term Use

Adverse consequences directly related to long-term codeine use include mood instability,[6] pupillary constriction (which impairs night vision), constipation, reduced libido, menstrual irregularity and certain types of respiratory impairment. Restlessness, tension and muscle twitches have been observed in chronic high-dose abusers.

Lethality

Deaths exclusively from overdose of codeine have been reported relatively infrequently. However, the potential for lethal overdose should not be underestimated. For example, 12 deaths in Los Angeles County were attributed to codeine overdose alone in a one-year period in 1979 and 1980. Codeine is also frequently identified in multiple-drug overdose deaths.

Severe overdose can result in seizures, delirium, coma, cardiac arrest and death, usually from respiratory arrest. The lethal dose in non-tolerant adults is estimated to be 0.5 to 1.0 gram (500 to 1,000 mg).

Large doses of codeine preparations containing ASA can also result in acute salicylate poisoning.

Tolerance and Dependence

Tolerance
When codeine is taken regularly and very frequently for an extended period, even in low to moderate doses, tolerance can develop gradually to its analgesic, cough-reflex

suppressant (antitussive) and mild euphoric effects. Higher daily doses may then become necessary to produce the desired effects.

Physical Dependence/Withdrawal

Physical dependence on codeine alone is not common. However, a withdrawal syndrome does occur upon abrupt termination of chronic high-dose abuse. Symptoms are similar to, but milder than, those observed during morphine withdrawal. Symptoms tend to appear about eight hours after the last dose, peaking in intensity by the second day and usually disappearing within less than a week. Early symptoms generally include anxiety, yawning, sweating, watering eyes, nasal discharge and a period of restless sleep. Later symptoms may include goose-flesh, dilated pupils, tremors, muscle twitches, alternations between chills and flushing, aching in the bones and muscles, and loss of appetite.

Psychological Dependence

Psychological dependence on codeine may occur when the drug is taken very frequently for extended periods, even at low daily doses. Psychologically dependent users continue to take the drug on a regular basis even after tolerance has developed to the effects of the usual daily dose. The user has a persistent craving for the drug, and may become preoccupied with ensuring that a sufficient supply of the drug is available. The user is likely to experience psychic distress if codeine is temporarily unavailable.

Patterns of Use

In Canada, codeine is the only opioid that can be obtained without prescription (in limited quantity per unit dose, and in combination with at least two other medicinal ingredients, in pain relief and cough suppressant products, as noted above). This ready availability contributes to its abuse by some individuals.

Codeine is also reported to be used, often in hazardously large quantities, by individuals physically dependent on heroin or other potent opioids. However, such users ordinarily resort to codeine only when they are attempting to postpone withdrawal sickness and their preferred drug is not sufficiently available. Although codeine is effective in at least partially suppressing heroin withdrawal sickness, the dose level required to achieve this effect may also produce tonic-clonic seizures (previously known as grand mal seizures) and possibly death due to respiratory arrest.

Potential for Abuse

Dependence Liability

The dependence liability of codeine is low. Its euphoric and analgesic effects are relatively mild. Although codeine phosphate can be injected, intravenous administration (the route preferred by those who inject opioids) can be hazardous.

Inherent Harmfulness

In low to moderate doses, adverse effects of codeine are usually both few and mild. However, the potential danger of CNS-stimulant effects at very high doses tends to limit use to amounts that generally do not produce the intensity of desired effects sought by experienced abusers of opioid drugs.

Availability

Codeine's potential for abuse is enhanced by the relative ease of obtaining the codeine-containing prescription products (and, probably to a lesser extent, by the availability of lower-potency OTC codeine-containing products). Many individuals who are dependent on more powerful opioids acknowledge that their earliest experiences with drugs in this class were with codeine.

Background Reading

Canadian Pharmaceutical Association. (1997). *Compendium of Pharmaceuticals and Specialties* (32nd edition). Ottawa: Canadian Pharmaceutical Association.

Reisine, T. & Pasternak, G. (1996). Opioid analgesics and antagonists. (Chapter 23). In J.G. Hardman, L.E. Limbird, P.B. Molinoff, R.W. Rudden & A.G. Gilman (Eds.), *Goodman and Gilman's The Pharmacological Basis of Therapeutics*. (9th edition). New York/Toronto: McGraw-Hill Health Professions Division.

Disulfiram

DRUG CLASS:	Antialcoholic, Alcohol Deterrant, Metabolic Inhibitor

Synopsis

Most commonly known by its trade name, Antabuse®, disulfiram is a drug taken daily by people with alcohol problems to deter the consumption of ethyl alcohol.[1,2] Disulfiram, which is taken orally, interferes with the normal metabolism of alcohol. When the user drinks alcohol, acetaldehyde, the intermediary metabolite of alcohol, rapidly accumulates in the bloodstream instead of being further metabolized. The acetaldehyde poisoning that results (i.e., the alcohol/disulfiram reaction) causes severe but temporary physical discomfort, which may last from 30 minutes to several hours. The severity of the reaction is proportional to the dose of disulfiram taken and to the amount of alcohol consumed. Some of the typical symptoms include weakness, vertigo, marked decrease in blood pressure, throbbing in the head and neck, extreme flushing of the face, headache, chest pain, labored breathing, nausea and vomiting.

For patients who reliably self-administer disulfiram, knowing that even small amounts of alcohol can prompt such a highly noxious reaction is sufficient to deter any alcohol consumption. For this reason disulfiram is sometimes referred to as a "psychological fence." Disulfiram therapy is generally viewed to be most beneficial to those patients who are simultaneously undergoing a comprehensive treatment and rehabilitation program.

When there is no alcohol in the body, disulfiram usually produces few and relatively mild side effects. In the presence of alcohol, only a small minority of patients suffer serious medical consequences resulting from the alcohol/disulfiram reaction. Because

---

[1]   Calcium carbimide (Temposil®) produces effects similar to those of disulfiram, but is no longer marketed in North America.

[2]   In this chapter, the term "alcohol" means ethyl (beverage) alcohol (ethanol).

most of these consequences involve the cardiovascular system, patients with a history of cardiovascular problems are normally excluded from disulfiram therapy.

Drug Source

Disulfiram is produced through chemical synthesis by the pharmaceutical industry.

Trade Names

Antabuse®.

Street Names

None.

Combination Products

None.

Physical Appearance

In its pure form, disulfiram is a white or off-white odorless powder that is very slightly soluble in water and soluble in alcohol. It is marketed in the form of white or off-white tablets.

Dosage[3]

Medical

Disulfiram should not be administered until the patient has abstained from alcohol for at least 12 hours. The initial oral dose is up to 500 mg of disulfiram administered

---

3   All doses refer to adults.

as a single daily dose, preferably in the morning, for a period of one to two weeks. The average maintenance dose is 250 mg daily, and ranges from 125 to 500 mg. The daily dose should never exceed 500 mg. Patients should be warned against drinking alcohol while taking disulfiram and informed that reactions can occur up to two weeks after they have stopped taking the medication. Ideally, patients being treated with disulfiram should carry a wallet card noting the signs and symptoms of the disulfiram-induced reaction, so that emergency medical personnel have access to this information.

Surgical implantation of disulfiram has been the subject of extensive clinical research, but the results have been generally disappointing. Experimental implantation of disulfiram usually involves a total quantity of approximately 1 gram (1,000 mg) in the form of a disc surgically inserted into the tissue of the abdomen once every several months. This formulation is currently not available in North America.

Non-medical
Not applicable.

Routes of Administration

Disulfiram is taken orally, usually in a daily single dose.

Effects of Short-Term Use: Low Doses[4]

In the absence of alcohol, a single dose of disulfiram usually does not produce noticeable effects, except for an initial two-week period in which the patient may experience drowsiness, lassitude and a metallic or garlic-like aftertaste.

Once present in the body, the effects of disulfiram on a person who ingests or inhales even small amounts of alcohol can be pronounced. The severity of the reaction increases with higher doses of alcohol. Mild to severe distress can result from ingesting a single dose of cough syrup containing alcohol, from inhaling rubbing

---

4   Single doses of 125 to 500 mg taken orally.

alcohol, perfume, nail polish or hair tonics, or from ingesting as little as 7 mL of ethyl alcohol (i.e., less than one-half of a standard drink).

Although the alcohol/disulfiram reaction is characteristically very unpleasant,[5] serious or life-threatening complications are unusual in otherwise healthy adults when they are carefully supervised by a physician. The typical syndrome occurs within a few minutes after alcohol is consumed, and can include the following symptoms.

CNS, behavioral, subjective: weakness, dizziness, blurred vision, drowsiness.

Cardiovascular: extreme flushing of the face, throbbing in the head and neck, palpitations, fainting, throbbing (possibly severe) headache, rapid and marked decrease in blood pressure, increased pulse rate, and chest pain.

Respiratory: gasping or labored breathing.

Gastrointestinal: dry mouth and throat, nausea and vomiting.

Other: sweating.

These effects may be experienced for a few hours, after which the exhausted patient typically falls asleep and, upon awakening, has usually completely recovered.

While severe reactions are unusual, they can include marked respiratory depression, cardiac arrhythmias, heart attack, extreme drop in blood pressure, acute congestive heart failure, obstruction of the coronary artery, coma and seizures.[6]

---

5   Effects are likely to be more intense after regular use of disulfiram has been established (i.e., usually a few days after the initial administration). Knowledge of these effects serves as a deterrent to alcohol use. Patients must be cautioned against any use of alcohol for up to two weeks after the termination of disulfiram therapy, since disulfiram is very slowly excreted from the body.

6   Careful medical screening, particularly to eliminate those patients with a history of cardiovascular disease or seizures, is essential, as is the continued supervision of those patients accepted for disulfiram therapy.

Effects of Short-Term Use: Higher Doses[7]

At higher doses of disulfiram drowsiness and fatigue are more pronounced than at low doses, and the alcohol/disulfiram reaction may be more intense.

Non-lethal overdose can produce elevated body temperature, lethargy, depression, inflammation of peripheral nerves, cerebellar dysfunction, impairment of intellectual functioning, and symptoms similar to parkinsonism.

Effects of Long-Term Use

With regular use, most side effects are mild and tend to disappear within a few weeks, although in some patients they can be quite severe. These side effects can include:

CNS, behavioral, subjective: fatigue, lassitude, morning drowsiness and difficulty in arising, sedation, tremor, restlessness and dizziness. While some patients report depression and anxiety, these symptoms may have been suppressed by alcohol use and merely unmasked by abstinence. Overt psychosis has also occasionally occurred, sometimes prompted by excessively high doses of disulfiram or interactions with certain other drugs. It may also represent the unmasking of latent psychosis.

Cardiovascular: headache.

Gastrointestinal: a variety of mild gastrointestinal disturbances, garlic breath, sometimes a metallic taste.

Other: skin eruptions, allergic dermatitis (which responds well to topical antihistamines), burning or itching sensations on the skin and reduced libido.

The rate of degradation of certain other drugs such as phenytoin (e.g., Dilantin®) and some anticoagulants may be considerably slowed in patients undergoing disulfiram treatment, thus prolonging duration of action of the other drug and requiring adjustments of the patient's dosage schedule.

---

[7] Single doses in excess of the therapeutic range, or lower doses in sensitive individuals.

Lethality

The alcohol/disulfiram reaction has occasionally caused cardiovascular collapse and death. A few cases of severe brain damage in very young children have resulted when they have accidentally taken disulfiram in large quantity.

Tolerance and Dependence

There is no evidence that tolerance develops to the effects of disulfiram. In fact, sensitivity to alcohol increases as the course of disulfiram therapy is prolonged.

Dependence on disulfiram does not occur.

Patterns of Use

Most experts now agree that the primary value of disulfiram is as an adjunct to a more comprehensive treatment program, particularly for patients who take the drug. Disulfiram treatment provides a means of deterring alcoholics from drinking while their other problems are being actively dealt with, for example, through Alcoholics Anonymous or professional counselling. Disulfiram is effective only if the user has a genuine desire to change the disruptive aspects of his or her lifestyle. In fact, there is no substantive evidence that disulfiram therapy, when undertaken without any additional treatment, is more effective than a placebo in deterring drinking once disulfiram therapy has been terminated.

Potential for Abuse

Disulfiram has no potential for abuse.

Background Reading

Canadian Pharmaceutical Association. (1997). *Compendium of Pharmaceuticals and Specialties* (32nd edition). Ottawa: Canadian Pharmaceutical Association.

Fastner, Z. (1977). Miscellaneous drugs. In M.N.G. Dukes (Ed.), *Side Effects of Drugs Annual I*. Amsterdam: Excerpt Medica.

Ethyl Alcohol
(Beverage Alcohol, Ethanol)

DRUG CLASS: Sedative/Hypnotic

Synopsis

Ethyl alcohol[1] is among the three most widely consumed non-medicinal drugs in the world — the others being caffeine and tobacco — and produces greater morbidity (health problems) and higher mortality (deaths) than all illicit drugs combined. While alcohol consumption has declined in recent years, the associated health and social costs remain enormous. However, research evidence from recent years also supports the view that middle-aged and older individuals who regularly consume small to moderate amounts of alcohol are at lower risk of some health problems, particularly coronary heart disease and ischemic stroke,[2] than are abstainers.

Alcohol is a central nervous system (CNS) depressant that is rapidly absorbed from the gastrointestinal tract and metabolized in the liver. Moderate doses produce disinhibition, while heavier doses produce cognitive and motor impairment and a decreased level of consciousness. Adverse effects of acute intoxication include blackouts, suicide, violence against persons and property, and trauma, including trauma from motor vehicle accidents.

Long-term excessive alcohol use is associated with numerous medical and psychiatric complications. Alcoholic liver disease is a major cause of illness and death in North America. Alcohol has diverse effects on the nervous system, including dementia, peripheral neuropathy, Wernicke-Korsakoff Syndrome and cerebellar degeneration. Cardiovascular effects of alcohol include high blood pressure (hypertension),

---

1   In this chapter, the terms ethyl alcohol, alcohol and ethanol are used interchangeably.

2   Ischemic stroke occurs when a blood clot travels to the brain, interrupting the supply of blood, depriving the cells of that area of oxygen and, as a result, causing them to die.

hemorrhagic stroke and cardiomyopathy. Alcohol is a carcinogen, increasing the user's risk of cancer of the esophagus, rectum, throat and possibly breast. Alcohol consumption during pregnancy can lead to fetal alcohol effects (FAE) or fetal alcohol syndrome (FAS).

Most people who drink alcohol do so moderately for social or ceremonial reasons and with low risk of problems. However, the abuse of alcohol by a minority of users causes great harm to individuals, families and society as a whole. Alcohol abuse is a major contributor to trauma, family disruption, lost productivity and crimes of violence such as spousal abuse and child abuse. Depression is a frequent and serious complication of alcohol abuse, and heavy drinkers are at high risk of suicide.

While a safe limit for alcohol consumption has not been established with certainty, current guidelines for low-risk drinking recommend a daily limit of no more than two standard drinks,[3] as well as weekly limits of 14 drinks for men and nine for women. In middle-aged and older people, moderate drinking is associated with lower total and cardiovascular mortality, but in young people mortality increases with the amount consumed (primarily due to deaths from suicide, accidents and violence). Moderate drinking has also been linked with breast cancer in women.

Alcohol problems occur along a spectrum of severity. "Problem drinkers" drink above the guideline limits and may have one or more alcohol-related problems, but do not have the clinical syndrome of alcohol dependence. They outnumber alcohol dependent individuals by a ratio of at least four to one. As a result, the bulk of alcohol-related morbidity and mortality occurs in the problem drinking group. Such individuals often respond to brief advice and reduced drinking strategies.

Alcohol dependence is a clinical syndrome characterized by very heavy alcohol consumption, continued drinking despite severe social or physical consequences, pre-occupation with alcohol, neglect of social responsibilities, difficulty moderating drinking behavior, and physical dependence (tolerance and withdrawal).

---

3   A standard drink = 341 mL (12 oz.) of regular-strength (5% alcohol) beer = 142 mL (5 oz.) of table wine (12% alcohol) = 43 mL (1.5 oz.) of spirits (40% alcohol) = 85 mL (3 oz.) of fortified wine, such as sherry or port (18% alcohol). Each of these portions contains approximately 17 mL (0.6 oz.) or 13.6 grams of pure (absolute) ethyl alcohol.

Tolerance to the effects of alcohol is due to behavioral adjustment, an increased rate of metabolism of alcohol and a neurological adaptation to the alcohol's sedative effects. Alcohol withdrawal produces symptoms of autonomic hyperactivity: tremors, sweating, vomiting, hypertension and rapid pulse. Complications of withdrawal include seizures, cardiac arrhythmias and delirium tremens.

The causes of alcohol dependence are complex. The probability of recovery is affected by individual characteristics such as social class, social supports, age, length of drinking history, co-morbid psychiatric conditions and addiction to other drugs besides alcohol. Treatment may include intensive inpatient or outpatient programs, participation in self-help groups such as Alcoholics Anonymous (AA), and anti-alcohol (alcohol-deterrent) drug therapy.

Drug Source

Beverage alcohol is made by fermenting and distilling fruit or grain products. Wines[4] and beers are direct products of fermentation, containing up to 14 per cent alcohol content. Spirits or liquor (rum, whisky, vodka, brandy and so on), which average 40 per cent alcohol by volume, and liqueurs, which range from 23 to 56 per cent alcohol by volume in Canada, are produced by distilling the product of fermentation to raise the alcohol content. The distillate is then adjusted (in most cases by adding water) to the desired alcohol concentration. Bitters are prepared by extracting certain plant materials with alcoholic or hydroalcoholic (i.e., alcohol mixed with water) solvents, and adjusting the alcohol content.

Trade Names

Beverage alcohol producers market their products using a distinctive brand name for each product. In some Canadian provinces, the provincial alcohol authorities bottle a few beverages purchased in bulk.

---

4   Fortified wines are wines that have been enriched in their alcohol content by addition of distilled neutral grape spirits.

Street Names

There are numerous street names and other popular terminology describing individual brands, types of alcohol beverage, or particular mixed drinks. More generic popular terms include:

- beer — brew, suds
- wine — vino, plonk
- spirits — booze, grog, hooch, moonshine, shine.

Combination Products

Alcohol beverages are combinations of alcohol, water and flavorings derived from the beverages' fruit or grain source, in some cases together with additives to improve their appearance, flavor or shelf life. Because alcohol is an excellent solvent, small amounts (typically 0.5 per cent) are included in many cough syrups and certain other orally administered medicinal products. Alcohol is also a constituent of mouthwashes, shaving lotions, perfumes and colognes and some aerosol sprays. These products often have a high alcohol concentration (40 per cent or more), and are sometimes abused by young people and impoverished alcoholics.

Medical Uses

Some physicians recommend the occasional use of alcohol to induce sleep, particularly for elderly patients. Such use has been reduced considerably with the introduction of safer and more effective hypnotic agents. In previous eras, when social use of alcohol was less acceptable in some sectors of the community, some physicians prescribed (or at least sanctioned) a small daily dose of an alcoholic beverage (often a fortified wine or an alcoholic beverage based on an extract of herbal principles) or a wine-based vitamin-containing "tonic" to improve appetite or aid digestion in some patients who were otherwise abstainers.

Physical Appearance

In pure form, ethyl alcohol is a clear, colorless, flammable liquid. The appearance of beverage alcohol depends on the particular diluents and additives with which it is combined.

Dosage[5]

Dosage levels of alcohol are typically described in terms of a given number of standard drinks, containing 13.6 grams of pure alcohol.

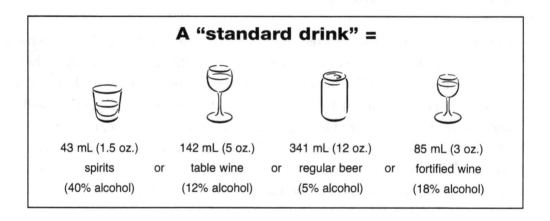

A "standard drink" =

| 43 mL (1.5 oz.) spirits (40% alcohol) | or | 142 mL (5 oz.) table wine (12% alcohol) | or | 341 mL (12 oz.) regular beer (5% alcohol) | or | 85 mL (3 oz.) fortified wine (18% alcohol) |

The degree of intoxication resulting from drinking alcohol does not depend on the type of alcoholic beverage but rather on the amount of absolute alcohol consumed. The amount of alcohol consumed during a single drinking episode might range from one to two drinks for light drinkers to 12 to 18 drinks for individuals with severe alcohol dependence.

Absorption and Metabolism (Biotransformation) of Alcohol

Alcohol is usually rapidly absorbed, partly through the stomach but predominantly through the small intestines. The rate of absorption is affected by the type of beverage, the stomach contents and whether the drinker's stomach is damaged. Very highly concentrated alcoholic beverages (e.g., brandy) can cause pylorospasm — an acute abnormal muscular contraction of the sphincter between the

---

5   All doses refer to adults.

stomach and the intestine, which prevents the stomach from emptying and thereby retards absorption of the alcohol. Similarly, if the stomach contains significant amounts of food, stomach emptying may also be retarded, and the absorption of the alcohol slowed. If the drinker has undergone a whole or partial gastrectomy (removal of stomach), however, alcohol will pass very rapidly into the intestines and the rise in blood alcohol level (BAL) will then be very dramatic. It should be emphasized that alcohol requires no digestion. It is absorbed unaltered directly into the bloodstream.

Absorbed alcohol is then transported in the blood to the liver, where it is metabolized first to acetaldehyde, then to acetate, and finally to water and carbon dioxide. No matter how much alcohol is consumed, or what blood level has been achieved, the liver metabolizes the alcohol at a constant rate of approximately 10 grams of ethanol per hour (slightly less than one standard drink, which contains 13.6 grams). Heavy drinkers metabolize alcohol somewhat more rapidly. The average man could thus drink a standard drink every hour without accumulating significant blood alcohol levels. A smaller person will be able to metabolize proportionately less alcohol per hour, and a larger-than-average person of normal weight for height will metabolize proportionately more.

Depending on body size and tolerance, an average man[6] will attain BALs of 30, 50 and 80 mg/100 mL[7] after consuming 1.5, 2.5 and 4 drinks respectively in an hour. Women will attain similar BALs with approximately two-thirds of this consumption. Women attain higher BALs because of several factors. Among these are their typically smaller volume of body water[8] through which consumed alcohol is distributed and possibly less activity of the enzyme alcohol dehydrogenase in the stomach lining.

Alcohol use may alter the biotransformation of some medications and vice versa. The presence of alcohol in the body along with the drug may slow, or occasionally increase, the rate of drug biotransformation. Chronic heavy use of alcohol may increase the liver's capacity to metabolize some drugs, whether or not alcohol is present at the same time, and the presence of some drugs reduces the rate of biotransformation of alcohol. For example, acute intoxication inhibits the metabolism of long-acting benzodiazepines, phenothiazines, tricyclic antidepressants and barbiturates. Long-term alcohol use increases the rate of metabolism of warfarin, diazepam and propranolol. Cimetidine and ranitidine inhibit gastric alcohol dehydrogenase, elevating blood alcohol levels.

---

6   Standard estimates of blood alcohol level are usually based on a man weighing 70 kg (154 lb.).

7   100 mL = 1 dL = 0.1 litres. Therefore, a blood alcohol level of 80 mg/100 mL may also be expressed as 0.08 g/dL or 0.08 per cent. Driving in Canada with a blood alcohol level in excess of this limit is an offence under the Criminal Code.

8   The amount of water in an individual's body is determined by the mass (weight) of the body and the proportion of the body that is water. Women typically have a smaller body mass, and a smaller proportion of water because of a higher fat-to-muscle ratio.

Effects of Short-Term Use: Low Doses[9]

Although alcohol is a CNS depressant, its usual early effects (after one to three drinks within approximately one hour) are heightened activity and disinhibition, resulting from depression of the inhibitory and behavioral control centres of the brain. This causes many drinkers to feel gregarious, expansive, jovial, relaxed and more self-confident, although some drinkers feel irritable, depressed or sleepy. Different individuals' emotional responses to alcohol vary widely, and can be greatly affected by the individual's mood before drinking and the drinking context.

Several perceptual and motor functions are impaired by low to moderate doses, including perception of distance and time, pain perception, reflex response and reaction time, and fine motor dexterity. Some people experience slurred speech and impairment of gross motor co-ordination. Observational studies have shown impaired driving performance at BALs as low as 30 mg/100 mL for infrequent drinkers.

Effects of Short-Term Use: Higher Doses[10]

Higher doses of alcohol produce exaggerated emotional responses, ranging from effusive conviviality to outright aggression. Thinking, memory, judgment, perception and motor function are highly impaired. Increasing doses cause drowsiness followed by stupor, coma and eventually death. A BAL of 500 mg/100 mL is considered lethal.

Adverse Effects of Short-Term Use

Blackouts

People who cannot remember some or all of the events that occurred during a bout of very heavy drinking are said to have experienced a "blackout." Individuals are

---

9   Alcohol differs from most other drugs of abuse in both its rate of administration and the rate at which it is metabolized. Unlike most other drugs administered orally, alcohol is typically consumed in very small "mini-doses" spread over a period of time (e.g., one might completely consume a serving of beer over a half-hour or so, although this time varies from drinker to drinker and setting to setting). Further, a standard dose (drink) of alcohol is completely metabolized in approximately one hour, a much shorter period than is required for the complete metabolism of many other psychoactive drugs. Therefore alcohol effects can best be described in relation to blood alcohol levels or both the dose and time over which the dose is consumed.

10   Generally more than two drinks for women and three drinks for men within one hour.

conscious during a blackout, but sometimes act in an uncharacteristic or even dangerous manner. Serious crimes have occurred during blackouts. Much more commonly, individuals wake up in a strange place unable to recall how they got there, or are informed of an argument or an embarrassing episode but cannot remember what happened.

Blackouts are frightening to many drinkers and sometimes lead them to seek help. Individuals being assessed for an alcohol problem should always be asked about blackouts, which are an early sign of a developing alcohol problem and may occur long before the individual develops tolerance or withdrawal.

Psychiatric Effects

Studies show that the mood changes produced by alcohol are different at different doses. As discussed above, moderate drinking (one to three drinks over the course of an hour) tends to cause relaxation and mild disinhibition, whereas heavy consumption (five drinks or more) is associated with three negative mood states: depression, anger or irritability, and over-sedation. These negative mood states, in combination with the impaired judgment, impulsiveness and reduced inhibition caused by intoxication, can lead to suicide or violence.

Drinking and Driving

Alcohol is a major cause of motor vehicle, work-related, household and recreational accidents. A recent Canadian survey found that 43 per cent of fatally injured drivers had alcohol in their blood, and 35 per cent were over the legal limit. The survey also found that one in five Canadian adults reports driving after drinking in the past month, with the highest proportion reported among males aged 25 to 45. The risk of a fatal motor vehicle accident occurring increases exponentially with increasing consumption. Compared with a driver with zero BAL, a driver with a BAL of 50 mg/100 mL (2.5 drinks in one hour for an "average" man) is twice as likely to be involved in a fatal motor vehicle accident. At 80 mg/100 mL (four drinks in one hour for a man), the risk quadruples.

Drivers should be reminded that their reaction time and judgment can be affected even if they "feel sober" after drinking. Even low levels of alcohol consumption are associated with slowed reaction time and decreased ability to handle complex driving situations. Teenage drivers who drink appear to have a greater risk of accidents than do older drivers who drink, perhaps because of driving inexperience, bravado and a lack of "behavioral tolerance" (see below).

Violence

Intentional violence against others is another consequence of intoxication. In a recent survey of violence experienced by Canadian women, the male involved in the violence had been drinking in more than 40 per cent of the episodes. Men who drank heavily (frequently consuming five or more drinks per occasion) were six times more likely to assault their wives than were men who did not drink. Assaults by men who were drinking were far more likely to cause physical injury than assaults by men who had not been drinking.

Other Physical Effects

Extremely heavy alcohol consumption can lead to respiratory depression, coma and death. Comatose drinkers can aspirate vomit into their lungs, causing severe pneumonia. Intoxication can also cause cardiac arrhythmias (irregularities of the heart rhythm).

Effects of Long-Term Use

CNS: Long-term, heavy alcohol use damages the axons (branches) of the neurons in the brain, resulting in fewer interconnections between neurons. This causes alcoholic dementia, the most important neurological complication of alcoholism. Dementia is a global decrease in cognitive functioning (brain functioning), which affects memory, judgment and abstract thinking. In contrast with Alzheimer's disease (the most common form of dementia in the elderly), alcoholic dementia is partially reversible in some cases. Repeated CAT (computerized axial tomography) scans over time have shown that the brains of alcoholics with dementia increase in size with prolonged periods of abstinence, suggesting that the axons partially regrow with time. Alcoholics in whom dementia is suspected should undergo neuropsychological testing to confirm or disprove the suspicion, and should be informed of the effects of alcohol on their cognitive functioning.

Alcohol increases the metabolism of vitamin B1 (thiamine). If an alcoholic does not eat a balanced diet with an adequate amount of thiamine, this can result in a serious condition known as Wernicke's encephalopathy, in which the individual becomes drowsy and confused, cannot walk properly and has abnormal eye movements. This is a medical emergency requiring an intravenous infusion of thiamine. If not treated appropriately, the individual may die or may develop Korsakoff's syndrome, a severe form of dementia characterized by almost total lack of short-term memory. Individuals with Korsakoff's are unable to remember events occurring just minutes earlier, although their long-term memory for events that occurred prior to developing Korsakoff's may be intact. This renders Korsakoff patients disoriented and incapable of understanding or interpreting their environment. Korsakoff patients frequently confabulate (make up stories about their lives) in order to make sense of what is happening to them. Their long-term prognosis is poor, and they often require institutionalization.

Alcohol also causes cerebellar degeneration. Individuals with this condition walk with a wide-based, staggering gait, as if they were intoxicated, even when they have not recently used alcohol.

Peripheral nervous system: Alcohol also damages the axons in the peripheral nervous system, resulting in peripheral neuropathy. Peripheral neuropathy is characterized by loss of feeling in the feet, sometimes accompanied by burning pain and difficulty in walking.

Cardiovascular: Alcohol elevates the blood pressure and interferes with clotting in the blood, putting hazardous drinkers[11] at an increased risk of hemorrhagic stroke (i.e., rupture and bleeding from a vessel that supplies blood to the brain). A small proportion of hazardous drinkers also develop cardiomyopathy (deterioration of the muscle fibres of the heart). Heavy drinkers are also at increased risk for cardiac arrhythmias and sudden death.

In contrast, middle-aged and older individuals who regularly consume small to moderate quantities of alcohol on a regular basis reduce their risk of coronary heart disease and ischemic stroke relative to abstainers.

Gastrointestinal: Alcohol irritates the lining of the stomach, causing inflammation and erosion, a condition called gastritis. Gastritis causes vomiting, decreased appetite and abdominal pain. Sometimes the irritation can damage the arteries underneath

---

11   Hazardous drinking has been defined as consumption of five or more standard drinks in any day, or three or more drinks on more than half the days of the week.

the stomach lining, resulting in internal bleeding. Gastritis can be fatal, but numerous effective medications are available for its treatment. Pancreatitis (inflammation of the pancreas) is an uncommon but serious complication of alcohol abuse, causing severe abdominal pain, vomiting and sometimes death.

Heavy drinking can also exacerbate ulcer symptoms, and can cause non-specific dyspepsia (upset stomach) and recurrent diarrhea.

Alcoholic liver disease, a major cause of morbidity and mortality in North America, occurs in three stages. In the first stage (fatty liver) liver cells accumulate fat, causing the liver to enlarge. Fatty liver is usually asymptomatic, and is reversible with abstinence from alcohol. In the next stage, alcoholic hepatitis, liver cells are damaged and the liver becomes inflamed. While a few individuals with alcoholic hepatitis develop severe or fatal liver failure, many individuals have no symptoms, and the condition is only detected through measurement of liver enzymes. With abstinence, hepatitis is reversible; the liver is one of the few organs in the body with the ability to grow new cells to replace damaged or dead cells.

Repeated or chronic alcoholic hepatitis leads to the final stage, cirrhosis. Cirrhosis of the liver is a major cause of illness and death in North America. In this stage, the liver's regenerative capacity has been overwhelmed by alcohol, and dead cells have been replaced by scar tissue. The portal vein, through which blood flows from the intestines to the liver, can be blocked by the scar tissue, causing blood to back up into veins in the esophagus. These veins then become engorged (esophageal varices) and sometimes burst, causing severe and frequently fatal internal hemorrhage. The blockage can also cause fluid to leak into the abdomen, giving the individual a swollen abdomen (ascites). People with severe cirrhosis have very little functioning liver left, and are prone to developing hepatic encephalopathy. In this condition, the liver is unable to metabolize dietary protein properly, and intermediate nitrogen-containing metabolites of protein build up in the bloodstream. Some of these metabolites are toxic to the brain, causing the individual to become drowsy and confused, and eventually to lapse into a coma and die.

The factors that put individuals at risk of developing cirrhosis are not completely understood. Women are more at risk than men, perhaps because they have higher blood alcohol levels than men after drinking the same amount of alcohol (see Absorption and Metabolism of Alcohol, above). Chronic viral hepatitis and cigarette smoking may also contribute to the development of cirrhosis.

Many people with cirrhosis have enough healthy liver tissue to function normally, but they should be advised that even small amounts of alcohol can contribute to the progression of their cirrhosis and that abstinence is the only safe course.

Cancer: Alcohol is a carcinogen that increases the risk of several cancers, including those of the esophagus, rectum, throat and breast.

Psychiatric: Alcoholics have a suicide rate six times that of the population average, and have a high rate of admission to psychiatric hospitals. Alcohol consumption contributes to psychiatric symptomatology in several ways: through direct pharmacological effects (as in depression), through adverse psychosocial consequences of drinking, and by interfering with treatment (non-compliance and missed appointments). Individuals with underlying psychiatric disorders, such as panic disorder, are more likely to abuse alcohol, relying on the sedative properties of alcohol to control their symptoms.

Like other sedative-hypnotics, alcohol can induce a depression that is very difficult to distinguish from a major affective disorder. Alcohol-induced depression resolves quickly with abstinence, usually in three to four weeks, although psychiatrists sometimes advise waiting up to two months of abstinence prior to initiating antidepressant therapy for patients who continue to be depressed.

Alcohol contributes to insomnia by suppressing REM sleep. Heavy drinkers commonly report that they feel poorly rested upon awakening.

Alcoholic hallucinosis is a syndrome that sometimes occurs in individuals with severe alcohol dependence. Hallucinations (usually auditory or tactile) may persist for months after the cessation of drinking.

Alcohol and Reproduction

Alcohol can cause impotence in men, both acutely (during a heavy drinking bout) and chronically (by suppressing testosterone production). Men with cirrhosis of the liver frequently exhibit a feminization syndrome, with testicular atrophy (reduction in the size of the testicles), loss of body hair and gynecomastia (growth of breasts).

Women who drink heavily may experience menstrual irregularities and infertility. Heavy alcohol consumption during pregnancy can cause fetal alcohol syndrome (FAS) in the child. FAS is characterized by behavioral abnormalities such as attention deficit disorder, developmental delays and mental retardation, growth deficiencies and facial abnormalities. These deficits persist into adulthood. FAS occurs in about one in 2,000 live births in North America. The risk of FAS is estimated to be 2.5 per cent in women who consume six drinks or more per day, particularly in the first trimester.

Children with fetal alcohol effects (FAE) have some but not all of the features of FAS. FAE is up to five times more common than FAS, and women who regularly consume two drinks or more per day during pregnancy are at risk. The effects of binge drinking (five drinks or more on a single occasion) on the fetus are unknown. Heavy drinking during pregnancy can also cause spontaneous abortion, low birth-weight and *abruptio placentae* (separation of the placenta from the uterus).

A safe level of alcohol consumption during pregnancy has not been established and abstinence is advised, although there is no evidence that the rare single drink during pregnancy causes adverse effects.

Low-Risk Drinking Guidelines

In Canada, low-risk drinking recommendations vary somewhat from country to country. The Royal College of Physicians and Surgeons recommends a maximum of two drinks per day for men, with one-third less for women, which translates into 14 drinks per week for men and 10 for women. In 1997, the Addiction Research Foundation and the Ontario Public Health Association recommended a maximum of two drinks per day, with weekly limits of 14 or fewer drinks for men and nine or fewer drinks for women. Lower levels are advocated for women because they reach a higher blood alcohol level than men for a given rate of alcohol consumption, and are more likely to develop alcohol-related liver disease.

A number of epidemiological studies have established that people who drink lightly or moderately have a lower mortality from coronary heart disease than do abstainers. Since coronary heart disease is by far the leading cause of mortality in the western world, moderate drinkers also have a lower total mortality than do abstainers.

Alcohol exerts its protective effect on the heart by inhibiting platelet aggregation (clumping), thereby lessening the risk of a heart attack, and by elevating blood levels of high-density lipoprotein (HDL), the form of cholesterol that protects against heart disease. Alcohol may also protect against ischemic stroke by the same mechanisms. Epidemiological studies suggest that the protective effect of alcohol may be achieved with as little as one drink every other day. The level of alcohol consumption that no longer protects against heart disease has not been established, but it may well be substantially higher than 12 to 14 drinks per week.

The beneficial effects of moderate drinking apply mainly to middle-aged men and women. In young people, alcohol consumption is associated with an increased total mortality due to accidents, violence and suicide. In women, several epidemiological studies have found that moderate drinking is associated with a slightly increased risk of breast cancer, although the mechanism for this is uncertain and further research is needed before the association can be confirmed.

Low-risk drinking recommendations usually advise that people who drink moderately, with no adverse effects, may continue to do so if they wish. Those who do not currently drink should not begin to do so just because of the cardioprotective effects of alcohol, especially because other lifestyle options, such as exercise and a low-fat diet, may be as cardioprotective as alcohol and far safer overall.

In certain situations, abstinence is advised for adults: during pregnancy, when taking medications that could interact negatively with alcohol, before driving or operating machinery, in the presence of medical conditions such as liver disease, which could be made worse by alcohol, and when previous attempts to moderate alcohol consumption have been unsuccessful.

Patterns of Use and Their Public Health Significance

Studies indicate a high prevalence of hazardous or problem drinking in the Canadian population. In a national survey conducted in 1994, 5.4 per cent of Canadian adults (9.1 per cent of men and 1.9 per cent of women) reported drinking once a week or more and usually consuming five or more drinks (i.e., frequent, heavy drinkers). In the same study, 3.3 per cent reported drinking less often than once a week, but usually five or more drinks on a drinking occasion (i.e., infrequent, heavy drinkers). Further, the survey found that hazardous drinking is most prevalent in men aged 24 and under.

A 1997 student survey found that 59.6 per cent of students in Grades 7 through 13[12] had used alcohol in the preceding 12 months. The study also found that 40.5 per cent of those who drank had consumed five or more drinks on a single occasion during the preceding four weeks, compared with 34.9 per cent in a similar 1995 survey.

---

12   Ontario's traditional Grade 13 has now been replaced by an Ontario Academic Credit (OAC) year in most Ontario schools. However, to facilitate comparison with surveys from previous years, the Ontario Survey and thus this text continue to use the term "Grade 13."

Alcohol consumption causes more harm to society than all illicit drug use combined. Tobacco is the only drug that causes greater illness and death. In Canada, almost 3,000 deaths were directly attributable to alcohol in 1988, while 14,000 deaths were indirectly attributable to drinking. In Ontario in 1990, alcohol was estimated to have cost $5.8 billion in health care, social assistance, law enforcement and lost productivity.

Despite the high social costs of alcohol, there is room for optimism. Alcohol consumption has declined by about one-third in the past decade, due in part to the aging of the population and a shift in society's attitudes. Intoxication is less socially acceptable, and there is a greater emphasis on healthy lifestyles.

Screening and Early Detection of Alcohol Problems

Given the prevalence of alcohol problems among the general population, health care professionals detect alcohol-related problems relatively infrequently, particularly among the elderly and women. In a health care setting, alcohol problems can be detected through the use of simple screening questionnaires such as the CAGE or the "problem" question. The CAGE is a mnemonic consisting of four questions:

C: Have you ever tried to CUT DOWN on your drinking?
A: Have you ever been ANNOYED by others telling you to cut down?
G: Have you ever felt GUILTY about your drinking?
E: Have you ever needed an EYE-OPENER in the morning?

Two out of four positive responses suggests a current or past alcohol problem. The CAGE has a sensitivity of 75 per cent in a general medical practice setting.

An even simpler alternative to the CAGE is to ask, "Have you ever felt you had a problem with alcohol?" Further research is needed to validate this question as a screening instrument. Laboratory measures such as the Gamma Glutamyl Transferase (GGT) and Mean Cell Volume (MCV) tests can provide additional evidence of an alcohol problem, and they can be useful in monitoring and counselling.

Heavy drinkers commonly seek health care for one or more of the following problems: trauma, hypertension (high blood pressure), gastrointestinal complaints such as gastritis and dyspepsia, and a full range of psychosocial and psychiatric problems.

Problem Drinking

Alcohol problems are thought to lie along a spectrum of severity, ranging from mild alcohol problems to severe alcohol dependence. There is no evidence that mild problems inevitably progress to alcohol dependence. On the contrary, many heavy drinkers moderate their alcohol use as they get older.

A "problem drinker" may be defined as someone who drinks above the safe limit, and may have one or more alcohol-related problems as a result, but who does not yet meet the criteria for alcohol dependence. Problem drinkers outnumber individuals with alcohol dependence by a ratio of at least four to one. Because of their larger numbers, members of this group account for most alcohol-related morbidity and mortality. For example, a recent study of individuals who had a motor vehicle accident after drinking and driving found that most were heavy weekend drinkers, but were not alcohol-dependent.

Problem drinkers often respond to brief advice and reduced drinking strategies, and may not require the intensive, abstinence-oriented treatment used to treat alcohol-dependent individuals.

Dependence, Tolerance and Withdrawal

Alcohol Dependence

Alcohol dependence is a clinical syndrome that may affect up to one to two per cent of the population. According to the *Diagnostic and Statistical Manual of Mental Disorders* (DSM-IV) published by the American Psychiatric Association, alcohol dependence is characterized by three or more of the following features occurring at any time in the same 12-month period:

- tolerance

- withdrawal

- consumption of alcohol in larger amounts or over a longer period than was intended: some alcohol-dependent individuals exhibit chronic, heavy daily drinking while others engage in "binge" drinking, in which drinking bouts lasting days or weeks alternate with periods of abstinence.

- a persistent desire or unsuccessful efforts to cut down or control use

- considerable time spent drinking, recovering from drinking and planning drinking opportunities

- "Important social, occupational, or recreational activities are given up or reduced because of alcohol use"; for example, individuals are frequently absent from school or work, and often neglect family responsibilities.

- Continued drinking "despite knowledge of a persistent or recurrent physical or psychological problem that is likely to have been caused or exacerbated [by alcohol]."

Physical Dependence

Physical dependence on alcohol is indicated by evidence of tolerance (reduced response to the intoxicating effects of alcohol) and/or withdrawal caused by abstaining from alcohol. Both components may contribute to continuation of excessive drinking. People who drink daily to achieve a "high" often need to drink larger and larger amounts to overcome their increasing tolerance to alcohol, leading to an escalation of drinking and alcohol-related problems. Those who have experienced withdrawal sometimes drink to prevent or relieve withdrawal symptoms. This commonly occurs in the morning, and is known as "relief drinking" or an "eye-opener." Tolerance and withdrawal are discussed below.

Tolerance

Three forms of tolerance to alcohol have been identified. "Behavioral tolerance" refers to experienced drinkers' learned ability to compensate for the intoxicating effects of alcohol by speaking and acting as if they were sober. "Metabolic tolerance" refers to the fact that chronically heavy drinkers metabolize alcohol more quickly than non-drinkers. "Neurological tolerance" is a neurological adaptation to regular alcohol use in which the nervous system "speeds itself up" to counteract the chronic sedative effects of alcohol. The neurological adaptation to alcohol is a more important factor in the development of tolerance than the increased metabolic rate.

Tolerance is a function of the amount of alcohol consumed and the duration of drinking. It can develop quickly (within a few days of heavy drinking) and it decreases with abstinence. Individuals vary greatly in their tolerance to alcohol. Cross-tolerance occurs between alcohol and other sedative/hypnotics and anxiolytics. As a result, heavy drinkers often show less response than abstainers or light drinkers to the effects of benzodiazepines and barbiturates even if they have not been previously exposed to these drugs.

A simple screening question to determine whether individuals are tolerant is to ask them how they feel after five drinks. If they reply that they still feel sober, they have likely developed tolerance.

Withdrawal

When drinking is abruptly stopped, the physically dependent drinker can experience alcohol withdrawal, a syndrome characterized by excessive activity of the autonomic nervous system (which may be indicated by sweating or racing pulse), tremors, insomnia, nausea or vomiting, hallucinations or illusions, agitation and anxiety. Withdrawal can begin within a few hours after the last drink (as the blood alcohol level declines) and may last from two to seven days, and interfere with usual life functioning.

Tonic-clonic (grand mal) seizures are the most common complication of alcohol withdrawal. They usually occur in the first 12 to 48 hours after the last drink, but later seizures have been reported. Other complications of withdrawal include cardiac arrhythmias, severe hypertension and hallucinations.

Delirium tremens ("DTs") is a late complication (occurring after six or more days) of untreated alcohol withdrawal. It is not common, but is extremely serious. Delirium tremens is characterized by confusion and disorientation, fluctuating levels of consciousness, fever, bizarre and frightening hallucinations, rapid pulse and high blood pressure. Death can occur from cardiovascular collapse.

Withdrawal can be effectively treated in the emergency room or a doctor's office with diazepam, a long-acting benzodiazepine. A "loading technique" is preferred, in which 20 mg of diazepam is given orally every hour until symptoms abate. Because of the long half-life of diazepam, take-home doses are not needed.

Causes of Alcohol Dependence

A number of factors can contribute to the development of alcohol dependence. Identical-twin and other studies suggest that genetics play a role, but it is not certain how a genetic predisposition translates into an increased risk. It has been suggested that a high genetic tolerance to the intoxicating effects of alcohol places individuals at greater risk for developing alcohol dependence. Males whose fathers were alcohol-dependent are at risk for developing severe dependence at an early age.

Social and cultural factors play a greater role than genetics in determining the risk of alcohol dependence. Cultures in which drunkenness is accepted behavior or in which daily consumption of alcohol with meals is the norm have higher rates of alcohol dependence and alcohol-related medical complications. Occupations in which alcohol consumption is tolerated or expected also place people at risk, as do social factors such as unemployment. Childhood sexual and physical abuse are increasingly being recognized as important etiological factors.

No single "addictive personality" has been identified, but the interaction of personality with environment certainly influences the development of alcohol dependence.

Prognosis and Treatment

The prognosis for alcohol dependence is not good. One year after treatment, only about 20 per cent of individuals remain abstinent. Higher social class, strong social supports, young age and relatively recent onset of heavy drinking are factors that are associated with successful treatment. Heavy drinkers who are polydrug abusers or have co-existing psychiatric problems are less likely to be successful in alcohol treatment.

No single treatment approach is appropriate for all individuals, and the treatment plan should be matched to the needs of the individual. Treatment consists of inpatient or outpatient alcohol rehabilitation programs, which may include a combination of group therapy, individual counselling and health education. There is no evidence that inpatient programs are more effective than outpatient programs. "Self-help" or mutual-help groups such as Alcoholics Anonymous, Women for Sobriety and Rational Recovery have not been extensively evaluated, but many members attribute their lasting sobriety to these groups. Anti-alcohol drugs such as disulfiram and naltrexone are not effective as sole agents for treating alcohol dependence, but they may be useful as supplements for selected cases. (For additional information on disulfiram and naltrexone, please refer to the individual chapters in Section 3.)

Potential for Abuse

Dependence Liability
Alcohol can rapidly produce a state of pleasurable intoxication and is highly effective in reducing tension. For these reasons, it is considered to have a moderate dependence liability, probably comparable to those of benzodiazepines or barbiturates.

Availability
The easy availability of alcoholic beverages also contributes to alcohol's abuse potential.

Background Reading

Addiction Research Foundation. (1997). *Alcohol and your health: Low-risk drinking guidelines*. Toronto: Addiction Research Foundation.

Adlaf, E., Ivis, F.J. & Smart, R.G. (1997). *Ontario Student Drug Use Survey, 1977-1997*. Toronto: Addiction Research Foundation.

American Psychiatric Association. (1994). *Diagnostic and Statistical Manual of Mental Disorders, DSM-IV* (4th edition). Washington: American Psychiatric Association.

Ashley, M.J., Ferrence, R., Room, R., Bondy, S., Rehm, J. & Single, E. (1997). Moderate drinking and health. Implications of recent evidence. *Canadian Family Physician, 43*, 687–694.

MacNeil, P. & Webster, I. (Eds.) (1997). *Canada's Alcohol and Other Drugs Survey 1994: A Discussion of the Findings*. Ottawa: Health Canada. Cat. No. H39-338/1-1994E.

O'Brien, C.P. (1996). Drug addiction and drug abuse (Chapter 24), in Hardman, J.G., Limbird, L.E., Molinoff, P.B., Rudden, R.W., & Gilman, A.G. (Eds.), *Goodman and Gilman's The Pharmacological Basis of Therapeutics*, (9th edition). New York/Toronto: McGraw-Hill Health Professions Division.

Single, E., Williams, B. & McKenzie, D. (1994). *Canadian Profile: Alcohol, Tobacco and Other Drugs, 1994*. Toronto: Canadian Centre on Substance Abuse/Addiction Research Foundation of Ontario.

Statistics Canada. (1993). *The Violence Against Women Survey*. Ottawa: Statistics Canada. Reported in *The Daily*. Ottawa: Statistics Canada, November 18, 1993.

Fentanyl

DRUG CLASS: Opioid

Synopsis

Fentanyl, a wholly synthetic opioid, is marketed under the trade names of Sublimaze® (injectable) and Duragesic® (transdermal patch). It is one of the most potent opioids in medical use today, and acts as an agonist at μ (mu) receptors. (Sufentanil®, an analogue of fentanyl, is even more potent — see Section 5.) Compared with morphine, fentanyl is about 80 to 100 times more potent as an analgesic. Fentanyl produces a profile of effects similar to other opioids, but appears less likely to cause vomiting than most opioids.

When injected intravenously, fentanyl acts almost immediately, although the duration of its analgesic activity is brief (30 to 60 minutes after a single dose of up to 100 mcg). When injected intramuscularly, the onset of analgesic action is more gradual (typically seven to eight minutes), and the duration of action is longer (up to two hours). Fentanyl is used by injection primarily as an analgesic during surgery. It may also be used pre- and post-surgically for control of pain, either by injection or, in the United States, by a lozenge, for delivery of the drug through the membranes of the mouth (i.e., transmucosally).

Fentanyl is also marketed in the form of a transdermal delivery system (i.e., a specially designed "patch" with an adhesive layer), which is applied to the skin to provide continuous delivery of fentanyl to the blood through the skin for up to 72 hours. These transdermal systems are available at various dose levels, with the higher doses, being contained in "patches" of larger surface area. This transdermal route of application is used primarily for management of pain in chronic cancer patients requiring continuous opioid analgesia.

Reports of fentanyl abuse have involved both individuals who used street opioids and health care personnel who had access to the drug in the course of their work. Deaths have been reported in opioid abusers who dissolved the contents of a (used and discarded) fentanyl patch and injected the liquid, or heated the contents of a patch and inhaled the fentanyl.

Drug Source

Fentanyl is produced through chemical synthesis by the pharmaceutical industry.

Trade Names

Sublimaze® (fentanyl citrate, injection); Duragesic® (transdermal patches); Fentanyl Oralet®[1] (buccal lozenge).

Street Names

None.

Combination Products

Innovar® (fentanyl citrate 50 mcg and droperidol 2.5 mg).

Medical Uses

Medical uses of fentanyl include providing short-duration pain relief during anesthesia as a pre-surgical medication, inducing anesthesia and managing pain in chronic cancer patients requiring continuous opioid analgesia.

---

[1]   Available in the United States.

Physical Appearance

Fentanyl citrate in pure form occurs as a white crystalline powder, soluble in water and slightly soluble in alcohol. The transdermal delivery system is composed of a protective layer, together with four functional layers: a backing layer, a gel layer of fentanyl, a membrane layer that controls the rate of drug release and an adhesive layer.

Dosage[2]

Medical

Dose levels are individualized, based on the patient's age, body weight, physical status, health problem and the type of anesthetic and surgical procedure. Typical doses include:

- pre-surgically: 50 to 100 mcg intramuscularly or up to 5 mcg per kilogram of body weight to a maximum of 400 mcg in buccal (transmucosal) lozenge form may be administered

- adjunct to anesthesia (total dose over the course of the surgical procedure): 2 to 50 mcg per kilogram of body weight

- post-operative pain management: 100 mcg epidurally.

- as an anesthetic: 50 to150 mcg per kilogram of body weight.

- control of chronic severe pain: transdermal delivery systems are designed to deliver fentanyl at a rate of 25 to 100 mcg per hour (i.e., 25 mcg per hour per 10 cm^2 surface).

Non-medical

- estimated at up to 1 mg.

---

[2]   All doses refer to adults.

Routes of Administration

By intravenous, intramuscular or epidural injection, or by transdermal patch to be worn for a 72-hour period.

Effects of Short-Term Use: Low Doses[3]

At low doses, fentanyl produces a spectrum of short-term effects (including euphoria) similar to those of other opioid analgesics. However, muscle rigidity (especially that of muscles involving respiration) and significant respiratory depression sometimes occur even at low levels. Muscle rigidity is most likely when fentanyl is rapidly injected via the intravenous route. Respiratory depression may last well beyond the period of analgesic activity; it also represents the principal danger upon overdose.

Minimum effective analgesic serum concentrations of fentanyl in opioid-naive individuals range from 0.2 to 2.0 ng/mL. Side effects increase in frequency at serum levels above 2 ng/mL.

CNS, *behavioral, subjective:* relief from and reduced emotional response to severe pain,[4] variously euphoria or anxiety, depression, drowsiness, confusion, dizziness, weakness, pupillary constriction, which may impair night vision, suppression of cough reflex.

Cardiovascular: reduction in blood pressure and possibly fainting on arising.

Gastrointestinal: nausea and vomiting (though less than other opioids), constipation.

Respiratory: dose-related slowing of breathing, constriction of bronchi and impairment of ventilation as a result of chest muscle rigidity (paralysis); the respiratory depressant effect persists longer than the analgesic effect; risk of respiratory depression is higher than for other opioids.

Other: sweating.

---

3   Single doses within the therapeutic range administered orally or by injection to non-tolerant persons. Symptoms tend to be similar to many of those produced by opioid analgesics.

4   A 100 mcg dose of fentanyl has an analgesic potency approximately equal to 10 mg morphine or 75 mg meperidine.

Effects of Short-Term Use: Higher Doses[5]

Intensification of fentanyl's low-dose effects may occur with administration of higher doses. These effects may include loss of consciousness and cessation of breathing (which can be treated by intravenous injection of naloxone, an opioid antagonist). The risk of respiratory depression and chest muscle paralysis increases as the dose is increased. At high doses, blood pressure is likely to be markedly increased, and heart rate may be increased.

Effects of Long-Term Use

When patients previously treated with other opioids are converted to fentanyl administered through transdermal delivery systems, the initial dose level of fentanyl should be conservative, supplementary analgesic provided as needed, and the dose reviewed and possibly increased after six days (i.e., two dosing periods).

Tolerance to the analgesic effect of fentanyl develops with long-term use. Individuals who are tolerant to fentanyl will also be cross-tolerant to other opioids. If patients are withdrawn from fentanyl, the dose should be gradually reduced to avoid withdrawal symptoms.

Lethality

Deaths from fentanyl overdose usually result from inadequate oxygen supply associated with the respiratory depressant effects of the drug, combined with paralysis of the chest muscles. Blood concentrations in a few fatalities have ranged from 2.7 to 15 ng/L. Because of the extremely rapid onset of respiratory paralysis after intravenous administration of high doses, some users have been found dead with the needle still present in their arm.

---

[5]   Single doses in excess of the therapeutic range (or lower doses in particularly sensitive individuals) administered by injection or inhalation from heated transdermal patch.

Tolerance and Dependence

With long-term use of fentanyl, tolerance to the euphoric effect and the slowing of respiration develops; however, episodes of slowed respiration may occur at any time. Both the minimum effective analgesic serum concentration and the concentration at which toxicity occurs increase with increasing tolerance. The rate of development of tolerance varies widely among individuals. In one reported case, the serum level of fentanyl in a chronic user reached 21 ng/mL with nausea and muscle stiffness, but without compromised cardiac or respiratory function.

Fentanyl produces physical and psychological dependence similar to morphine, but dependence rarely develops in patients being treated for control of severe chronic pain.

Patterns of Use

Reports of fentanyl abuse have involved both individuals who used street opioids and health care personnel who had access to the drug in the course of their anesthesia-related work. Deaths have been reported in opioid abusers who dissolved the contents of a (used and discarded) fentanyl patch and injected the liquid, or heated the contents of a patch and inhaled the fentanyl.

Potential for Abuse

Dependence Liability
The dependence liability of fentanyl appears to be as great as that of heroin. The effects are similar to those of morphine, but the extremely rapid onset of action after intravenous administration increases fentanyl's dependence liability.

Inherent Harmfulness
Fentanyl shares the harmfulness of morphine and heroin, but presents a higher risk of breathing cessation, as a function of its respiratory depressant effects and paralysis of chest muscles.

Availability

Legally produced fentanyl is controlled in the same manner as morphine, and in its injectable form is available mainly in health facilities that provide anesthesia. Its availability, therefore, is largely restricted to health care personnel, except when such supplies are stolen and diverted to the illicit market. However, fentanyl is also produced in illicit laboratories for street distribution.

The increasing use of the transdermal delivery system has given rise to abuse of discarded used "patches" that still contain a substantial reservoir of fentanyl. In response to this abuse, health care facilities have developed strict policies and procedures for disposal of used "patches."

Background Reading

Berens, A.I.L., Voets, A.J. & Demedts, P. (1996). Illicit fentanyl in Europe. *The Lancet, 347* (May 11), 1134–35.

Canadian Pharmaceutical Association. (1997). *Compendium of Pharmaceuticals and Specialties.* (32nd edition). Ottawa: Canadian Pharmaceutical Association.

DeSio, J.M., Bacon, D.R. & Lema, M.J. (1993). Intravenous abuse of transdermal fentanyl therapy in a chronic pain patient. *Anesthesiology, 79,* 1139–1141.

Jeal, W. & Benfield, P. (1997). Transdermal fentanyl. A review of its pharmacological properties and therapeutic efficacy in pain control. *Drugs, 53 (1),* 109–138.

Marquardt, K.A. & Tharratt, R.S. (1994). Inhalation abuse of fentanyl patch. *Clinical Toxicology, 32 (1),* 75–78.

McEvoy, G. (1997). *American Hospital Formulary Service (AHFS) Drug Information.* (pp. 1565–1569), Bethesda, MD: American Society of Health-System Pharmacists.

Reisine, T. & Pasternak, G. (1996). Opioid analgesics and antagonists. (Chapter 23). In J.G. Hardman, L.E. Limbird, P.B. Molinoff, R.W. Rudden & A.G. Gilman (Eds.), *Goodman and Gilman's The Pharmacological Basis of Therapeutics* (9th edition). New York/Toronto: McGraw-Hill Health Professions Division.

Heroin

DRUG CLASS: Opioid

Synopsis

Heroin (also called diamorphine and diacetylmorphine) is a powerful semi-synthetic opioid produced by chemical modification of morphine. Because of its powerful euphoric and analgesic effects, heroin has the greatest potential for producing dependence of any of the common opioids. Although the drug can be administered by several routes — injection, sniffing, smoking or swallowing — North American heroin-dependent users prefer to inject it intravenously ("mainlining"). This method results in more immediate and more intense effects than administration by any other route. However, many individuals who are not accustomed to intravenous drug use or to heroin prefer to use this drug for the first few times by inhaling it through the nose ("snorting"), injecting it just under the skin ("skin popping") or smoking it ("chasing the dragon," — heating the heroin until a vapor is given off, then "chasing" the smoky tail of the liquid with a tube and inhaling it, so that it is absorbed through the lungs). In many instances, these early experiences are unpleasant: nausea and vomiting are quite common. Gradually the desired effects are more fully appreciated as the user develops tolerance to these adverse effects. Tolerance, however, to the desired effects such as euphoria, tranquillity and analgesia can also develop rapidly. To compensate for the developing tolerance, users typically increase their daily dose, and/or change to another route of administration such as intravenous injection, so that more drug is made available to the brain more rapidly. Both types of change increase the user's risk of dependence.

Although severely distressing, the withdrawal sickness that users experience after abruptly terminating heroin use is rarely fatal. In many respects, it resembles a case of moderately severe flu, and most observable symptoms disappear within seven to 10 days.

The principal cause of death from heroin overdose is respiratory arrest as a result of severe depression (slowing of the functions) of the brain centres that control breathing.

Drug Source

Heroin is produced in the laboratory by reacting the naturally occurring opioid morphine with acetic anhydride.

In the United Kingdom, heroin is produced commercially for pain management and for carefully monitored maintenance programs for individuals who are heroin-dependent. Supplies of heroin required for medical use in Canada are imported from the United Kingdom. In North America, heroin may be produced under special licence in very small quantities for research purposes.

Street heroin is produced in illicit laboratories in many parts of the world.

Generic Names

Diamorphine, diacetylmorphine.

Trade Names

Not applicable.

Street Names

Dust, "H," horse, junk, smack, scag, black tar.

Drug Combinations

Heroin is sometimes encountered on the illicit market in combination with amphetamines (bombitas) or with cocaine (dynamite, speedball, whizbang).

Medical Uses

Until early in this century, heroin was widely employed in North America as a powerful analgesic. However, in Canada and the United States, heroin's high dependence liability and the increasing availability of synthetic opioid alternatives led to its replacement by other opioids in medical practice, and to changes in federal regulation to effectively prohibit its manufacture and importation. In contrast, physicians in the United Kingdom continued to use heroin in maintenance treatment programs for opioid-dependent patients.

In the mid-1980s some Canadian physicians and members of the public campaigned actively to have heroin made available by a physician's prescription for control of intense pain, especially for patients with terminal cancer. As a result, Canadian drug regulations were changed to permit authorized importation, and arrangements were made to obtain supplies from a U.K. manufacturer. However, current levels of legitimate medical use are extremely low — much lower than anticipated during the campaign to "reintroduce" heroin for the control of pain. Meanwhile, the U.S. ban on heroin use for medicinal purposes continues.

Although heroin is more potent than morphine, this greater potency refers only to the quantity of drug needed to control pain. It does not mean that heroin is a more effective analgesic agent. Double-blind studies of pain management have shown that heroin possesses no real advantage over morphine (to which it is rapidly converted in the body). However, heroin is somewhat more soluble. It has been argued, therefore, that heroin is easier to administer (by injection) to the severely ill, emaciated patient.

Physical Appearance

In pure form, heroin is a fine, white, bitter-tasting crystalline powder that is soluble in water. It is usually diluted for sale on the illicit market with a variety of non-opioid substances such as milk, sugar, dextrose or quinine. Heroin from certain parts of Asia and Mexico is brown in color because of the impurities present.

Dosage

Medical

When administered by intramuscular injection, 5 to 8 mg of heroin produces the same analgesic effect as 10 mg of morphine.

Non-medical

Inexperienced users may be introduced to the drug at dosages of 2 to 3 mg or less. In contrast, some dependent users, who have developed a high degree of tolerance to the drug, claim to take as much as 200 to 300 mg per day.

Variable Quality of Street Heroin

Many heroin-dependent persons do not use as much of the drug as they believe, because they over-estimate the concentration of heroin in their purchased product. In the 1960s, reports indicated that samples of street heroin from major U.S. centres on the Eastern seaboard often contained as little as three per cent heroin, while street samples from major Canadian centres typically had a higher concentration, often 10 to 20 per cent. However, since that time the concentration in products obtained by individual users has increased considerably. In some cases, individual users have been able to secure product containing more than 90 per cent heroin. The remainder of the product may include impurities and diluents; the most common diluents are sugars such as lactose and dextrose, substances such as quinine, which are added to contribute to a bitter taste suggestive of a high-potency product, and sometimes talc, which is insoluble in water and can give rise to problems at the site of injection and in the lungs. The street heroin-dependent user, having no way to reliably estimate the amount of heroin in a bag when making a purchase, is vulnerable to being cheated ("burned").

Reports from low-income chronic heroin users suggest that the amount of drug they take from day to day varies considerably, depending on how much money they have available to buy the drug. On some days they may use very low doses or none at all. As a result, some low-income users who develop psychological dependence may not develop a high degree of physical dependence because their use, although chronic, has been at relatively low dose levels.

Routes of Administration

Most commonly, the heroin powder is dissolved in water and injected, either subcutaneously, intramuscularly or intravenously. Experienced users generally prefer the intravenous route ("mainlining"), as it produces the most rapid and intense response to the drug.[1] Occasionally heroin is sniffed or taken orally,[2] although oral consumption is not the route of choice for dependent users, since immediately after heroin is absorbed from the small intestine, it must pass through the liver, where much of it is destroyed and thus wasted. Smoking of heroin was reported to be very common among military personnel engaged in the Vietnam War, since the drug was relatively freely available and inexpensive by western standards. It may be added to regular cigarettes or marijuana. When smoked, its effects are more potent than those of smoked opium.

Effects of Short-Term Use: Low Doses[3]

CNS, *behavioral, subjective:* Effects of heroin use include suppression of the sensation of pain, euphoria, mental clouding, heightened feelings of well-being, relaxation and drowsiness in some, and in others talkativeness and activity. After administration users experience a drowsy, dreamy, mild dozing state referred to as a "nod" (owing to the characteristic lolling of the head). Often users also experience decreased physical activity, inability to concentrate, apathy, pupillary constriction, droopy eyelids, reduced visual acuity and impaired night vision. Inexperienced users may react with giddiness and dizziness or fearfulness and anxiety. Often users must administer the drug several times, usually with the encouragement of peers, before they experience the desired effects fully.

---

[1]   Heroin produces a more intense "rush" than the same intravenous dose of morphine, apparently because the greater fat solubility of heroin enables it to penetrate the brain more rapidly than morphine. Once in the brain, heroin is rapidly metabolized to monoacetyl morphine and subsequently to morphine; this conversion is necessary for it to produce its effects. (For further discussion of the significance of solubility, see the discussion on absorption in Section 1.)

[2]   When taken orally, heroin may be put into bread, empty capsules or even small twists of tissue paper to mask its bitter taste.

[3]   Single doses of 3 to 4 mg, taken by injection in non-tolerant users.

Respiratory: slowing of the respiratory rate, which becomes more pronounced at higher doses.

Gastrointestinal: nausea and vomiting (very common among inexperienced users), reduced appetite, deceased gastric motility and constipation.

Other: reduced libido, itching or burning sensation on the skin, increased urinary output, slightly lowered body temperature, sweating.

Effects of Short-Term Use: Higher Doses[4]

Intensification of heroin's low-dose effects typically occurs with administration of higher doses. The duration of effects also increases with higher dosage. As the dose increases, the user's sensitivity and emotional response to painful stimuli decrease, the ability to concentrate is increasingly impaired, the probability of sleep increases, breathing becomes progressively slower and more shallow, heart rate gradually slows and blood pressure decreases.

The most desired effect is referred to as a "rush." It occurs almost immediately following intravenous injection, and the subjective experience has been described as akin to an intense orgasmic sensation in the abdomen.

In very high doses (i.e., overdose), heroin can produce deep sleep that may progress to stupor or coma, low blood pressure, slow and irregular heart rate, cyanosis, shallow and marked depression of respiration, low body temperature, flaccid skeletal muscles, cold and clammy skin, and pinpoint pupils.

Effects of Long-Term Use

When heroin- or morphine-dependent users have been provided with daily maintenance doses of heroin under medical supervision, marked physiological deterioration or significant psychological impairment has not been observed. In fact, most of the

---

4   Single doses of 10 to 25 mg or higher by injection in non-tolerant users, or lower doses in particularly sensitive individuals.

serious adverse consequences of chronic heroin use seem to be related to lifestyle and factors related to needle administration. The adverse consequences that are directly related to long-term heroin use itself are similar to those produced by other opioids: mood instability due to the relatively short duration of action of the drug, reduced libido, constipation, pupillary constriction (which adversely affects night vision), menstrual irregularity and certain types of respiratory impairment.

Heroin and Pregnancy

Pregnant heroin-dependent women have a high infant-mortality rate, due primarily to high rates of prematurity and low birth weight. Low birth weight has been attributed to the direct effects of heroin on the fetus, as well as to poor nutrition, smoking and inadequate prenatal care. Opioid withdrawal can trigger uterine contractions, which may lead to spontaneous abortion in the first trimester and premature labor in the third trimester.

Infants born to physically dependent heroin users sometimes go into withdrawal. Neonatal withdrawal is characterized by poor feeding, irritability, sweating, tremors, vomiting and diarrhea. Seizures and death have been reported with severe, untreated withdrawal. Withdrawal usually begins shortly after birth and generally within 24 hours, and may last up to several weeks. Treatment consists of supportive care in a neonatal unit, and administration of phenobarbital, morphine or paregoric.

Lifestyle and Chronic Needle Use

Infections at injection sites and collapsed veins resulting from repeated injections are very common. Tetanus, viral hepatitis (which is a common cause of regular heroin users' admission to hospital medical services), acquired immune deficiency syndrome (AIDS), endocarditis,[5] pneumonia and other pulmonary complications including tuberculosis all occur more frequently among heroin addicts than in the general population. Although there is no evidence of permanent CNS impairment specifically due to chronic heroin use, diminished oxygen intake resulting from a large overdose may result in brain damage. Malnutrition, poor housing, untreated illness and frequent use of and physical dependence on other psychoactive drugs, together with heroin dependence, are likely to result in a generally poor state of health and lowered resistance to disease.

---

5   Infection of the membrane lining of the interior of the heart.

Lethality

Severe overdose, usually self-administered and unintentional, results in very slow, shallow and irregular respiration, flushing, pinpoint pupils, cyanosis, markedly decreased blood pressure and coma. Administration of an opioid antagonist[6] that can reverse the acute effects of overdose of heroin (or other opioids) is an essential part of emergency treatment under these conditions. Death, when it occurs, usually results from respiratory arrest or other respiratory or cardiovascular complications.

Death from Other Causes

Although heroin overdose is the most frequently reported cause of death among dependent users, many deaths can also be linked to a heroin-centred lifestyle. In one study of causes of death among 1,400 addicts, it was estimated that up to 40 per cent might have been caused by violence, often murder. The rates of suicide and death from infectious diseases, including AIDS and viral hepatitis, among heroin users are considerably higher than among the general population.

Tolerance and Dependence

Tolerance

Most intravenous users of heroin who use the drug frequently and at substantial dose levels rapidly develop a high degree of tolerance to most of the drug's effects. However, such tolerance is less likely to develop with infrequent or intermittent use at lower doses and with administration by other routes (see "chipping" below). As tolerance develops, increasingly higher doses are required to produce satisfactory analgesic, sedative and euphoric effects. Tolerance also develops to heroin's respiratory-depressant and nauseating effects. However, tolerance has not been reported to develop to the pupillary-constricting or constipating effects.

As tolerance develops with chronic use and the user gradually increases the dose to achieve the desired effects, a dose plateau is reached where no amount of the drug is sufficient to produce the intensity of effects desired. When this level is achieved, dependent users continue to administer the drug, but now largely for the purpose of delaying withdrawal sickness, which typically commences six to 12 hours after the last dose.

---

6   See the chapter on naloxone in Section 3.

Some chronic, highly tolerant users claim that they continue to experience a mild rush immediately after intravenous injection. It is difficult to determine whether this is linked to the user's expectations or is an actual drug effect.

Users may attempt to reduce the cost of their habit by deliberately undergoing withdrawal (medically supervised or otherwise) and then abstaining from all opioids for a few weeks. Abstaining reduces the user's drug tolerance level, so that they can once again afford the (now-lower) doses needed to produce the desired effects. However, tolerance is quickly regained once users resume regular heroin use.

Physical Dependence/Withdrawal

Powerful physical and psychological dependence can also develop very rapidly for the regular high-dose user. The severity of withdrawal sickness, which follows abrupt cessation of use, is related to several factors: how long the person has regularly used the drug and at what dosage, the user's general health and the conditions under which withdrawal occurs.

Early symptoms: With onset typically occurring six to 12 hours after the last dose, symptoms include watering eyes, "runny nose," yawning and sweating. This stage is characteristically followed by a phase sometimes referred to as the "yen," which is an agitated sleep that may last for several hours. Upon wakening, agitation continues, accompanied by depression, loss of appetite, goose-flesh, dilated pupils and tremors.

Peak intensity: Peak symptom intensity usually occurs 36 to 72 hours after last administration of heroin. Usually, bouts of chills and shivering alternate with bouts of flushing and excessive sweating. Goose-flesh is highly prominent.[7] Other signs and symptoms during the peak period include increased irritability, insomnia, continued loss of appetite, violent yawning and sneezing, continued watering of the eyes and runny nose, vomiting, nausea, intestinal spasms, diarrhea, elevated heart rate and blood pressure, abdominal cramps, pains in the bones and muscles, muscle spasms and uncontrolled kicking movements.[8] General weakness, increasingly severe agitation and emotional depression also occur.

---

[7]   The skin is reported to resemble that of a plucked turkey — hence, probably, the expression "cold turkey" for abrupt cessation of drug use by physically dependent users.

[8]   It has been suggested that the expression "kicking the habit" is derived from these muscle spasms and uncontrolled kicking movements.

Secondary effects, resulting from not taking food or fluids (combined with vomiting, sweating and diarrhea), include weight loss, dehydration and disturbance of the acid/base balance.

Severity of the syndrome gradually decreases, and most observable symptoms are no longer present five to 10 days after the onset of withdrawal sickness.

At any point during the course of withdrawal sickness, even at its peak, administration of a suitable amount of heroin or another opioid[9] will result in the reduction or complete disappearance of the withdrawal effects. That opioids other than heroin have the ability to partially or completely (depending on the amount of the dose) suppress heroin withdrawal is an example of the more general phenomenon of cross-dependence among opioid drugs.[10]

"Chipping"

It is popularly believed that even occasional use of heroin will inevitably lead to dependence as described above. However, not all heroin users develop significant tolerance or become physically dependent on the drug. Some heroin users seem to be able to engage in "chipping" — using the drug infrequently or on a regular intermittent basis (e.g., on weekends) and at relatively low doses, without significantly increasing the dose level or frequency of use. Nevertheless, it should be kept in mind that the vast majority of physically dependent heroin users once mistakenly believed that they could continue to use heroin only occasionally without escalating the dose or frequency of use or becoming physically dependent.

Psychological Dependence

The profound impact of heroin dependence can persist long after the signs of withdrawal sickness have disappeared and despite continuing medical and psychological intervention. Chronic depression, anxiety, insomnia, loss of appetite, periods of agitation and a continued craving for the drug may last for periods of months and even years. Rates of recidivism (resuming drug use after stopping once) are higher

---

9   It is usually impractical to use low-potency drugs such as codeine and propoxyphene to suppress heroin withdrawal, for they have serious side effects at very high doses.

10   An individual tolerant to an effect of one opiate or opioid will also be cross-tolerant to this effect in other drugs of this class.

among users of opioids than among users of other drugs. Even participants in medically supervised methadone maintenance programs report cravings for heroin, although their recidivism rate is considerably lower than for users who try to stop heroin use without treatment assistance.

Such symptoms are often reported to be indicators of psychological dependence. However, a purely psychological explanation may be an oversimplification. Much remains to be understood about the complex physiological changes that occur with opioid dependence and about the disruption of these adaptive changes when drug use is terminated.

The Vietnam Experience

Following the Vietnam War, opioid dependence among American military personnel became a high-profile issue in the drug abuse field. Large numbers of American veterans became dependent on heroin while serving in Vietnam, and it was widely feared that they might present a major health and social problem when they returned to the United States. However, follow-up surveys at one year and three years after discharge found that almost 90 per cent of these veterans were no longer heroin-dependent. The large majority of those surveyed experienced a remission, without relapse, throughout the three-year period — in many cases, with little or no treatment.

It remains uncertain why the rate of recovery was so much greater among these veterans than any other group of heroin-dependent people. However, an interesting explanation has been advanced. Vietnam presented to soldiers an unusual set of circumstances: an extremely stressful environment — an unpopular war, far from home, with a high rate of casualties — in which drugs such as heroin were cheap, easily available and of high purity. Furthermore, in some periods the risk of apprehension was not great. It is understandable that under these exceptional circumstances (and with considerable peer support) many soldiers turned to compulsive drug use as a means of coping.

Discharge meant separation from the stressful environment and from peer support for drug use. Furthermore, it signalled an end to easy access to cheap, high-potency drugs (which were simply not available in the United States). For most, heroin dependence was uniquely linked to the conditions in Vietnam. When the conditions were left behind, the main motivations for compulsive drug use were also eliminated. These situational factors, coupled with an intensive military program of treatment assistance, may account for the much lower rates of dependence among this group than had been anticipated.

Patterns of Use

A 1996 survey found that 1.1 per cent of Ontario adults had used heroin in their life-time. Among Ontario students in Grades 7 through 13, a 1997 survey found that 1.8 per cent had used heroin in the preceding 12 months, with more males than females reporting use. Although the survey methods differed, so that comparisons of the findings must be approached with caution, the results appear consistent with an increased incidence of heroin use in recent years.

Although heroin-dependent individuals come from all walks of life, it has long been recog-nized that the highest concentration of regular users in North America tends to be in the central areas of large cities. Earlier in this century, use was particularly high in major cities on the east and west coasts of the United States and the West Coast of Canada. However, as Montreal, Halifax and Toronto have developed into major centres of international commercial traffic, they have joined Vancouver as Canadian centres with a high rate of heroin use. Although some generalizations about the typical progression and characteristics of users can be made, they should be interpreted with considerable caution, for they by no means apply to all heroin-dependent people.

A disproportionately high number of those who become heroin dependent are from lower socioeconomic and disadvantaged minority groups. First-time users tend to be young (in their teens). They have almost always had at least some (and, in many instances, considerable) experience with other drugs of abuse, and are likely to associate with other drug users, among whom some have at least occasionally used heroin or other opioids. Often first-time heroin users have experienced considerable family disorganization, and their performance and interest in school are generally low.

A user's first experience with heroin often results from both curiosity and peer-group pressure. Early and irregular use is usually through "snorting" (nasal inhalation) or "skin-popping" (subcutaneous injection). Graduation to intramuscular or intravenous injection tends to result from the desire to achieve a quicker and more intense "high." It may also be an early sign of increasing tolerance to and dependence on the drug. With each progressive step — increasing the dosage, using a more direct route of administration and increasing the frequency of administration — the risk of dependence increases. Ultimately, most of those who proceed to "mainlining" (intravenous injection), which results in the most rapid and intensely pleasurable response, can be viewed as having achieved a high degree of both physical and psychological dependence.

Maintaining and supporting heroin addiction can be very expensive, and enormous fluctuations in cost can occur literally overnight and without any notice. Consistent with the laws of street drug supply and demand, a major drug "bust" (police seizure) can result in a dramatic increase in price as supplies are suddenly limited. Most users from lower socioeconomic groups routinely engage in criminal activities to support their habit. Such activities often include small-scale trafficking in illicit substances, possession and sale of stolen property, forgery of prescriptions, pimping and soliciting for purposes of prostitution. However, violent offences represent a very small fraction of such activity. Heroin users from higher socioeconomic groups typically have greater financial resources to support their habit in the face of fluctuating prices, but may be drawn ultimately into fraudulent business or professional activity because of the promised financial returns.

"Polydrug" abuse (concurrent abuse of more than one drug) is remarkably high among heroin-dependent individuals. Among the drugs widely abused by such individuals are other opioids, cannabis, sedative/hypnotics such as barbiturates, anxiolytics, alcohol, amphetamines and cocaine. The use of other opioids is often a function of their availability and a preference for prescription opioids because of the reliability of their purity and intensity of effect. Further, if heroin is unavailable, other opioids will serve as adequate substitutes to prevent withdrawal. Barbiturates can produce a pleasurable state of intoxication in those who have achieved such a high level of tolerance to heroin that they can no longer experience even a mild "high" from it.[11] However, neither barbiturates nor other sedative/hypnotics can delay or reduce the intensity of heroin withdrawal sickness. Although anxiolytics and alcohol may be used merely as part of a lifestyle, they may also be used effectively as self-medication to deal with the stresses of a heroin-focused lifestyle. Finally, stimulants such as amphetamines and cocaine are often used in combination with heroin to achieve a heightened drug experience. This seeking of an enhanced heroin experience may have been the basis for heroin-dependent individuals being among the early adopters of cocaine when it re-emerged in the 1960s as a popular drug of abuse, after several decades of obscurity. This latter phenomenon may also be linked to cocaine's greater availability to heroin users because of their street drug connections.

---

11   Combining heroin and such CNS depressants as barbiturates is a practice that can prove fatal, as both present a risk of significantly depressed respiration, and the combination can result in death from respiratory arrest.

Potential for Abuse

Dependence Liability

The dependence liability of heroin is among the greatest of the opioids in common use, including morphine. This characteristic results from both its extremely powerful euphoric and analgesic effects and its solubility. The drug enters the brain extremely rapidly after intravenous injection to permit immediate and intense gratification.

Inherent Harmfulness

In low to moderate doses, the adverse effects of heroin are relatively mild (e.g., nausea and vomiting) and frequently not sufficiently distressing to dissuade the inexperienced user from continuing use of the drug. However, higher doses of heroin — in excess of the levels to which the user has developed tolerance — can be life-threatening. Street users are especially at risk because they cannot be sure of the size of the dose they are injecting. Nevertheless, because of the powerful dependence-producing properties of heroin, and despite first-hand knowledge of deaths from overdose, street users continue to accept this risk.

Availability

In the early 1900s, when heroin was more freely available, it was widely abused. Today, possession and manufacture of heroin are completely banned in most countries,[12] and a concerted international effort has been made under the auspices of the United Nations to prevent illicit manufacture and distribution. However, despite widespread legal, social and moral sanctions against heroin use, the drug continues to be widely available on the street.

---

[12]   In 1985, tightly controlled medical use of heroin (e.g., in the treatment of severely ill cancer patients) was resumed in Canada. See Medical Uses above.

Background Reading

Canadian Pharmaceutical Association. (1997). *Compendium of Pharmaceuticals and Specialties.* (32nd edition). Ottawa: Canadian Pharmaceutical Association.

Finnegan, L.P. (1978). *Management of Pregnant Drug-Dependent Women.* New York: New York Academy of Sciences.

Finnegan, L.P. & Weiner, S.M. (1993). Drug withdrawal in the neonate. In G.B. Merenstein & S.L. Gardner (Eds.), *Handbook of Neonatal Intensive Care.* (3rd edition). (pp. 40–54). St. Louis: Mosby Year Book Inc.

Reisine, T. & Pasternak, G. (1996). Opioid analgesics and antagonists. (Chapter 23). In J.G. Hardman, L.E. Limbird, P.B. Molinoff, R.W. Rudden, & A.G. Gilman (Eds.), *Goodman and Gilman's The Pharmacological Basis of Therapeutics* (9th edition). New York/Toronto: McGraw-Hill Health Professions Division.

Hydromorphone

DRUG CLASS: Opioid

Synopsis

Hydromorphone (dihydromorphinone) is a powerful semi-synthetic opioid. Its primary clinical uses are to relieve severe pain and to suppress severe cough. When it is administered by subcutaneous injection (the most common medical route of injection), its analgesic potency is estimated to be seven to eight times greater than that of morphine. In low doses, the side effects of hydromorphone such as nausea, vomiting and drowsiness are both less common and milder than those of most other powerful opioid drugs. However, because of hydromorphone's powerful depressant effect on the centres of the brain that control respiration, a lethal dose of hydromorphone is smaller than a lethal dose of most other opioids.

Tolerance to the effects of hydromorphone tends to develop gradually. Nevertheless, powerful physical dependence can develop rapidly with high-dose abuse. The withdrawal syndrome that occurs after abrupt abstinence from hydromorphone is similar to but less intense than that produced after abrupt abstinence from heroin or morphine, with symptoms resembling those produced by a case of moderately severe flu. The euphoric potency of hydromorphone is lower than that of most other powerful opioids, and when chronically injected, the drug also produces more pain and tissue irritation. However, because of its relatively easy availability by prescription and its low cost when compared with street heroin, hydromorphone is desirable to opioid abusers.

Drug Source

Hydromorphone is a semi-synthetic drug produced by the pharmaceutical industry through chemical modification of morphine.

Trade Names

Dilaudid®, Dilaudid-HP®, Dilaudid-HP-Plus®, Dilaudid-XP®, Dilaudid Sterile Powder®, Hydromorph Contin®, PMS-Hydromorphone®.

Street Names

"Juice" (a common street name for all cough syrups containing opioids), dillies, DS.

Combination Products

Dilaudid® cough syrup (hydromorphone, guaifenesin and alcohol 5%; available in the United States only).

Medical Uses

Medical uses of hydromorphone include the relief of moderately severe and severe pain, and suppression of severe cough.

Physical Appearance

In pure form, hydromorphone occurs as a fine, white, odorless crystalline powder that is soluble in water and slightly soluble in alcohol.

Dosage[1,2]

Medical

- for moderate to severe pain — 2 to 4 mg orally every four to six hours as necessary; 2 mg by subcutaneous or intramuscular injection every four to six hours as necessary, increased up to 4 mg to treat very severe pain; 3 mg by rectal suppository for longer duration of relief, particularly at night

- for cough — 1 mg every three to four hours.

Non-medical

The use of doses up to 100 mg per day has been reported.

Routes of Administration

Orally in solution or tablet form; also by subcutaneous, intramuscular or intravenous injection and by rectal suppository.

Effects of Short-Term Use: Low Doses[3]

CNS, behavioral, subjective: Effects of hydromorphone use include suppression of the sensation and emotional response to pain,[4] mild euphoria, occasional drowsiness, lethargy, relaxation, difficulty in concentrating, lightheadedness, mild anxiety or fearfulness, suppression of cough reflex and pain at the site of injection (due to hydromorphone's tendency to irritate local tissue when injected). Pupillary constriction does not occur.

---

[1]   All doses refer to adults.

[2]   Hydromorphone 1.5 mg injected intramuscularly or 7.5 mg administered orally is approximately equivalent in analgesic potency to 10 mg of morphine injected intramuscularly.

[3]   Single doses of 2 to 4 mg taken either orally or by subcutaneous or intramuscular injection in non-tolerant persons, up to 20 mg per day.

[4]   Hydromorphone 1.5 mg is equivalent in analgesic potency to 10 mg of morphine when both are given intramuscularly.

Respiratory: slightly reduced respiratory rate.

Gastrointestinal: mild nausea, vomiting, appetite suppression and constipation.

Other: sweating, reduced libido and slight drop in body temperature.

Effects of Short-Term Use: Higher Doses[5]

Intensification of hydromorphone's low-dose effects may occur with administration of higher doses. Duration of effects also increases with increased dosage. As the dose increases:

- sensitivity and emotional response to painful stimuli decrease
- probability of sleep increases
- ability to concentrate is increasingly impaired
- breathing becomes progressively slower and more shallow
- heart rate gradually slows and blood pressure decreases
- the degree of euphoria produced increases, but this euphoria is not as intense as that produced by morphine or heroin.

In very high doses (i.e., overdose), hydromorphone can produce deep sleep, which may progress to stupor or coma; low blood pressure; slow heart rate; cyanosis; shallow and markedly reduced rate of breathing; low body temperature; flaccidity of skeletal muscles and cold and clammy skin.

Effects of Long-Term Use

Chronic subcutaneous injection of hydromorphone in any particular area, e.g., the forearm, tends to produce pronounced pain, tissue irritation and hardening of the tissue under the skin, as does injection of most other common opioids. Other long-term effects are also similar to those produced by other opioids such as morphine and heroin.

---

5   Single doses above the therapeutic range administered, whether orally or by injection, in non-tolerant persons.

Other adverse consequences directly related to chronic hydromorphone use include mood instability,[6] constipation, reduced libido, menstrual irregularity and certain types of respiratory impairment.

Lethality

Because of the intensity of hydromorphone's respiratory-depressant effect, an overdose that can be lethal to a non-tolerant individual is smaller than a lethal dose of most other opioids. It has been estimated to be as low as 100 mg. Severe overdose results in coma, cessation of breathing, circulatory collapse, cardiac arrest and death.

Tolerance and Dependence

Tolerance

Generally, tolerance to the main effects of hydromorphone develops more gradually than tolerance to the effects of most other potent opioids. However, tolerance to the euphoric, sedative, analgesic and respiratory-depressant effects clearly does develop. As is the case with many other opioids, as tolerance develops with chronic use and the user gradually increases the size of the dose to achieve the desired effects, a dose plateau is reached where further increases cannot produce the intensity of effect desired. Attempts to go above this plateau can be lethal because of hydromorphone's pronounced respiratory-depressant effect at higher doses. Dependent users who continue to administer the drug after reaching this plateau do so primarily to prevent withdrawal symptoms.

Physical Dependence/Withdrawal

After long-term administration of hydromorphone, abruptly stopping use or abruptly reducing the dose substantially will result in withdrawal symptoms similar to those associated with morphine. Early symptoms may appear as few as three hours after the last dose, but while these symptoms are qualitatively similar to those produced by morphine or heroin withdrawal, they tend to be less severe.

---

6   Mood instability is due to the relatively short duration of action of hydromorphone. The effects of a therapeutic dose last for approximately five hours.

In chronic high-dose users, early withdrawal symptoms include exaggerated autonomic responses (e.g., rapid heart rate), runny nose, anxiety, "goose-flesh," tremor, yawning, insomnia, elevated temperature, watering eyes and restlessness. Later withdrawal symptoms include nausea, vomiting, diarrhea, severe abdominal pain, loss of appetite, elevated heart rate and blood pressure, severe agitation, insomnia, pains in the muscles and joints, muscle spasms and uncontrolled kicking movements.

The severity of the syndrome gradually declines, and most observable symptoms disappear within approximately one week.

Psychological Dependence

Symptoms of long-term dependence on hydromorphone (and other opioids) are often observable for extended periods after the classical phase of withdrawal sickness has ended. Depression, anxiety, insomnia, loss of appetite, periods of agitation and a craving for the drug may persist for several weeks or months. Such symptoms are often considered indicative of psychological dependence. However, such an explanation based purely on psychological factors may be an oversimplification. More research is needed into the possibly complex physiological adjustments that may result from opioid dependence and about the fate of these adjustments after withdrawal.

Patterns of Use

Because hydromorphone is available in many forms and in higher strengths for parenteral administration, it is useful in hospitals for relief of extreme pain, such as that experienced by cancer patients. Furthermore, because of its powerful suppressant effect on the cough reflex, hydromorphone is also effective in the management of severe cough.

Until the 1980s, hydromorphone did not appear to be widely popular among street opioid abusers. However, more recent evidence suggests that hydromorphone has gained considerable favor and is now an important drug of abuse. In fact, many users of heroin and other opioids have switched to oral or intravenous hydromorphone when their drug of choice has been in short supply.

Hydromorphone's current popularity among drug users is due to its ability to produce euphoria when injected or taken orally and its availability through thefts from pharmacies and forged prescriptions. It is relatively inexpensive compared with heroin, and is of known strength and purity. Users who take hydromorphone orally by prescription may experience less of a social stigma than do users of heroin.

Potential for Abuse

Abuse Liability

Although hydromorphone has powerful analgesic properties, researchers report that when it is injected its euphoric effects are not as intense as those of other powerful drugs in this class, such as heroin and morphine. When hydromorphone is taken orally, the intensity of its euphoric effects is further diminished because compared with injection, orally administered hydromorphone takes longer to reach the target sites in the brain.

Inherent Harmfulness

Chronic injection of hydromorphone produces tissue irritation and pain. Therefore, the various routes of injection tend in the long run to be less preferable than oral administration. Because of the drug's highly potent effects on brain centres controlling respiration, high-dose users risk potentially lethal effects.

Availability

Hydromorphone's current popularity appears to be related to its relatively easy availability, its relatively low cost and (unlike illicitly produced opioids) its high degree of purity. In addition, dependence on a drug such as hydromorphone does not carry the same social stigma as heroin dependence. For these reasons, regular users of hydromorphone appear to be willing to forgo the more immediate and intense effects of injected opioids.

Background Reading

McEvoy, G. (Ed.), (1997). *American Hospital Formulary Service (AHFS) Drug Information.* (pp. 1295–1297). Bethesda, MD: American Society of Health-System Pharmacists.

Portenoy, M.K. & Payne, R. (1992). Acute and chronic pain. In J.H. Lowinson, P. Ruiz, R.B. Millman & J.G. Langrod (Eds.), *Substance Abuse — A Comprehensive Textbook.* (2nd edition). Baltimore: Williams and Wilkins.

Reynolds, J.E.F. (Ed.) (1996). *Martindale's The Extra Pharmacopeia.* (31st edition). London: Royal Pharmaceutical Society.

Isopropyl Alcohol

DRUG CLASS: Topical Antiseptic and Rubefacient, Poison

Synopsis

Isopropyl alcohol (isopropanol, 2-propanol) is a synthetic chemical used in iso-propanol rubbing compounds ("rubbing alcohol") and in certain cosmetics such as hand lotions and aftershave lotions. In these products isopropyl alcohol functions as an antiseptic agent, a rapidly evaporating solvent, a preservative and a rubefacient (by stimulating blood flow to the skin). It possesses mild CNS-depressant properties and produces a state of mild intoxication when swallowed, but is more toxic than ethanol. Isopropyl alcohol is a highly toxic poison. Poisoning occurs as a result of the conversion of isopropyl alcohol to acetone, which is a CNS depressant. The accumulation of acetone in the body can cause kidney impairment, coma and frequently death from respiratory arrest. The lethal dose of isopropyl alcohol has been estimated at somewhat less than 250 mL. A few impoverished alcoholics have been reported not only to deliberately ingest isopropyl alcohol but also to express a *preference* for it over ethyl (beverage) alcohol, despite their awareness of its hazards. In most cases, however, skid-row alcoholics consume isopropyl alcohol out of desperation, without knowing what they are drinking or that it is potentially lethal.

Drug Source

Isopropyl alcohol is produced through chemical synthesis.

Trade Names

Isopropyl alcohol is marketed as an antiseptic under names such as Isopropanol 99% and Isopropyl Alcohol U.S.P. [1]

Street Names

None in common use.

Combination Products

Isopropanol rubbing compounds contain 70 per cent alcohol diluted with water. Sometimes colors and perfumes are added to make rubbing compounds. Isopropyl alcohol is also a component of skin cleansers, hand lotions, aftershave lotions and similar cosmetics, antifreeze solutions and quick-drying inks.

Skid-row alcoholics sometimes combine isopropyl alcohol with ethyl alcohol.

Physical Appearance

In pure form, isopropyl alcohol is a clear, colorless, volatile liquid with a slightly bitter taste and a characteristic odor.

Dosage[2]

Medical

In products intended for application to unbroken skin, for the chemical's antiseptic and cooling effects, the concentration of isopropyl alcohol may range from 50 to 99 per cent.

---

[1]   The suffix U.S.P. indicates that the formulation meets the specifications of the *United States Pharmacopoeia*.

[2]   All doses refer to adults.

Non-medical

Isopropyl alcohol has been purposely ingested by some chronic alcoholics in the form of rubbing compounds, aftershave lotions or other products, sometimes combined with beverage alcohol.

While single doses of 250 mL are normally fatal, there is at least one documented case report of a chronic alcoholic surviving after ingesting approximately 310 mL of pure isopropyl alcohol.

Routes of Administration

Individuals who drink isopropyl alcohol are usually unaware of its toxic properties.

Inhaling isopropyl alcohol vapors in a poorly ventilated area can produce toxic effects.

Effects of Short-Term Use: Low Doses[3]

Effects of the short-term use of low doses of isopropyl alcohol include the following.[4]

CNS, behavioral, subjective: mild inebriation, dizziness, mild impairment of motor co-ordination, and other relatively mild nervous and muscular disturbances.

Cardiovascular: mild to moderate drop in blood pressure and prolonged headache.

Gastrointestinal: diarrhea, painful gastritis, nausea and vomiting.

---

[3]   Approximately 30 mL (1 oz.) or less taken orally by non-tolerant users.

[4]   Effects are generally experienced for a longer period than those associated with comparable amounts of ethyl alcohol, because isopropyl alcohol is metabolized more slowly.

Effects of Short-Term Use: Higher Doses[5]

An intensification of low-dose effects may occur with the use of higher doses of isopropyl alcohol, as well as any of the following effects.

CNS, behavioral, subjective: confusion, possibly marked impairment of motor co-ordination, stupor and coma.[6] The clinical picture may be complicated by the presence of other ingredients in products that contain isopropyl alcohol, particularly volatile aromatics (e.g., camphor, naphthalene). Such combinations can result in a syndrome of CNS stimulation with motor restlessness, extreme apprehension, hallucinations and disorientation.

Cardiovascular: marked drop in blood pressure, slow pulse, sometimes circulatory collapse and shock.

Respiratory: respiratory depression.

Gastrointestinal: gastrointestinal pain and hemorrhage, nausea and vomiting, and diarrhea.

Other: low body temperature, possibly severe kidney impairment.

Effects of Long-Term Use

Even among impoverished alcoholics, isopropyl alcohol is rarely used on a regular basis. As a result, and because of user's typically heavy ethyl alcohol use, chronic effects directly attributable to isopropyl alcohol are not fully known. However, severe kidney and liver impairment is likely.

---

5   Approximately 60 mL (2 oz.) or more taken orally by non-tolerant users, or lower doses in particularly sensitive individuals.

6   Prolonged inhalation of concentrated vapors of isopropyl alcohol in poorly ventilated areas can produce deep coma.

Lethality

The lethal potential of isopropyl alcohol is much higher than that of ethyl alcohol and somewhat lower than that of methyl alcohol. Doses of 250 mL of isopropyl alcohol can kill an adult, and much lower doses can kill a small child. In cases of lethal overdose, death is generally preceded by extremely low blood pressure and deep coma, and results from respiratory arrest.

Because even small doses of isopropyl alcohol can be fatal for small children, care must be taken to store this substance out of their reach. Isopropyl alcohol has also been implicated in both successful and unsuccessful suicide attempts.

Hemodialysis is useful for removing isopropyl alcohol from the body.

Tolerance and Dependence

Researchers have reported that the few impoverished alcoholics who regularly drink isopropyl alcohol appear to develop tolerance to its inebriating effects.

Patterns of Use

A small number of impoverished alcoholics actually express a preference for isopropyl alcohol and other toxic alcohols over ethyl alcohol. Research interviews clearly indicate that all of these regular users are aware of the toxic effects of the non-beverage alcohols. However, service providers to impoverished alcoholics have reported that many resort to isopropyl alcohol only occasionally. They are most likely to do so out of desperation when they are on the threshold of withdrawal and cannot buy or otherwise obtain ethyl alcohol.

Potential for Abuse

Because of the known toxicity of isopropyl alcohol, it is very rarely abused except by impoverished alcoholics.

Background Reading

Klaassen, C.D. (1996). Nonmetallic environmental toxicants: Air pollutants, solvents and vapors, and pesticides. (Chapter 67). In J.H. Hardman, L.E. Limbird, P.B. Molinoff, R.W. Rudden & A.G. Gilman, (Eds.), *Goodman and Gilman's The Pharmacological Basis of Therapeutics*, (9th edition). New York/Toronto: McGraw-Hill Health Professions Division.

LSD
(Lysergic Acid Diethylamide)

DRUG CLASS: Hallucinogen

Synopsis

LSD (lysergic acid diethylamide) is the most powerful of the known hallucinogens. In doses as small as 25 to 50 micrograms (0.025 to 0.05 mg), it can produce mild changes in perception, mood and thought. As doses increase, the effects become more intense, and at 100 micrograms may include visual hallucinations and distortions that the user usually knows to be unreal. Users may experience synesthesia — the paradoxical perception of the senses melding together — believing, for example, that they are "seeing" music or "hearing" visual patterns. Normal boundaries of identification between the self and the environment frequently disappear under the influence of LSD, and there may be distortions of body image, space and time (minutes may seem to pass as slowly as hours).

These experiences may be accompanied by periods of deep introspection, in which the users may feel they are gaining great insights or may feel alienated from themselves and their environment. Any given LSD "trip" may produce a sense of wonder and joy, as well as sensations of feeling "high," or a sense of anxiety, fearfulness or even panic. Even users who have experienced the drug positively on some occasions may have an adverse episode, or "bad trip," on other occasions.

There have been reports that LSD has induced severe (although usually brief) psychotic episodes in a very small minority of users who have not manifested these symptoms previously. These symptoms may persist for a few days after the drug has been eliminated from the body. A psychotic episode may be characterized by bizarre behavior, delusional thinking, terror and true hallucinations (i.e., hallucinations that the user believes to be real). In cases of more long-lasting psychosis after taking LSD, it would appear that schizophrenia was unmasked by LSD, rather than caused by the drug. Some users experience flashbacks (hallucinogen persisting perception disorder [HPPD]) for a period of months or years after use ceases.

LSD, like certain other hallucinogens, cannot be taken continuously for more than a few days without losing its psychic potency in that individual. Tolerance (tachyphylaxis) develops quickly, and the user must abstain for at least a few days in order to regain sensitivity to the desired effects. Physical dependence is not known to occur.

Drug Source

LSD is produced through chemical synthesis in illicit laboratories, except for a small amount that is legally produced exclusively for research purposes.

Trade Names

Not applicable. LSD is not used medically except for research.

Street Names[1]

Acid, barrels, blotters, California sunshine, cube, domes, flats, frogs, lids, wedges, windowpane.

Drug Combinations

Unknown to the purchaser, LSD combinations encountered on the street most often contain PCP (phencyclidine).[2] A combination of MDMA ("ecstasy") and LSD is called "X and L" or "flip-flops." Some street drug preparations in earlier years included amphetamines. LSD has been occasionally added to alcoholic beverages.

LSD users sometimes take benzodiazepines or other CNS depressants together with LSD to combat the anxiety that may be experienced during an LSD trip.

---

[1]   Street drugs alleged to contain a different substance often contain LSD. A noteworthy example of such mislabelling or misrepresentation is the sale of LSD as mescaline.

[2]   Street-drug preparations alleged to contain LSD often contain additional drugs or are in fact different drugs.

Medical Uses

There is currently no generally accepted medical use for LSD. However, clinical research with LSD has resumed with a goal of better understanding the drug's effects on the brain. Research evidence suggests that LSD exerts its effects by interacting with serotonin receptors, but the drug also binds to dopamine receptors.[3] A better understanding of LSD activity at these molecular levels may lead to the recognition of potential medical uses of LSD and the design of more selective LSD-like drugs and drugs that reverse the hallucinogenic effects of LSD.

Physical Appearance

When pure, LSD tartrate is a white, odorless crystalline material that is soluble in water. However, LSD is so potent that an effective dose of pure drug is so small as to be virtually invisible. As a result, it is diluted with other materials before distribution in capsule, tablet or solution form. Alternatively, drops of LSD solution are dried on gelatin sheets, pieces of blotting paper or sugar cubes, which release the drug when they are swallowed, sucked or placed in water.

Dosage

Medical
There is no current medical use for LSD.

Non-medical
Street-drug preparations usually range from 40 to 500 micrograms (0.04 to 0.5 mg) per individual dose.

---

[3]   To date, there is evidence of LSD agonist action at 5-HT2, 5-HT1A and 5-HT1C receptors, as well as at D1 and D2 dopamine receptors.

Routes of Administration

LSD may be taken orally, inhaled or injected.

Effects of Short-Term Use[4]

CNS, behavioral and subjective: Early CNS effects may include numbness, muscle weakness, muscle twitching, rapid reflexes, tremulousness, and impairment of motor skills and co-ordination. Often there is early anxiety or sometimes exhilaration; the latter is likely due to the user's expectations, as it may occur prior to the onset of hallucinogenic actions. Seizures have also occurred, although rarely.

The typical "psychedelic" or "hallucinogenic" effects usually begin 30 to 45 minutes after LSD is taken. There is a fairly wide variation among users in the perceptual, cognitive and emotional experiences produced by LSD. In addition to the size of the dose, drug effects are also influenced by the setting and the user's expectations, past drug experiences and personality. It is not unusual for a user to experience differing reactions to LSD during different drug-taking episodes.[5] The typical effects include the following:

- There may be vivid perceptual (usually visual) distortions such as "pseudo-hallucinations" and "pseudoillusions," in which the user is aware that the experience is not real.

- The user's perception of time may be distorted (minutes may seem to pass as slowly as hours).

---

4   One hundred micrograms taken orally by non-tolerant users. Increasing doses of LSD tend to produce quantitative changes (i.e., greater intensity) rather than qualitative changes (i.e., different symptoms). It has been demonstrated that "between the dose ranges of 1 - 16 micrograms per kg, the intensity of the psychophysiological effects of LSD is proportional to the dose." For instance, this dose range for a 73 kg (160 lb.) person would be between approximately 70 and 1,100 micrograms.

5   Individuals being treated with antidepressant medications face special risks of interaction of LSD with their drug therapies. Similarly, patients experiencing LSD-related HPPD may react atypically to some antipsychotic drugs. Research has shown that individuals who have been treated with a serotonin reuptake inhibitor (SSRI) for several weeks prior to taking LSD have a much reduced response, or even a virtually complete lack of response to LSD, while those who have been treated chronically with tricyclic anti-depressants or lithium show an increased response to LSD. However, SSRI agents have also been found to provoke or worsen LSD flashbacks in patients treated for depression. Similarly, treatment with the antipsychotic drug risperidone has been found to worsen the panic and visual disturbance of patients with HPPD.

- Space perception may be distorted, which can prove hazardous if the user is driving or in some other potentially dangerous situation.

- Users' perceptions of their bodies may be distorted. Some users feel heavy and "pulled down" by gravity, while others experience sensations of weightlessness and floating.

- Users' perception of recognized boundaries between self and environment is diminished and may be lost completely. For some users, this generates a feeling of oneness with the universe, but for others it can be terrifying, as anchors in both internal and external reality may appear to be no longer present. The term "depersonalization" refers to a state in which the user feels that the mind has left the body, and is looking at the body from a distance.

- Control over thinking processes and concentration can be markedly diminished.

- Synesthesias, in which one sensory modality is melded with another, occur frequently. For example users may think they can "see" music or "hear" colors.

- Recent or even long-forgotten memories can vividly resurface and possibly blend with current experience.

- Otherwise insignificant thoughts may seem to take on deep meaning.

- Parts of the user's body or trivial objects may be the subject of careful and prolonged scrutiny and may also take on magnified importance or meaning.

- All sensory experiences tend to be heightened; the user perceives brighter colors, sharper definition of objects, increased hearing acuity, more sharply distinguished taste and so on.

- Different emotions may appear to exist simultaneously, or rapidly follow each other.

- Some users withdraw and appear to be indifferent to their surroundings; others may become hypervigilant; many alternate between these states.

- Users may feel that they are undergoing a profound mystical, religious or "cosmic" experience — for some users perhaps the most desired effect.

Such effects typically subside within six to eight hours.

The earliest effects, occurring 15 to 45 minutes after a dose has been taken by mouth, are physical effects resulting from stimulation of the sympathetic nervous system. They resemble the effects of adrenaline or amphetamine and include the following.

Cardiovascular: increased blood pressure and heart rate.

Respiratory: abnormally rapid and deep breathing.

Gastrointestinal: nausea and vomiting, suppression of appetite.

Other: elevation of body temperature and sweating, which may alternate with chills and shivering.

Adverse Reactions ("Bad Trips")

Many users have experienced unpleasant reactions to the effects of LSD. Fearfulness, anxiety and depression may occur even in experienced users who have had no prior adverse reactions. Some users undergo highly adverse reactions to LSD's effects (i.e., "bad trips"). Users can experience panic reactions, feeling that they are losing their identity, or fearing that they are disintegrating into nothingness and reality does not exist. "Pseudohallucinations" may give way to terrifying true hallucinations. Acute paranoid states may occur, and bizarre delusions may be manifested in such extreme behavior as violent, homicidal or suicidal actions. Severe confusion and disorientation may also provoke highly inappropriate behavior. These symptoms usually rapidly decline in intensity and disappear after the drug is metabolized and excreted from the body. However, a long-lasting psychotic state may continue in vulnerable individuals. Some users have been reported to experience prolonged after-images (palinopsia) as a chronic visual complication of LSD use. This problem may persist for several years after drug use ends.

Because adverse effects are particularly common among new users, early LSD "trips" are usually taken in the company of experienced users who are familiar with the effects of the drug and therefore can often forestall acute panic reactions.

The frequency of adverse reactions to LSD that were serious enough to cause users to seek medical intervention declined significantly through the 1980s. In some areas, however, the frequency of such serious reactions has increased in the 1990s. During the late 1960s and early 1970s, there were no more than a handful of documented reports of LSD-related extreme violence (e.g., bizarre homicides, suicides and self-mutilations). Nonetheless, extensive media coverage and political statements in the

United States regarding unpredictable and dangerous behavior during LSD episodes suggested to many that such phenomena were widespread and also posed a potential threat to society. The much more common serious reactions to LSD included severe anxiety, panic and other symptoms of severe psychic distress, but in the overwhelming majority of these cases, there was neither violence nor any threat to society. However, LSD-related violent behavior appears to have increased during the 1990s.

The effects of hallucinogens on users are strongly associated with the users' expectations and attitudes (their "emotional set") as well as the predominant attitudes and beliefs of their culture. In the 1960s, the prevailing societal perception of LSD was highly negative. The drug was viewed as dangerous and was thought to routinely cause people to become psychotic and/or to behave in bizarre and violent ways. While many LSD users professed to disbelieve these claims, sensational and widely publicized cases, as well as "authoritative" medical opinion regarding the hazards of LSD, undoubtedly adversely affected the expectations of users. Furthermore, in the late 1960s many LSD users were self-selected "fringe" members of society: dropouts, hippies and others with unconventional lifestyles. A tendency toward emotional problems was undoubtedly greater for members of this group than for those young people in the general population who did not use LSD and who identified more closely with traditional societal norms. Conflicting expectations and emotional instability among the users of LSD during the 1960s probably increased their vulnerability to bad trips.

The users of the 1980s appeared to be more within the mainstream of North American life than their predecessors. They were also somewhat better tolerated and their behavior (although still unacceptable) was not viewed as quite so deviant. Therefore, they were not exposed to the sort of virulent societal hostility directed toward LSD users in the past.

Furthermore, significantly more information was available to more recent users regarding means of effectively combating adverse reactions. For example, they knew that LSD should be taken only in the company of trusted and experienced users who could "talk down" those who might experience excessive anxiety or fearfulness. Many users also recognized the value of benzodiazepines to calm distress and had a supply of them available as self-medication. Finally, many learned to avoid busy hospital emergency departments, because their atmosphere can exacerbate such symptoms as panic and paranoid thinking. However, the apparent increase in the 1990s in LSD-related emergency-room visits and violent behavior has suggested that today's adolescent may be destined to relearn the lessons about LSD learned by a previous generation.

Clinical Use of LSD

LSD had been used medically almost exclusively as an experimental drug in psychotherapy and in the treatment of alcoholism. Some medical researchers began early investigations with LSD in the hope that it would reduce psychological disturbance in their patients by inducing greater insight and self-acceptance. It was reasoned that the LSD experience should help patients to temporarily detach their conscious mind from reality and be more able to deal with repressed painful experiences and modify their perception of themselves and their external reality. As a result, LSD was used experimentally with a spectrum of emotional conditions, ranging from alcoholism to fear of death in terminally ill patients. Unfortunately, such treatment was not found to have lasting impact. However, some researchers and physicians continue to claim that not enough research was undertaken and that the negative conclusions regarding the potential of LSD therapy were premature. Such voices generally support the recent resumption of clinical research with LSD.

Effects of Long-Term Use

Flashbacks (Hallucinogen Persisting Perception Disorder)

Perhaps the persistent phenomenon most frequently associated with LSD use is "flashbacks" — spontaneous recurrences of specific experiences that originally occurred during an LSD episode. Typically flashbacks are brief, lasting only a few minutes or less. Their recurrence is not predictable, nor are they experienced by most LSD users. They may occur shortly after an LSD episode or, in some cases, up to four or five years later. They are frequently elicited by the use of other psychoactive drugs, such as cannabis. They can occur after entering a dark room, or they may be triggered by emotional distress, fatigue or even exercise. Some users acknowledge having experienced only one flashback while others report several. At one extreme, some report the experience to be pleasant (referring to it as a "free trip"), whereas others feel acute panic. Regular users are more likely to experience flashbacks than those who have taken a single LSD "trip." Generally, the greater the number of LSD experiences, the greater the probability of experiencing flashbacks. However, there is no evidence that LSD users who experience flashbacks are more psychologically disturbed than users who do not. Nor is there any evidence to suggest an association between flashbacks and brain damage.

Visual images are by far the most frequently reported form of flashback, ranging from formless colors to frightening hallucinations. However, true hallucinations (which the individual believes to be real) are much less common than pseudohallucinations (which the individual knows are not real). Pseudohallucinations involving geometric patterns are the most common sort of flashback. Prolonged after-images (palinopsia) have been reported for several years after the last use of LSD. Less frequently, flashbacks involve other senses including taste, smell, hearing, touch, body sensations and balance. They may also recur in the form of distortions of time, space, body image or reality. Their physiological basis is unknown.

Amotivational Syndrome

An "amotivational syndrome" has been observed in some users of LSD as well as of marijuana. The common manifestations of this syndrome are increasing apathy and decreasing interest in both one's environment and social contacts, loss of effectiveness, passivity, diminished tolerance for frustration, and lack of interest in planning ahead. Affected users also often appear to disregard typical social conventions such as appropriateness of dress and public comportment. In the case of cannabis, many clinical researchers now regard the amotivational syndrome as a form of chronic toxicity that usually clears up once cannabis use stops and the cannabis metabolites are cleared from the body. In the case of LSD, this explanation seems less probable. Although it may be tempting to suggest that these behaviors result exclusively from chronic LSD use, a causal relationship of this nature is extremely difficult to demonstrate because of the numerous factors involved. It has been proposed that this syndrome may, in many instances, be more realistically attributed to certain aspects of a lifestyle adopted by many young people during the 1960s and early 1970s, rather than solely to drug use. Conservatively, it may be suggested that in some respects, the use of LSD and other drugs may serve to foster a lack of motivation in some users, while a lack of motivation as a lifestyle may serve to foster the use of LSD and other drugs in others.

LSD-Precipitated Psychosis

Acute psychotic episodes caused by a single dose of LSD ordinarily last for several hours. However, both a single dose and chronic use have resulted in a protracted period of psychosis for some individuals. This psychosis resembles paranoid schizophrenia in many respects and is characterized by true hallucinations (mainly visual[6]), delusional thinking and bizarre behavior. Although many of those who experience LSD-related psychosis are believed to have been latent psychotics prior to their use of the drug, a few had previously exhibited little or no obvious personality disturbance.

---

6   However, paranoid schizophrenics more often experience auditory hallucinations.

The issue is yet to be fully resolved as to whether chronic psychosis precipitated by LSD is a diagnostic entity distinct from schizophrenia, although the weight of evidence suggests that such a distinction is probably not warranted. Indeed, there are many more similarities than differences between these two groups.

Other Effects

Although LSD has been associated with chromosomal breaks in some laboratory studies, research evidence to date does not support claims that chronic LSD use causes genetic disorders. There appears to be a higher risk of spontaneous abortion and congenital abnormalities in offspring of women who have regularly used LSD during pregnancy. However, because most of these mothers had also used other drugs during their pregnancies, the causal relationships are difficult to determine. While there has also been concern about the possibility of brain damage in chronic users, again causality has not been established. On the whole, studies have found no consistent differences between LSD users and non-users in tests designed to diagnose brain impairment.

Lethality

No deaths in humans resulting exclusively from acute LSD overdose have been reported. However, cases of suicide during or following LSD intoxication have occasionally occurred. Other results of violent or hazardous behavior have included accidental (sometimes bizarre) fatalities and very infrequently homicides and self-mutilations.

Tolerance and Dependence

Tolerance develops particularly rapidly to the subjective effects of LSD[7] and to its effect on blood pressure, pupils and reflexes. With consecutive daily doses, often by the third or fourth day no amount of the drug can produce the desired effects. After three to four days' abstinence, normal sensitivity usually returns. Once tolerance to LSD develops, the effects of several other hallucinogens, including psilocybin, mescaline and other lysergic derivatives, also cannot be experienced until after a period of abstinence from LSD. This phenomenon is referred to as "cross-tolerance."

---

7   See the discussion of tolerance and tachyphylaxis in Section 1.

Chronic use of LSD does not appear to result in physical dependence and no withdrawal sickness after termination of use has been reported.

The degree to which psychological dependence on LSD develops varies considerably among users. For some regular users, LSD plays a central role in their lives and they experience a compulsive need to continue using the drug. For them, temporary unavailability of LSD can result in anxiety or even feelings of panic. These users rarely discontinue their drug use voluntarily. However, this group represents a small minority of LSD users, who, in the street vernacular, are derogatorily referred to as "acid heads" or "acid freaks."

Patterns of Use

LSD is not typically used on a daily basis. Since tolerance to the subjective effects develops rapidly, continued daily use is pointless. Many regular LSD users are "weekend trippers," who restrict their use to no more than a day or two each week. Many others report using the drug even less frequently. Surveys also indicate that LSD is unlikely to be the exclusive drug of use. LSD users are also likely to use cannabis, in some cases together with other drugs. However, many users of other drugs have experimented with LSD once or twice, primarily for the experience and without continuing to use it.

Most reports suggest that LSD remains inexpensive and fairly easy to obtain in most areas of North America. This is reflected in the drug's use by high school students.

Today's typical LSD users probably take the drug less frequently and tend to remain "high" for shorter periods than did users of the previous generation. Also, primary motives for LSD use have changed. Whereas many LSD users of the 1960s were engaged in psychic exploration and seeking greater insight, many current users report taking LSD in order to get "high." LSD is simply one of a number of drugs that can be taken for this purpose, and it no longer has special symbolic meaning for young users.

A 1993 survey of Ontario students from Grades 7 to 13[8] reported levels of LSD and other hallucinogen use that were significantly higher than those reported in a similar survey in 1991. LSD was found to be the second most common illicit drug, used by

6.9 per cent of students. It was also found that significantly more males than females used LSD (8.1 per cent males versus 5.7 per cent females). Of those who reported LSD use, 28 per cent used it 10 or more times during the 12 months prior to the survey. The level of overall use was similar in 1997, when 7.6 per cent reported use in the preceding year.

In a survey of Toronto street youth, LSD was also reported to be the second most commonly used illicit drug. Fifty-nine per cent of the sample of 217 youths reported using LSD in the previous year.

Potential for Abuse

Abuse Liability

LSD does not have direct "reinforcing effects" — it does not stimulate the brain's "reward system." Experimental animals that will voluntarily self-administer heroin, cocaine or nicotine will not do so with LSD. Therefore, the drug's intrinsic abuse potential is low, and humans generally must learn to like its effects through repeated trials in "safe" settings, usually in the company of experienced users.

Physical dependence on LSD does not occur, and only a small fraction of users become psychologically dependent on it.

Inherent Harmfulness

LSD can cause severe psychic distress (the "bad trip") in some users, and such occurrences cannot be predicted. "Flashbacks," which users can experience unexpectedly at any later point, often after use of cannabis, can also be quite distressing. Many potential users have probably been deterred by hearing about these negative effects and by the adverse publicity that LSD has received for a variety of reasons, often without sound evidence.

8　　The traditional Grade 13 has been replaced by an Ontario Academic Credit (OAC) year in Ontario schools. However, the Ontario survey, and thus this text, has continued to use "Grade 13" to facilitate comparison with previous survey data.

Availability

The availability of LSD tends to vary with its popularity on the street. When the drug is in fashion, it is usually quite easy to obtain. At other times it can be very difficult to find. Other substances, such as PCP, are frequently sold as LSD to the unsuspecting buyer.

Background Reading

Abraham, H.D. & Aldridge, A.M. (1993). Adverse consequences of lysergic acid diethylamide. *Addiction, 88,* 1327–1344.

Adlaf, E.M., Smart, R.G. & Walsh, G.W. (1993). *Ontario Student Drug Use Survey, 1977-1993.* Toronto: Addiction Research Foundation.

Adlaf, E.M., Ivis, F.J. & Smart, R.G. (1997). *Ontario Student Drug Use Survey 1977-1997.* Toronto: Addiction Research Foundation.

Kawasaki, A. & Purvin, V. (1996). Persistent palinopsia following ingestion of lysergic acid diethylamide (LSD). *Archives of Ophthalmology, 114 (1),* 47–50.

Markel, H., Lee, A., Holmes, R.D. & Domino E.F. (1994). LSD flashback syndrome exacerbated by selective serotonin reuptake inhibitor antidepressants in adolescents. *Journal of Pediatrics, 125 (5),* 817–819.

O'Brien, C.P. (1996). Drug addiction and drug abuse. In J.G. Hardman, L.E. Limbird, P.B. Molinoff, R.W. Rudden & A.G. Gilman (Eds.), *The Pharmacological Basis of Therapeutics,* (9th edition). New York/ Toronto: McGraw-Hill Health Professions Division.

Schwartz, R.H. (1995). LSD. Its rise, fall, and renewed popularity among high school students. *Pediatric Clinics of North America, 42 (2),* 403–413.

Smart, R.G., Adlaf, E.M., Walsh, G.W. & Zdanowicz, Y.M. (1992). *Drifting and Doing: Changes in Drug Use Among Toronto Street Youth, 1990 and 1992.* Toronto: Addiction Research Foundation.

Ungerleider, J.T. & Pechnick, R.N. (1992). Hallucinogens. In J.H. Lowinson, P. Ruiz, R.B. Millman & J.G. Langrod (Eds.), *Substance Abuse — A Comprehensive Textbook* (2nd edition). Baltimore: Williams and Wilkins.

MDA
(Methylenedioxyamphetamine)

DRUG CLASS: Hallucinogen with Stimulant Properties

Synopsis

MDA (3,4-methylenedioxyamphetamine) is a hallucinogenic drug with properties similar to those of both LSD and the amphetamines.[1] Because it is alleged to produce emotional closeness to others, serenity and relaxation, street users have termed it the "love drug." However, in higher doses MDA has been associated with serious adverse effects, including death. There is no medical use for MDA, although it was investigated for use in facilitating psychotherapy. MDA was widely used in North America until its restriction by law in the late 1960s in Canada and the early 1970s in the United States.

Drug Source

MDA is produced through chemical synthesis, almost exclusively in illicit laboratories.

Trade Names

Not applicable.

Street Names

Love drug. MDA was also known as "ecstasy" until the emergence of MDMA as a street drug in the 1980s.

---

[1]   MDA is a member of the family of hallucinogenic drugs sometimes referred to as the ring-substituted amphetamines.

Combination Products

None known.

Medical Uses

There are no approved medical uses for MDA. It was patented in 1956 as a cough suppressant and in 1961 as an anorexiant (i.e., diet aid), although apparently it was never used clinically for such purposes. MDA was used as an adjunct to psychotherapy and a few anecdotal reports and open trials were reported in the medical literature in the 1960s and early 1970s. Therapeutic use stopped when MDA was classified as a restricted substance and rendered effectively illegal.

Physical Appearance

MDA hydrochloride in its pure form is a white powder, but on the street it ranges from white through yellow to brown depending on its state of purity.

Dosage[2]

Medical
Not applicable.

Non-medical
Typically 100 to 200 mg.

Routes of Administration

MDA is usually taken orally.

---

[2]   All doses refer to adults.

Effects of Short-Term Use: Low to Moderate Doses[3]

While increasing doses in the low to moderate range generally result in correspondingly greater intensity of effects, users may have individual differences in sensitivity. Subjective experiences vary among individual users, possibly as a result of factors such as the user's mental attitude and expectations. The short-term use of low to moderate doses of MDA can result in the following effects.

CNS, *behavioral, subjective*: feelings of peacefulness, tranquillity, joy, empathy and emotional closeness to others (hence the street name "love drug"); aesthetic enjoyment; intuitive insight and a heightened state of consciousness, self-awareness and increased spirituality.

At moderate doses, MDA's effects tend to approximate those of LSD even more closely, but do not include its hallucinations and perceptual distortions. Intensification of feelings, heightened but not distorted sensory awareness, spontaneous recalling of events long past and a belief of greater awareness and self-insight are among the more commonly reported effects.

Mild to moderate adverse effects include confusion, fatigue, anxiety or panic, and decreased concentration.

Additional effects include decreased appetite, dilation of the pupils, periodic tensing of the neck and jaw muscles, and, at moderate doses, teeth grinding.

***Cardiovascular*:** increased blood pressure and heart rate.

***Gastrointestinal*:** dryness of the mouth, throat and nose.

***Other*:** increased body temperature and sweating.

---

3   Single doses between 60 and 150 mg.

Effects of Short-Term Use: Higher Doses[4]

At high doses, many symptoms produced by MDA are similar to those of the major amphetamines at high doses.

Certain hallucinogens, such as LSD, are relatively benign in terms of their physical effects, even at higher doses. In contrast, high single doses of MDA have been observed to produce undesirable and/or very harmful effects in some users. Short-term use of high doses of MDA can result in the following effects.

CNS, behavioral, subjective: widely dilated and non-reactive pupils; twitching of the lips; rigid extension of the neck and extremities; hyperactive deep-tendon reflexes; extreme reflex hyperexcitability to auditory, visual and tactile stimuli; agitation; hallucinations; delirium; seizures and coma.

Cardiovascular: rapid pulse; disseminated intravascular coagulation (an acute life-threatening blood coagulation disorder).

Respiratory: labored breathing associated with muscle spasm; respiratory distress syndrome.

Other: erection of body hair, very high body temperature, profuse sweating and rhabdomyolysis (breakdown of muscle tissue).

Effects of Long-Term Use

Effects of long-term use are not known. Repeated MDA use in animals causes destruction of certain brain cells. The dose that produces this effect is only about twice as large as the hallucinogenic dose in humans. As a result, there is the possibility of neurotoxicity in humans. A particular problem in gathering accurate information about the specific effects of chronic MDA abuse is that many people who use MDA are also likely to use other drugs concurrently.

---

4   Doses of 300 to 500 mg have produced these effects in some users.

Lethality

Deaths associated with MDA use have been documented in the medical literature, including a report of five deaths in Ontario. Such deaths have resulted from seizures, hyperthermia, disseminated intravascular coagulation and cardiac arrest.

Tolerance and Dependence

Little information is available regarding the development of tolerance to and/or dependence on MDA. Clinical investigation of the effects of MDA on humans has been quite limited.

Patterns of Use

MDA appeared as a recreational drug in the 1960s, and was known as the "love drug." It was widely used in the United States until it was restricted in 1973. It has been a restricted drug in Canada since 1969. The current extent of use of MDA is unknown.

Potential for Abuse

Abuse Liability
The abuse liability of MDA is unknown. In laboratory studies, animals have been shown to continue to infuse themselves with MDA, which suggests that the drug has some reinforcing properties.

Inherent Harmfulness
In the low to moderate dose range, adverse effects tend to be relatively mild. However, higher doses may produce significantly hazardous effects including neurotoxicity and fatal reactions.

Availability
The popularity of MDA appears to have waned with the emergence of MDMA, which now appears to be more widely used as a street drug.

Background Reading

Buchanan, J.F. & Brown, C.R. (1988). "Designer drugs": A problem in clinical toxicology. *Medical Toxicology, 3,* 1-17.

Cimbura, G. (1972). 3,4-Methylenedioxyamphetamine (MDA): Analytical and forensic aspects of fatal poisoning. *Journal of Forensic Science, 17,* 329-333.

Climko, R.P., Roehrich, H., Sweeney, D.R., Al-Razi, J. (1987). Ecstasy: A review of MDMA and MDA. *International Journal of Psychiatry in Medicine, 16 (4),* 359–372.

Davis, W.M., Hatoum, H.T. & Waters, I.W. (1987). Toxicity of MDA (3,4-methylenedioxyamphetamine) considered for relevance to hazards of MDMA (ecstasy) abuse. *Alcohol and Drug Research, 7,* 123–134.

Naranjo, D., Shulgan, A.T. & Sargent, T. (1967). Evaluation of 3,4-methylenedioxyamphetamine (MDA) as an adjunct to psychotherapy. *Medicina et Pharmacologia. Experimentalis (International Journal of Experimental Medicine), 17,* 359–364.

Richards, K.C. & Borgstedt, H.H. (1971). Near fatal reaction to ingestion of the hallucinogenic drug MDA. Journal of the American Medical Association, *218 (12),* 1826-1827.

Riedlinger, T.J. & Reidlinger, J.E. (1994). Psychedelic and entactogenic drugs in the treatment of depression. *Journal of Psychoactive Drugs, 26 (1),* 41-55.

MDMA
("Ecstasy"; 3,4 methylenedioxymethamphetamine)

DRUG CLASS: Hallucinogen with Stimulant Properties

Synopsis

MDMA ("ecstasy") is one of a number of hallucinogens related to amphetamine.[1] Often called a "designer drug," MDMA has actually been "rediscovered" by producers of designer drugs. (For more information on "designer drugs," see the chapter on hallucinogens in Section 2.) MDMA was first produced (but not marketed) by pharmaceutical researchers in 1912, as an appetite suppressant. It was not until the 1970s that the drug was used in a few cases to facilitate psychotherapy. In the 1980s, MDMA gained popularity as a recreational drug, and the emergence of MDMA for sale on the street resulted in its complete restriction in the United States in 1985. MDMA has been a restricted drug in Canada since 1976.

Drug Source

MDMA is produced through chemical synthesis in both clandestine and authorized research laboratories.

Trade Names

Not applicable.

---

[1]   These hallucinogens are sometimes referred to as ring-substituted amphetamines.

Street Names

Ecstasy, XTC, Adam, euphoria, X, MDM, M&M, rave, hug drug.

Combination Products

Mixing other drugs, especially LSD, with MDMA is referred to as "candy-flipping." The combination of MDMA and LSD may also be referred to as "X & L."

Medical Uses

There is no approved medical use for MDMA.

Physical Appearance

MDMA is sold illegally as a loose white powder or in gelatin capsules or tablets.

Dosage[2]

Medical
Not applicable.

Non-medical
MDMA is generally taken in doses of 50 to 200 mg.

Routes of Administration

MDMA is usually taken orally.

---

[2]   All doses refer to adults.

Effects of Short-Term Use: Low to Moderate Doses

CNS, *behavioral, subjective*: mild intoxication; euphoria; a great sense of pleasure, emotional insight or empathy; enhanced self-esteem; increased sociability or closeness and communication with others (also described as the opposite of paranoia); mild alterations in visual perception (not true hallucinations); blurred vision; depression and/or anxiety and panic attacks.

Cardiovascular: increased blood pressure and heart rate.

Gastrointestinal: loss of appetite, nausea and vomiting.

Other: muscle aches or stiffness, sweating, teeth grinding or jaw clenching.

Symptoms that may persist into the next day include insomnia, fatigue, sore jaw muscles, loss of balance and headache. Some users have reported symptoms of confusion, depression and anxiety lasting for several weeks after taking a single dose. There have also been reports of prolonged psychotic reactions.

As is the case with other drugs, MDMA's effects may be related to the underlying characteristics of the user, including psychological problems or heart disease.

MDMA and Psychotherapy

Prior to its classification as an illegal substance, a few psychotherapists in the United States used MDMA as an adjunct to psychotherapy. These clinicians/researchers reported that, by reducing the fear associated with exploring emotions, MDMA allowed patients to reassess aspects of their lives while maintaining feelings of security. Some users of MDMA claim that carefully planned experiences have provided lasting spiritual or therapeutic benefits without continued use of the drug. These reports are limited to a few uncontrolled trials and anecdotal reports.

It is worth remembering that other recognized drugs of abuse were once falsely reported to be safe and to possess tremendous therapeutic potential. Sigmund Freud, for example, endorsed the use of cocaine.

Concerns about the use of MDMA in humans are based on: (1) the potential neurotoxicity (damage to brain cells) caused by the drug and (2) the drug's chemical similarity to the already-restricted drug MDA (MDA is a metabolite of MDMA.) In 1985, the U.S. Drug Enforcement Agency placed MDMA in the most restricted drug category, a decision that generated considerable controversy. In Canada, MDMA has been a restricted drug since 1976. One result of this restriction has been difficulty in obtaining approval to conduct controlled clinical studies on the use of MDMA as a psychotherapeutic agent.

Effects of Short-Term Use: Higher Doses[3]

In addition to intensification of the low-dose effects described above, use of higher doses of MDMA may result in the following effects.

CNS, *subjective, behavioral*: possible neurotoxicity[4]; distortion of perception, thinking or memory; hallucinations and lasting psychological effects, such as anxiety or depression, in susceptible users.

In general, higher doses of MDMA do not appear to enhance the desirable effects; in other words, "more is not better."

Effects of Long-Term Use

The effects of long-term MDMA use in humans have not been well documented. Regular users have reported increased physical discomfort, or "hangovers," as well as weight loss, exhaustion, "flashbacks," irritability, paranoia, depression, psychosis and loss of desired drug effects. Repeated use may cause jaundice and liver damage. The neurotoxic effects discussed above are thought to be related to frequency of MDMA use.

---

[3]   These hallucinogens are sometimes referred to as ring-substituted amphetamines.

[4]   As mentioned above, controversy surrounds the possible neurotoxic effects of MDMA. The drug has been shown to have toxic effects on certain brain cells (the serotonergic system) in animals (including primates). This neurotoxicity appears to be dose- or frequency-related and some, but not complete, recovery occurs over several months. The dose required to produce this toxicity in animals is only two to four times the doses used in humans, and the resulting risk is perceived to be high enough to restrict use of the agent in human studies. It is not clear if this toxicity occurs in humans, although the possibility is supported by some preliminary evidence.

Lethality

MDMA has been implicated as a cause of death. The deaths reported have mostly been associated with kidney or cardiovascular failure induced by hyperthermia (dangerously high body temperature) and dehydration. MDMA users who participate in vigorous all-night dance sessions called "raves" may fail to drink enough fluids to replace those lost to the hot environment at these events, thus increasing their risk of toxicity from MDMA. There have been reports of the following conditions after physical exertion in combination with the use of MDMA:

- seizures

- hyperthermia

- disseminated intravascular coagulation (a life-threatening blood-clotting disorder)

- rhabdomyolysis (breakdown of muscle tissue)

- acute renal failure.

Other causes of MDMA-related deaths, including ventricular arrhythmia (abnormal heart rhythm) and liver failure, have also been reported. Other deaths have resulted from MDMA use in the presence of underlying conditions such as coronary heart disease, cardiomyopathy or other heart disease, or have occurred as a result of drug-related accidents. A few reported deaths were apparently caused by allergic reactions.

Tolerance and Dependence

It has been reported that with continued use, tolerance to MDMA develops rapidly. Some users increase their dosage over weeks or months of use. Little information is available regarding MDMA's ability to produce dependence or withdrawal symptoms once regular use has stopped.

Patterns of Use

There appear to be two types of MDMA users, distinguished by their reasons for using the drug. Many report that they use MDMA for therapeutic or spiritual reasons and claim to derive long-term benefits from even infrequent use of the drug. Others are more recreationally oriented and use MDMA for the euphoric experience. In the 1980s and 1990s, MDMA gained popularity as a recreational drug. There are reports of increasing frequency and size of "rave" parties where MDMA is used. Rave parties are a phenomenon that originally developed in England and spread to the United States after a clamp-down by British authorities. In Ontario, use of MDMA by students in grades 7 to 13[5] increased from 0.6 per cent in 1993 to 1.8 per cent in 1995.

Potential for Abuse

Abuse Liability

In animal studies, MDMA, unlike most other hallucinogens, was self-administered by the test animals, which indicates that the drug has some reinforcing properties. The rapid development of tolerance and the increase in unpleasant "after-effects" may be important in limiting long-term abuse of MDMA.

Inherent Harmfulness

Serious adverse reactions have been reported, but the incidence of these reactions relative to the extent of MDMA use is unknown. The influence of knowledge of the harmful effects of MDMA on the use of the drug is also unknown.

Availability

MDMA has been restricted since 1976 in Canada and since 1985 in the United States. However, MDMA is available illicitly, as evidenced by the number of students who reported having tried it.

---

[5]   The traditional "Grade 13" has now been replaced by an Ontario Academic Credit (OAC) year in most Ontario schools. However, the Ontario survey and thus this text, has retained the term "Grade 13" to facilitate comparison with surveys from previous years.

Background Reading

Beck, J. & Rosenbaum, M. (1994). *Pursuit of Ecstasy*. Albany: State University of New York Press.

Climko, R.P., Roehrich, H., Sweeney, D.R. & Al-Razi, J. (1987). Ecstasy: A review of MDMA and MDA. *International Journal of Psychiatry in Medicine, 16 (4)*, 359–372.

Dowling, G.P., McDonough, E.T. & Bost, R.O. (1987). "Eve" and "Ecstasy": A report on five deaths associated with the use of MDEA and MDMA. *Journal of the American Medical Association, 257 (12)*, 1615-1617.

Fahal, I, Sallomi, D.F., Yaqoob, M. & Bell, G.M. (1992). Acute renal failure after ecstasy. *British Medical Journal, 305*, 29.

Fidler, H., Dhillon, A., Gertner, D. & Burroughs, A. (1996). Chronic ecstasy (3,4 methylene-dioxymethamphetamine) abuse: A recurrent and unpredictable cause of severe acute hepatitis. *Journal of Hepatology, 25 (4)*, 563-566.

Henry, J.A., Jeffreys, K.J. & Sawiling, S. (1993). *The Lancet, 340*, 384-387.

McCann, U.D. & Ricaurte, G.A. (1991). Lasting neuropsychiatric sequelae of (+/-) methylene-dioxymethamphetamine ("Ecstasy") in recreational users. *Journal of Clinical Psychopharmacology, 11*, 302–305.

Milroy, C.M., Clark, J.C. & Forrest, A.R. (1996). Pathology of deaths associated with "ecstasy" and "eve" misuse. *Journal of Clinical Pathology, 49 (2)*, 149–153.

Randall, T. (1992). Ecstasy-fueled "rave" parties become dances of death for English youths. *Journal of the American Medical Association, 268 (12)*, 1505–1506.

Riedlinger, T.J. & Reidlinger, J.E. (1994). Psychedelic and entactogenic drugs in the treatment of depression. *Journal of Psychoactive Drugs, 26 (1)*, 41–55.

Screaton, G.R., Cairns, H.S., Sarner, M., Singer, M., Thrasher, A. & Cohen, S.L. (1992). Hyperpyrexia and rhabdomyolysis after MDMA ("ecstasy") abuse. *The Lancet, 399*, 667-668.

Watson, L. & Beck, J. (1991). New age seekers: MDMA use as an adjunct to spiritual pursuit. *Journal of Psychoactive Drugs, 23 (3)*, 261–270.

Meperidine

DRUG CLASS: Opioid

Synopsis

Meperidine (also called pethidine) is a synthetic opioid that acts on μ (mu) receptors. Its principal clinical use is to relieve moderate to severe pain. The analgesic potency of meperidine administered by injection is substantially less than that of morphine. However, meperidine is more efficiently absorbed than morphine after oral administration. Tolerance develops to its analgesic and, to some extent, respiratory-depressant effects.

Both physical and psychological dependence can develop with long-term use, even at low daily doses. When meperidine is chronically administered by injection, significant local irritation of tissue occurs and continued needle use may become increasingly painful. The principal toxic effects of meperidine when administered in high doses are respiratory depression and, to a lesser degree, circulatory depression. These toxic effects can be lethal. High doses given frequently may produce CNS (central nervous system) excitation, as evidenced by twitches, tremors and agitation and, in very high doses, in convulsions and hallucinations. For these reasons, and because the intensity of euphoria produced by meperidine is less than that of heroin or morphine, meperidine is usually not the drug of choice among street users. However, because of its availability in health care settings, meperidine is a commonly reported drug of abuse among health care workers who are dependent on opioids.

Drug Source

Meperidine is produced through chemical synthesis by the pharmaceutical industry.

Alternative Non-Proprietary/Generic Names

Pethidine, isonipecaine.

Trade Names

Demerol®.

Street Names

None in common use.

Medical Uses

The primary medical use of meperidine is for relief from moderate to severe pain, including pain associated with childbirth and dental procedures.

Physical Appearance

In pure form, meperidine occurs as tiny white crystals that are very soluble in water and soluble in alcohol. Meperidine is slightly bitter to the taste.

Dosage[1,2]

Medical

Meperidine is used clinically for relief of pain at doses of 50 to 150 mg administered orally or by subcutaneous or intramuscular (or occasionally intravenous) injection, at three- to four-hour intervals as necessary.

---

[1]   All doses refer to adults.

[2]   Meperidine hydrochloride 75 to 100 mg administered parenterally is approximately equal in analgesic potency to morphine 10 mg injected intramuscularly.

Non-medical

Typical single doses for a chronic abuser may exceed 200 to 300 mg, and drug use may occur as frequently as every three hours or less. Use of as much as 3 to 4 grams per day has been reported.

Routes of Administration

Orally or by subcutaneous, intramuscular or intravenous injection (the last route is preferred by many abusers).

Effects of Short-Term Use: Low Doses[3]

CNS, behavioral, subjective: Effects of meperidine use include suppression of the sensation of pain and of emotional response to it (with slightly faster onset and slightly shorter duration than with morphine); euphoria; some clouding of mental function; drowsiness; lightheadedness; dizziness; in some cases, mild depression, anxiety and agitation; visual disturbances.

Cardiovascular: increased or decreased heart rate, drop in blood pressure.

Respiratory: reduction in respiratory rate.

Gastrointestinal: dry mouth, nausea, vomiting, constipation, spasm of smooth muscles in the biliary tract, loss of appetite.[4]

Other: sweating, itchy or prickly skin, urinary retention, reduced libido.

---

[3] Single doses within the therapeutic range administered orally or by injection to non-tolerant users.

[4] Smooth muscle spasms and constipation may be less severe with meperidine than with doses of morphine that provide the same level of pain relief.

Effects of Short-Term Use: Higher Doses[5]

Intensification of meperidine's low-dose effects may occur with administration of higher doses. As the dose increases, the following symptoms may be experienced:

- decreased sensitivity to painful stimuli

- sleepiness

- inability to concentrate

- progressively slower and more shallow breathing

- slower heart rate and lower blood pressure

- at higher doses, especially at frequent intervals, CNS excitation evidenced in muscle twitches and tremors, and agitation.

At very high doses (i.e., overdose), meperidine can produce disorientation, hallucinations, convulsions, deep sleep possibly progressing to stupor or coma, shallow and markedly slowed breathing, slow heart rate, low blood pressure, cyanosis, low body temperature, flaccidity of skeletal muscles, and cold and clammy skin.

Effects of Long-Term Use

Chronic subcutaneous injection of meperidine is both considerably more painful and more irritating than that of most other common opioid analgesics. Round scars on the skin and numerous hardened areas beneath the skin are commonly observed on the arms of abusers of injectable meperidine. Despite the discomfort associated with chronic needle use, users must administer the drug more often than do heroin- or morphine-dependent users, as the duration of action of meperidine is shorter. Withdrawal symptoms may begin as early as three hours after the last dose.

Users of high daily doses of one to three grams (1,000 to 3,000 mg) of meperidine often experience persistent muscular twitches and tremors, hyperactive reflexes, exaggerated startle responses, agitation, and sometimes seizures and toxic psychosis (including hallucinations).

---

[5]   Single doses above the therapeutic range in non-tolerant users, or lower doses in particularly sensitive individuals.

Other effects resulting from long-term use of meperidine are mild and similar to those produced by most other opioid analgesics.

Lethality

Severe overdose, particularly after intravenous injection, can result in very slow, shallow and irregular breathing, circulatory collapse, cardiac arrest and death from respiratory arrest. The lethal dose for a non-tolerant adult is estimated to be one gram (1,000 mg).

Tolerance and Dependence

Tolerance

Tolerance to the analgesic effect of meperidine develops with repeated, frequent use. Those who abuse the drug for these effects must, therefore, frequently increase their daily dose. Tolerance to meperidine's respiratory-depressant effects also develops to some extent, but even after protracted use of high doses, tolerance to its CNS excitation effects does not appear to develop.

Physical Dependence/Withdrawal

Physical and psychological dependence can develop with frequent use, even at low daily doses. However, the severity of dependence increases with chronicity of use and with increasingly higher daily doses. Withdrawal symptoms begin earlier after the last dose and have a shorter duration than withdrawal associated with morphine or heroin. Early withdrawal symptoms (as soon as three hours after the last dose) typically include restlessness, muscle twitches, sweating and anxiety. These symptoms peak in intensity within eight to 12 hours. In some cases the symptoms may be as severe as in morphine withdrawal, but may involve less nausea, vomiting and diarrhea. The intensity of symptoms declines gradually, and they usually disappear by the fourth or fifth day.

Psychological Dependence

The impact of long-term dependence on meperidine (and other opioids) is often observable long after the classic signs of withdrawal have disappeared. Depression, anxiety, insomnia, loss of appetite, agitation and a craving for the drug may persist for extended periods. Although such symptoms have often been interpreted as indications of psychological dependence, they are likely associated with complex physiological adjustments after withdrawal.

Patterns of Use

Meperidine is widely used in health care settings for relief of severe pain, and this availability has made it subject to abuse by health care workers. Its use in oral tablet form for pain control in patients treated in community settings allows for its potential diversion to the illicit market.

Potential for Abuse

Dependence Liability

Meperidine can produce drug dependence similar to that produced by morphine, although its effects profile may make its abuse somewhat less likely. When meperidine is administered intravenously, its effects are experienced more rapidly than those of morphine, but both its euphoric potency and analgesic potency are considerably less. However, when administered orally, meperidine retains a greater degree of its potency than many other common opioid analgesics, including morphine and heroin.

Inherent Harmfulness

Because meperidine is highly irritating to local tissue when injected, chronic needle administration can be very painful to the user. Furthermore, when meperidine is abused in high daily doses, very harmful effects such as agitation, toxic psychosis and convulsions can occur.

Availability

Although commonly used in hospitals (and to a lesser degree by patients treated in community settings), meperidine is infrequently encountered on the street. It appears that the relatively moderate degree of euphoria produced by meperidine together with its inherently harmful effects when abused make it less appealing to street users than other opioid analgesics.

Background Reading

Canadian Pharmaceutical Association. (1997). *Compendium of Pharmaceuticals and Specialties.* (32nd edition). Ottawa: Canadian Pharmaceutical Association.

Kaiko, R.F., Foley, K.M., Grabinski, P.Y., Heidrich, G., Rogers, A.G., Inturrisi, C.E. & Reidenberg, M.M. (1983). Central nervous system excitatory effects of meperidine in cancer patients. *Annals of Neurology, 13 (2)*, 100–185.

Reisine, T. & Pasternak, G. (1996). Opioid analgesics and antagonists. (Chapter 23). In J.G. Hardman, L.E. Limbird, P.B. Molinoff, R.W. Rudden & A.G. Gilman (Eds.), *Goodman and Gilman's The Pharmacological Basis of Therapeutics* (9th edition). New York/Toronto: McGraw-Hill Health Professions Division.

Mescaline

DRUG CLASS: Hallucinogen

Synopsis

Mescaline is a naturally occurring hallucinogen derived from the Mexican peyote cactus (*Lophophora williamsii*) and the San Pedro cactus found in Peru and Ecuador. This drug produces a spectrum of effects similar to those of LSD and psilocybin, including vivid visual "pseudohallucinations" and distortions (which are known to the user to be unreal) and synesthesias (the paradoxical melding of the senses so that, for example, music may appear to be "seen"). Alterations in the perception of time, space and body image also frequently occur.

The individual's emotional response to these psychic effects may range from joy and exhilaration to extreme anxiety and even terror. There is no way to accurately predict how any user will react to mescaline on any given occasion. Even seasoned users who usually experience the desired pleasant effects may at times experience intense distress.

Mescaline has been used for centuries for its alleged propensity to induce profound mystical experiences. Until recently, members of the Native American Church had the legal right to use mescaline-containing peyote in a religious ritual, but a 1990 decision by the U.S. Supreme Court gave states the right to prohibit such religious use.

The legendary reputation of this drug is the principal reason for the widespread practice on the street of selling other drugs such as PCP (phencyclidine) or LSD as mescaline. In fact, mescaline is rarely found outside Mexico and the southwestern United States.

Drug Source

Mescaline naturally occurs in the peyote cactus, *Lophophora williamsii,* which is found in Mexico and parts of the southwestern United States, and the San Pedro cactus, found in Peru and Ecuador. It can also be produced in a laboratory by chemical synthesis.

Trade Names

Not applicable.

Drug Combinations

Peyote (peiotl) buttons, which contain mescaline, also contain more than a dozen other alkaloids including a respiratory stimulant, a reflex excitant and a convulsant.

A combination of mescaline, LSD and cannabis has occasionally been used in some areas of North America. Its street name is TMA.[1]

Medical Uses

There is no current medical use for mescaline. In the past, researchers had explored the possibility of using the drug in facilitating psychotherapy.

Physical Appearance

In its pure form, mescaline sulphate is a white crystalline material. Synthetic mescaline often appears as a white or colored powder. "Organic" or "natural" mescaline is the name sometimes used to describe dried, ground peyote buttons, which are usually distributed in capsule form. On the street, however, preparations alleged to be natural

---

[1] The name "TMA" is an acronym based on the constituents tetrahydrocannabinol (from cannabis), mescaline and acid (i.e., LSD). However, the drug trimethoxyamphetamine, a synthetic hallucinogen related to MDA, is also known as TMA.

mescaline have almost invariably been found to be some other drug such as LSD and/or PCP, which are sometimes combined with ground seeds or other plant material.

Routes of Administration

Mescaline is most frequently administered orally in the form of a powder, tablet, capsule or liquid. Peyote buttons, although they have a very unpleasant taste, can be chewed to obtain the desired effects. Peyote buttons are sometimes ground and smoked with a leaf material, such as cannabis or tobacco. In its pure form, mescaline can be injected in solution, but this route is used much less frequently than the oral route.

Dosage[2]

Medical
Not applicable.

Non-medical
The usual oral dose of mescaline ranges between 300 and 500 mg (approximately equivalent to the amount contained in three to six peyote buttons). This dose level produces effects roughly similar to those of 50 to 100 micrograms (0.05 to 0.1 mg) of LSD or 10 to 20 mg of psilocybin.

Effects of Short-Term Use[3]

The short-term use of mescaline produces the following effects.

CNS, behavioral, subjective: Mescaline produces perceptual, cognitive and emotional experiences that vary widely among users. Drug effects are influenced by the

---

2   All doses refer to adults.

3   Three hundred to 500 mg taken orally by non-tolerant users. The chemical structure of mescaline bears a resemblance to norepinephrine and amphetamines. At hallucinogenic doses the somatic symptoms produced by mescaline are similar to those produced by small amounts of these substances. At higher doses there may be reduced blood pressure and heart and respiratory rate. Psychic effects at higher doses tend to be more intense.

size of the dose, the setting and the user's expectations, personality and past drug experiences. It is not unusual for the user to experience differing reactions to mescaline during different drug-taking episodes. Early somatic effects[4] can include numbness, tension and anxiety, rapid reflexes, muscle twitches and muscle weakness, impaired motor co-ordination, tremulousness, dizziness and dilation of the pupils. Later effects can include the following.

- Users may experience vivid perceptual (primarily visual) distortions, such as "pseudohallucinations" and "pseudoillusions," which they know to be unreal. Often the user "sees" brightly colored lights, geometric patterns, animals or occasionally humans.

- The user's perception of time may be distorted (minutes may seem to pass as slowly as hours).

- Space perception may be distorted.

- Users' perceptions of their bodies may be distorted. Some users feel heavy and "pulled down" by gravity, while others experience sensations of weightlessness and floating.

- Synesthesias, in which one sensory modality is melded with another, occur frequently. For example, users may think they can "see" music or "hear" colors.

- Users may experience a partial or complete loss of recognized boundaries between self and the environment, which may produce reactions ranging from intense pleasure to terror.

- All sensory experiences tend to be heightened. Users experience brighter colors, sharper definition of objects, increased hearing acuity, more sharply distinguished taste and so on. These heightened experiences may alternate with sensory impairment.

- Users often experience difficulties in concentrating, thinking and maintaining attention.

- Although memory may also be impaired, it is not unusual for past and possibly repressed experiences to be vividly recalled and sometimes melded with current experiences. The user's sense of the present reality (the "here and now") may also be temporarily lost.

---

4   Occurring within the first hour after administration.

- Users may be preoccupied with otherwise trivial thoughts, experiences or objects, which take on magnified importance.

- Users may feel that they are undergoing a profound mystical, religious or "cosmic" experience, which for many may be the most desired effect.

- Some users may experience a highly adverse reaction, or "bad trip," characterized by the following symptoms: frightening hallucinations, confusion, disorientation, fear of non-existence or disintegration of self, inability to distinguish between reality and unreality, paranoid thinking, possibly severe agitation and/or depression, and panic or even terror.

These subjective effects of mescaline are experienced within one to two hours and typically disappear gradually 10 to 12 hours after administration.

Physical effects of the short-term use of mescaline can include the following.

Cardiovascular: increased blood pressure and heart rate.

Gastrointestinal: intense nausea and vomiting and suppression of appetite are extremely common early effects.

Other: Early effects include elevated body temperature and sweating, which may alternate with chills and shivering.

Effects of Long-Term Use

Because of the rapid development of tolerance to the effects of mescaline, chronic daily use is very unlikely (see Tolerance and Dependence, below).

Animals subjected to regular administration of mescaline have shown an increased risk of birth defects in their offspring. However, preliminary research on the frequency of chromosomal abnormalities in Mexican Indians did not find any significant differences between those who traditionally use peyote and those who do not.

Mescaline has occasionally precipitated a protracted psychotic state similar to paranoid schizophrenia. However, some observers have suggested that this is likely to occur only in those users who were latent psychotics prior to the psychosis-inducing event.

Lethality

Although very high doses of mescaline can produce severe, but temporary, sensory disturbances, no reports of life-threatening effects have been directly attributable to the drug. However, PCP or PCP/LSD combinations are frequently sold as mescaline. In severe overdose, these drugs can result in death. The dramatic increase in heart rate and blood pressure associated with mescaline use might be also expected to be life-threatening to individuals with pre-existing cardiovascular problems.

Tolerance and Dependence

Tolerance to the effects of mescaline develops rapidly with repeated daily use of hallucinogenic doses of mescaline, ordinarily within three to six days.[5] Cross-tolerance to such other hallucinogenic drugs as LSD and psilocybin also occurs. As a result, without a period of abstinence from mescaline and these other drugs, no amount of any of them will produce the desired effects in the tolerant user. After several days of abstinence, however, the desired sensitivity is restored.

There is currently no evidence of physical dependence (i.e., of a withdrawal syndrome upon cessation of use). While psychological dependence is possible, it has not been reported.

Patterns of Use

Mescaline is a name frequently mentioned on the street drug market, but real mescaline is rarely available in most areas of North America. Drug analyses by Canadian and U.S. laboratories reveal that an overwhelming percentage of alleged mescaline samples are actually such other drugs as PCP or PCP/LSD combinations. Therefore, the apparently increasing use of mescaline reported by North American adolescents in surveys (e.g., in adolescent treatment programs and student populations) must be interpreted with caution.

---

[5]   See the discussion of tolerance and tachyphylaxis in Section 1.

Although ingestion of mescaline-containing peyote is a traditional ritual of the Native American Church of North America, which claims to have approximately 250,000 members of Native American ancestry in the United States and Canada, the U.S. Supreme Court ruled in 1990 that states may prohibit the use of peyote for religious purposes.

Potential for Abuse

Dependence on mescaline is not known to occur, and whatever harm the drug may cause does not appear to be a significant deterrent to its use.[6] As the drug is rarely available in most North American communities, its abuse potential is currently extremely low.

Background Reading

Adlaf, E.M., Ivis, F.J. & Smart, R.G. (1997). *Ontario Student Drug Use Survey 1977-1997*. Toronto: Addiction Research Foundation.

Bullis, R.K. (1990). Swallowing the scroll: Legal implications of the recent Supreme Court peyote cases. *Journal of Psychoactive Drugs, 22 (3)*, 325–332.

Dorrance, D.L., Janiger, O. & Teplitz, R.L. (1975). Effect of peyote on human chromosomes. *Journal of the American Medical Association, 234*, 299–313.

Schultes, R.E. & Hofmann, A. (1980). *The Botany and Chemistry of Hallucinogens*. (2nd edition). Springfield, IL: Charles C. Thomas Publisher.

Schwartz, R.H. (1988). Mescaline: A survey. *American Family Physician, 37 (4)*, 122–124.

Ungerleider, J.T. & Pechnick, R.N. (1992). Hallucinogens. In J.H. Lowinson, P. Ruiz, R.B. Millman & J.G. Langrod (Eds.), *Substance Abuse — A Comprehensive Textbook* (2nd edition). Baltimore: Williams and Wilkins.

---

6   Nonetheless, there is some danger of a psychotic reaction in a small percentage of users.

Methadone

DRUG CLASS: Opioid

Synopsis

Methadone is a synthetic opioid similar in potency to morphine. For medical purposes it has certain advantages over the opioids morphine and heroin. Because the effects of methadone are longer lasting, it can be administered less frequently, and since it is highly effective when administered orally, methadone is more convenient to use. Moreover, because it is administered orally, methadone presents less of a risk that users will associate its effects with the ritual-like injection of drugs. These factors explain why methadone is used widely to treat opioid dependence. In methadone maintenance programs, an oral methadone preparation is substituted for the user's usual opioid(s) to allow dependent users to achieve more productive lifestyles and avoid medical complications of drug use, such as AIDS, hepatitis and endocarditis.

Unfortunately, methadone has a high dependence liability. In the past it was subject to widespread abuse, and deaths among street users were attributed to methadone overdose. More recently, however, strict controls — over the production of methadone preparations, which are difficult to use by injection, and over their distribution — appear to have resulted in considerably less street abuse. Nonetheless, because even oral preparations of methadone, if taken in sufficient amounts, can suppress withdrawal symptoms resulting from abrupt abstinence from heroin (or other powerful opioids) use, they continue to retain value to the street drug abuser.

Drug Source

Methadone is produced through chemical synthesis by the pharmaceutical industry.

Trade Names

In Canada, methadone is marketed under its non-proprietary name.

Street Names

Dollies (from the trade name Dolophine® under which it is marketed in some countries, but not in Canada), meth.[1]

Combination Products

Experimental oral combinations containing methadone and an opioid antagonist[2] such as naloxone have been tested in clinical trials. When this combination is taken orally, the opioid antagonist is ineffective, but when it is injected, the opioid antagonist almost immediately causes a withdrawal reaction. Such combination products are designed to be useless if diverted to the street market for injectable methadone.

Benzodiazepines, cocaine, opioids and alcohol are among the drugs most frequently abused by methadone maintenance patients. Many such patients report that large doses of benzodiazepines in combination with methadone produce a "high" or an enhanced methadone effect.

Medical Uses

Methadone is used clinically as a substitute drug in opioid dependence therapy and as a long-acting analgesic for moderately severe to severe pain.

---

[1]   It is important to note that the term "meth" is also used in some circles as a short-hand term for methamphetamine.

[2]   See the chapter on naloxone in Section 3.

Physical Appearance

In pure form methadone is a white crystalline powder that is soluble in water and freely soluble in alcohol. When used in opioid dependence programs it is usually dissolved in an orange-flavored drink.

Dosage[3]

Medical[4]

The dose range for a single oral administration for relief of pain is 5 to 15 mg. The dose range for subcutaneous injection is usually 5 to 10 mg. As an analgesic, methadone's potency is similar to that of morphine; 7.5 to 10 mg of methadone have an equivalent analgesic effect to 10 mg of morphine.

Methadone Maintenance Programs[5]

The dose levels of methadone used in methadone maintenance programs have varied considerably over time. In initial methadone trials, daily doses considerably in excess of 100 mg for stabilized clients were deemed appropriate. The rationale was to achieve a methadone level that would serve as a "blockade" against the effects of any supplementary opioid such as heroin, which the client might use contrary to program rules. Later, so-called low-dose methadone programs were developed, in which doses were typically in the range of 40 mg.

Many existing programs have developed a more flexible approach in which the clinical team's perception of client needs rather than fixed program rules determines the maximum dose level. The initial oral daily dose is typically quite low, often 15 to 30 mg, usually taken as a single dose. The daily dose is gradually increased as tolerance develops and as the client's symptoms and signs are monitored, until a stabilization (or maintenance) dose level is achieved. Thereafter, the patient is typically maintained on a single daily oral dose at the stabilization level, without

---

3   All doses refer to adults.

4   In Canada, physicians must obtain authorization from Health Canada to prescribe methadone for pain relief.

5   In Canada, methadone may be prescribed for opioid maintenance treatment only by medical practitioners who have received special authorization from Health Canada.

further increases. Some clients do well on daily doses as low as 20 to 30 mg, but most are stabilized in the 50- to 120-mg range. Research suggests that clients receiving daily doses greater than 60 mg (and possibly 80 mg) are more likely to remain in treatment and to reduce or eliminate their use of illicit drugs.

Routes of Administration

Methadone as a maintenance drug for opioid-dependent individuals is usually formulated for oral administration in a fruit-flavored drink. Methadone prescribed for pain relief is administered orally or, less frequently, by subcutaneous injection. Abusers generally prefer intravenous injection if an injectable form is available.

Effects of Short-Term Use: Low Doses[6]

CNS, *behavioral, subjective*: Effects of methadone use include suppression of the sensation of and emotional response to pain, euphoria or anxiety, lightheadedness, dizziness, sedation, relaxation, weakness, drowsiness, pupillary constriction, impaired visual acuity and impaired night vision.

***Cardiovascular*:** flushing.

***Respiratory*:** slightly reduced respiratory rate.

***Gastrointestinal*:** nausea and vomiting, constipation, suppression of appetite and dry mouth.

***Other*:** sweating, slight drop in body temperature, reduced libido, itchy skin and urinary retention.

---

6   Single doses of 2.5 to 15 mg in non-tolerant users by subcutaneous injection, up to 45 mg per day; 15 to 30 mg initial oral daily doses in opioid-dependent individuals.

Effects of Short-Term Use: Higher Doses[7]

Intensification of methadone's low-dose effects may occur with administration of higher doses. Duration of effects also increases with progressively higher doses. As the dose increases, the user's sensitivity and emotional response to painful stimuli decrease; the probability of sleep increases; the ability to concentrate is progressively impaired; breathing becomes progressively slower and more shallow; the heart rate gradually slows and blood pressure decreases.

At very high doses (i.e., overdose), markedly shallow and slow breathing, deep sleep possibly progressing to stupor or coma, pinpoint pupils, cyanosis, flaccidity of skeletal muscles, low blood pressure, slow heart rate, and cold and clammy skin occur.

Deaths have been associated with initial doses of methadone exceeding 60 mg in non-tolerant patients. Some of these patients had chronic hepatitis, which probably limited their capacity to metabolize the drug to inactive compounds.

Effects of Long-Term Use

In North America, long-term use of methadone occurs mainly in methadone maintenance programs in the treatment of people who are physically dependent on opioids. Treatment facilities with a special licence or authorization provide dependent users with methadone as a substitute for such other opioids as heroin, morphine and oxycodone (e.g., in Percodan®). Users can be maintained on methadone for extended periods, in some cases for decades.

Methadone was selected for North American programs as the most appropriate drug because it possesses important advantages over most other opioid analgesics, including the following:

- Methadone is sufficiently potent to suppress the withdrawal symptoms of other powerful opioid analgesics.

---

[7] Doses above the medically recommended level in non-tolerant users, or lower doses in particularly sensitive individuals.

- In many users, methadone can also suppress chronic "drug hunger" (intense craving) for these other drugs. Some clinicians and researchers believe "drug hunger" to be the major reason why many dependent users relapse after periods of abstinence. Tolerance to methadone's ability to suppress craving does not appear to develop. Patients routinely report that an adequate maintenance dose of methadone helps them to feel "normal."

- Unlike many other powerful opioids, methadone administered orally retains much of its efficacy in relieving "drug hunger" and withdrawal symptoms, but does not produce euphoria in those users already tolerant to the euphoric effect of other powerful opioids.[8]

- Methadone's effectiveness when administered orally helps to extinguish gratification previously associated with needle administration.

- Methadone has a longer period of action than most other common powerful opioids, and therefore can be administered less frequently. In most cases a single daily dose (usually between 50 and 120 mg) is sufficient.

- Long-term maintenance on methadone does not appear to produce any significant health problems other than physical dependence and chronic constipation. On the contrary, health often improves when needle use is terminated.

Methadone maintenance programs that provide methadone in combination with counselling have proven to be effective in improving the quality of life in individual patients. The longer patients remain in treatment, the fewer crimes they commit, the more likely they are to be employed, the less likely they are to be receiving social assistance, the less likely they are to suffer from serious medical conditions, the less likely they are to use illicit opioids and the less dysfunctional are their families.[9]

However, some unpleasant side effects are directly associated with chronic methadone use. These include constipation, pupillary constriction (which may impair night vision), blurred vision, excessive sweating, reduced libido, menstrual irregularity, urinary retention, sleep disturbance, certain types of respiratory impairment and occasionally pains in the joints and bones.

---

8   A result of the high degree of cross-tolerance among opioids.

9   Methadone maintenance programs are not without their critics. These criticisms are discussed in the chapter on opioid analgesics and antagonists in Section 2.

In some methadone treatment programs clients who have achieved stability in their life are gradually withdrawn (i.e., tapered) from methadone. The purpose of this dose tapering is to help the methadone-dependent client achieve a drug-free state without suffering the distress of abrupt withdrawal. However, many tapering clients find that they experience extreme discomfort (withdrawal symptoms) in the final stages of tapering, when their daily dose of methadone is reduced below 10 mg.

Methadone and Pregnancy

Methadone maintenance treatment can be used to improve the outcome of pregnancy in heroin-dependent women. The normally high rate of infant mortality in such cases, resulting from prematurity and low birth weight, is reduced in methadone-treated women. Lower rates of infant mortality among women in methadone treatment result from the avoidance of withdrawal-induced uterine contractions, improved prenatal care including counselling about smoking and nutrition, and anticipation of the need for intensive care of the newborn infant.

Within 72 hours of birth, infants exposed to methadone in the uterus experience a withdrawal syndrome characterized by irritability, sleep disturbances, tremors, poor feeding, vomiting and occasionally seizures. Although these signs may persist for several weeks or months, evidence suggests that there are no long-term effects. These neonatal withdrawal effects can be effectively treated by careful dosing with an opioid preparation such as morphine or paregoric.

Lethality

Symptoms of methadone overdose include coma, cyanosis, pinpoint pupils, severe respiratory depression and circulatory collapse. Death usually results from respiratory arrest, and in some cases from cardiac arrest.

The minimum lethal dose in non-tolerant adults is estimated to be 60 mg. Doses as small as 10 mg have been reported to be fatal to children. Because of these relatively low lethal dose levels, methadone maintenance program clients who have take-home dose privileges must be counselled carefully concerning safe storage of methadone in the home.

Overdose in methadone maintenance clients may result from use of excessive doses of methadone (although deaths in such cases are rare), or from injecting other opioids in an attempt to "shoot over" their methadone.

Tolerance and Dependence

Tolerance

When methadone is taken regularly in high doses by abusers, substantial tolerance to the euphoric, analgesic and sedating effects can develop rapidly, within one to two weeks. Therefore users must increase their daily dose just to maintain their subjectively pleasurable experiences. However, this rapid development of tolerance is a positive feature of methadone for maintenance programs: clients who are maintained at a stable dose level do not experience a "high," but only the absence of withdrawal symptoms. Tolerance to other effects develops more gradually with methadone than with morphine. These effects include nausea, loss of appetite, pupillary constriction, and particularly respiratory depression. Users develop a partial tolerance to methadone's constipating effects.

Physical Dependence/Withdrawal

Chronic high-dose use can lead to powerful physical and psychological dependence. Early symptoms of withdrawal after abrupt termination of use are usually not observed until 24 to 48 hours after the last dose. These include loss of appetite, insomnia, abdominal pain, flushing alternating with chills, excessive sweating, headache and pains in muscles and bones. Nausea and vomiting, as well as increases in body temperature, blood pressure, pulse, respiratory rate and pupillary size, also occur. The intensity of these symptoms peaks at 72 hours after the last administration and symptoms typically continue at this level for at least two weeks. The syndrome declines very gradually, and signs are no longer evident by about the sixth or seventh week.

When clients of methadone treatment programs are gradually withdrawn from methadone as part of their treatment plan, through periodic small reductions in daily dose (tapering), the withdrawal typically occurs over several months, and in some programs, up to a year. However, much more rapid withdrawal (i. e., over one to three weeks) has been widely employed in the United States, especially for young clients who are thought to be less heavily dependent on heroin or other opioids, and in many correctional facilities. In some treatment programs, clients who violate program rules, especially by use of street drugs, are withdrawn over a similar period prior to involuntary discharge. The recidivism rate among this latter group is exceptionally high (see Patterns of Use, below).

Psychological Dependence

After withdrawal from methadone is complete, users typically experience some craving for opioids that may persist indefinitely. In addition, many former users complain of fatigue, weakness, sleep disturbances, and anxiety and/or depression. Such symptoms are thought by some people to be indicative of psychological dependence. However, such an explanation may be an oversimplification. More research is needed into the possibly complex physiological adjustments that may result from opioid analgesic dependence and withdrawal.

Patterns of Use

In the early 1970s, in the core of large U.S. cities abuse of methadone via intravenous injection was extremely high. In fact, in 1973 the number of deaths believed to be related to methadone abuse in New York City exceeded the number of deaths attributed to heroin abuse. Since that time, however, with more stringent control over distribution and the greater use of methadone preparations that make injection less attractive, widespread street abuse has substantially diminished. Nevertheless, because of its considerable effectiveness in suppressing withdrawal from other opioids, methadone continues to be valued on the street.

In North America during the past two decades, hundreds of thousands of clients have been treated in programs that provide methadone maintenance and/or methadone-assisted withdrawal on either a rapid or gradual basis. A small fraction of these clients have been treated in Canada, where methadone treatment is provided almost exclusively on an outpatient basis. The number of Canadian programs and their total caseload grew quite rapidly in the early 1970s, but decreased in the late 1970s and early 1980s. However, these numbers increased again over the next decade. A number of factors appear to have influenced these shifts:

- Prior to 1972, abuse of methadone (diverted from licit sources) in Canada was found to be increasing. Primarily for this reason, the federal *Narcotic Control Act* was amended to place stricter controls over methadone's availability and use.

- Some physicians who originally prescribed methadone were disappointed by the results and/or frustrated by the problems and risks they faced in treating these clients, and turned to other approaches to treat heroin-dependent persons.

- After their initial excitement about a new treatment for opioid dependence, many patients were dissatisfied with methadone. They reasoned correctly that methadone, like heroin, is highly addictive, and that withdrawal from methadone can be even more difficult and protracted. Many also complained of methadone-associated constipation and loss of sex drive.

- Patients objected to what they viewed as excessively strict conditions imposed by some clinics, and also to staff who were inflexible and insensitive to their needs. Program staff, in turn, became frustrated with the behaviors of clients despite their clear statement of terms and conditions for treatment and the intensive counselling provided. Staff burn-out became a significant problem.

- Prior to the 1970s, most addicts chose to use heroin exclusively or almost exclusively, and they were heavily dependent on it. However, beginning in the early 1970s, both the availability and quality of street heroin began to decline, mainly due to greater police enforcement. Reduced heroin supplies resulted in a greater price for an inferior product. Users increasingly relied on other illicit substances to supplement their weak heroin habit. The extent of their physical dependence on heroin was thus not nearly so great as it had been in the past. Cocaine, in particular, gained favor among heroin users; however, its high cost left users with less money for heroin.

- However, after the assignment of large numbers of military personnel to Asia, and the increases in direct trade between opium-producing and North American countries, alternative methods were developed for importing higher-quality heroin. By the 1980s at least some populations of users had access to heroin of much higher purity; therefore once again a population of more heavily dependent clients emerged.

- As the philosophy of harm reduction began to take hold in Canada in the 1990s, new models of methadone treatment programming were developed, with less rigid rules concerning supplementary drug use. This not only created more client capacity, but made treatment more attractive to users who had complained about program rigidity.

- At the same time, the 1980s and '90s saw a new generation of physicians develop an interest in treating opioid-dependent patients, and a few developed practices specializing in the treatment of these patients.

In summary, the shifts in numbers of treatment programs and clients reflect changes in the numbers of opioid-dependent users, public and institutional policy, heroin availability, physician commitment to this population, and client acceptance of methadone as a treatment and of methadone program policies and procedures.

On average, patients in long-term methadone maintenance programs and gradual withdrawal programs (i.e., with periodic dose reductions planned over several months) remain in treatment for significantly longer periods than do patients in rapid withdrawal programs. Most data indicate a positive relationship between length of stay in methadone treatment and favorable outcome. (Favorable outcome is usually defined as remaining free of substance abuse, decreasing criminality and participating in productive activity such as employment or education.) However, caution is warranted in interpreting the results of treatment outcome studies: clients who remain in treatment for longer periods, and have more successful outcomes, may have quite different characteristics compared with those who drop out of treatment much earlier.

A recent study of pre-treatment characteristics as predictors of treatment outcome found that younger age and more serious legal problems were predictive of poorer performance and shorter stays in treatment. In contrast, severity of psychopathology was a strong predictor of good outcome in respect to overall substance use, and opioid use in particular, but not of retention in the program. One possible interpretation of this finding is that clients with psychiatric symptoms had been using opioids as self-medication, and that methadone filled this role. Two other findings of this study contrast with findings of other researchers, and require further investigation — that pre-treatment employment problems forecast less frequent opioid use, and that pre-treatment frequency of cocaine use is not a predictor of cocaine use in treatment.

Recent research has shown that clients receiving methadone maintenance treatment, even without counselling or with very little counselling, are more likely to be free of heroin, less likely to be involved in deviant criminal behavior and more likely to be employed than individuals receiving no treatment or only assisted withdrawal. More successful outcomes have been associated with methadone dose levels of more than 70 mg. One recent study found that outcomes are improved when a broader array of psychosocial modalities is included in the methadone-based treatment program, but this finding was not supported by another study.

Potential for Abuse

Dependence Liability

Methadone in its pure form has a dependence liability similar to that of morphine.[10] This reflects both its euphoric and analgesic properties and its solubility. The high fat-solubility of methadone permits immediate and intense gratification, since the drug enters the brain very rapidly after intravenous injection.

Inherent Harmfulness

In low to moderate doses, methadone ordinarily does not produce hazardous effects in adults. However, nausea and vomiting are common and the user must be willing to continue using the drug until tolerance to these side effects develops. In the past, when methadone was more easily available to street users in injectable preparations, many deaths were attributed to methadone overdose.

Availability

In Canada, only specially authorized physicians can prescribe methadone. Currently, the methadone formulations used legally in treatment programs make injection very difficult.

---

10   When each drug is injected subcutaneously, experimental subjects report an intensity of euphoria similar to that of morphine.

Background Reading

Brands, B. (Ed.) (1997). *Methadone Maintenance: A Clinician's Manual.* Toronto: Addiction Research Foundation.

Hartel, D.M., Schoenbaum, E.E., Selwyn, P.A., Kline, J., Davenny, K., Klein, R.S. & Friedland, G.H. (1995). Heroin use during methadone maintenance treatment: The importance of methadone dose and cocaine use. *American Journal of Public Health, 85 (1),* 83–88.

McLellan, A.T., Arndt, I.O., Metzger, D.S., Woody, G.E. & O'Brien, C.P. (1993). The effects of psychosocial services in substance abuse treatment. *Journal of the American Medical Association, 269 (15),* 1953–1959.

Saxon, A.J., Wells, E.A., Fleming, C., Jackson, T.R. & Calsyn, D.A. (1996). Pre-treatment characteristics, program philosophy and level of ancillary services as predictors of methadone maintenance treatment outcome. *Addiction, 91 (8),* 1197–1209.

Reisine, T. & Pasternak, G. (1996). Opioid analgesics and antagonists. (Chapter 23). In J.G. Hardman, L.E. Limbird, P.B. Molinoff, R.W. Rudden & A.G. Gilman (Eds.), *Goodman and Gilman's The Pharmacological Basis of Therapeutics* (9th edition). New York/Toronto: McGraw-Hill Health Professions Division.

Methyl Alcohol
(Methanol)

DRUG CLASS: Poison

Synopsis

Methyl alcohol (methanol, wood alcohol) is used chiefly as an industrial solvent and as a constituent in some antifreezes, paint removers, cleaning solvents and special purpose fuels. It is also used as an adulterant, or "denaturant," to make certain non-beverage products that contain ethyl alcohol undrinkable. In the human body, methyl alcohol is transformed into formaldehyde and formic acid, which can cause blindness, nerve damage and a state of severe chemical imbalance known as acidosis. Drinking methyl alcohol in sufficient quantity, absorbing excessive amounts through the skin or being exposed to its vapors for a prolonged period can cause coma and possibly seizures and death from respiratory arrest. Desperate impoverished alcoholics who are unable to obtain alcoholic beverages have occasionally consumed methyl alcohol deliberately. However, most cases of poisoning with methyl alcohol result from accidental consumption by individuals who are unaware of the methyl alcohol content of the product they are consuming.

Drug Source

Methyl alcohol is produced through chemical synthesis. It was formerly produced by chemical treatment of wood, which is the origin of its names "wood alcohol," "wood spirit" and "wood naphtha."

Trade Names

Not applicable. Methyl alcohol has no medical use. It is used in pure form as a chemical solvent or as a component in combination products.

Street Names

None in common use.

Combination Products

Specifically denatured alcohols,[1] paint removers, cleaning solvents (for use in the restoration of paintings, in printmaking and in industry), antifreeze solutions, liquid fuels and Sterno®. The term methylated spirit refers to a mixture of ethyl alcohol and methyl alcohol in a specified ratio.

Physical Appearance

Methyl alcohol is a clear, colorless volatile liquid. It is almost odorless when freshly distilled.

Dosage[2]

Medical
Methyl alcohol has no medical use.

Non-medical
The concept of "dose" is not recognized for methyl alcohol because as little as a teaspoonful (5 mL or 0.14 oz.) can produce toxic effects.

Routes of Administration

Most cases of methanol poisoning result from drinking methanol-containing products. Users are typically unaware of the product's toxicity. People who work with

---

[1]   SDAG No. 1-A and SDAG No. 1-E under regulations of the *Canadian Excise Act*.

[2]   All doses refer to adults.

methanol-containing products such as pain removers, solvents and shellacs in improperly ventilated areas may inhale a sufficient amount to cause medical problems. Methanol can be absorbed through the skin.

Effects of Short-Term Use

Methyl alcohol is a less potent inebriant than ethyl alcohol. Unless large quantities are consumed or unless ethyl alcohol is consumed simultaneously, inebriation may not be an obvious effect. However, a state of impairment characterized by mild euphoria, loss of inhibitions and impaired muscle co-ordination may be noted shortly after ingestion.

Methyl alcohol acts as a poison in three ways:

- Methyl alcohol causes some depression of the central nervous system similar to but less marked than that caused by ethyl alcohol.

- Methyl alcohol is metabolized in the body to formic acid and other acids that give rise to a state of acidosis.[3]

- One of the products of metabolism of methyl alcohol (probably formic acid) has a directly toxic effect on the retinal cells of the eye.[4]

Since the toxicity of this substance is largely attributable to the products of its bio-transformation, symptoms of methyl alcohol poisoning may not be apparent for a period of several hours, or possibly more than a day, after its ingestion. Symptoms of methyl alcohol poisoning include the following effects.

CNS, *behavioral, subjective:* blurred vision and other visual disturbances, which may proceed to partial or total blindness; headache; restlessness; dizziness and vertigo.

Cardiovascular: headache, weak and rapid pulse, cold and clammy extremities and cyanosis.

Respiratory: rapid and shallow breathing.

---

3   A state of reduced alkali reserve in the blood and other body fluids.

4   As little as 15 mL (0.5 oz.) of methyl alcohol can cause blindness.

Gastrointestinal: severe abdominal pain, nausea and vomiting, and sometimes diarrhea.

Other: severe acidosis, severe back pain and impaired kidney function.

Life-threatening overdose can result in severe agitation and delirium, seizures (occasionally), coma, very slow and labored breathing, and very slow pulse.

When methyl alcohol and ethyl alcohol are ingested together, the metabolism of methyl alcohol is slowed down so that the toxic metabolites are not produced as rapidly and toxic effects are delayed and/or reduced. Based on the same principle, treatment of a person who has recently consumed methyl alcohol may include administration of ethyl alcohol.

Effects of Long-Term Use

Visual impairment or blindness may result from repeated ingestion of even very small quantities of methyl alcohol, or from regular exposure to its vapors in an enclosed atmosphere.

Lethality

Death can occur after ingestion of less than 30 mL (1 oz.) of methyl alcohol, and consumption of 70 to 100 mL (2.4 to 3.4 oz.) is usually fatal.[5] Death can be sudden or it may follow a coma lasting for several hours, and is almost invariably preceded by blindness (i.e., lack of pupillary response to light). Terminal symptoms include gasping, spasms and seizures, and death usually results from respiratory arrest. Methyl alcohol has been deliberately ingested in both successful and unsuccessful suicide attempts.

The prognosis in methanol overdose can be favorable if treatment is rapidly instituted before vision is impaired. With early detection, effective treatment is possible; such

---

[5]   Very small doses of methyl alcohol can be lethal to small children. Hence it is essential to store methyl alcohol products out of their reach.

treatment may include hemodialysis and the administration of both a sodium bicarbonate solution, to counterbalance the acidosis, and ethyl alcohol.[6]

Tolerance and Dependence

Methyl alcohol is so toxic to the body that a pattern of sustained use, which might provide a basis for development of tolerance and dependence, is not possible.

Patterns of Use

Occasionally, desperate impoverished alcoholics and people who are attempting suicide deliberately consume methyl alcohol. In most cases, including those involving young children or household pets, ingestion is inadvertent.

Potential for Abuse

Because of its toxicity, methyl alcohol has little or no abuse potential.

Background Reading

Klaassen, C.D. (1996). Nonmetallic environmental toxicants: Air pollutants, solvents and vapors, and pesticides. (Chapter 67). In J.H. Hardman, L.E. Limbird, P.B. Molinoff, R.W. Rudden & A.G. Gilman, (Eds.), *Goodman and Gilman's The Pharmacological Basis of Therapeutics*, (9th edition). New York/Toronto: McGraw-Hill Health Professions Division.

---

[6]   The mechanism for ethanol and methanol metabolism is based on alcohol dehydrogenase. When ethanol and methanol are present together, ethanol is preferentially metabolized. Methanol can be removed by physical means such as dialysis or by administering ethanol through a continuous intravenous drip and increasing urine flow to eliminate the methanol via the kidneys. Typically, ethanol should be continued until the methanol blood level has fallen to zero and has remained at zero for a few hours. If ethanol treatment is stopped too early, a rebound methanol effect may occur.

Methylphenidate

DRUG CLASS: CNS Stimulant, Amphetamine-like Drug

Synopsis

Methylphenidate is chemically related to the amphetamines but has a less potent stimulant effect on the central nervous system. For this reason, it is preferable to other stimulants in the treatment of attention-deficit hyperactivity disorder (ADHD) in children, which is its primary medical use. At higher doses, methylphenidate and the amphetamines produce similar effects. Methylphenidate shares with other CNS stimulants the potential for abuse, and both tolerance and dependence have been documented.

Drug Source

Methylphenidate is produced through chemical synthesis by the pharmaceutical industry.

Trade Name

Ritalin®.

Street Names

Rits. Most stimulant drugs are also referred to on the street as "uppers."

Combination Products

Methylphenidate has been subject to abuse in combination with the opioid pentazocine (Talwin®). This combination is referred to by street users as "Ts & Rs" or "Ts and Ritz."

Medical Uses

Methylphenidate is used in the treatment of attention-deficit hyperactivity disorder (ADHD) in children. ADHD is a syndrome characterized by a short attention span, distractibility, abnormally high levels of usually dysfunctional and non-directed activity, impulsiveness and low frustration tolerance. Methylphenidate is also used to treat narcolepsy in adults.

Physical Appearance

In its pure form, methylphenidate is a white, odorless, fine crystalline powder that is practically insoluble in water and soluble in alcohol.

Dosage[1]

Medical
- for ADHD in children over the age of six — beginning with 5 to 10 mg orally once to three times per day and increased as needed, but not exceeding 60 mg daily

- for narcolepsy in adults — initially 20 to 60 mg orally per day in divided doses, with adjustment as needed.

---

1   All doses refer to adults, unless otherwise specified.

Non-medical

There have been reports of heavily dependent abusers taking several hundred milligrams per day. Abusers then increase their daily dose as they develop tolerance to the drug's desired effects.

Routes of Administration[2]

Methylphenidate is taken orally. Abusers may crush the tablets and prepare them in a solution for injection, sometimes in combination with pentazocine, or "snort" the powdered tablets intranasally.

Effects of Short-Term Use: Low Doses[3]

Methylphenidate produces both desired and adverse effects similar to, but less intense than, those of amphetamines in comparable doses.

CNS, behavioral, subjective: insomnia, suppression of appetite, dizziness, nervousness, heightened alertness or drowsiness, euphoria, postponement of fatigue, impairment of voluntary movement.

Cardiovascular: headache and rapid and/or irregular heartbeat.

Gastrointestinal: nausea and vomiting.

Other: skin rash.

Effects of Short-Term Use: Higher Doses

Intensification of methylphenidate's low-dose effects may occur at higher doses, as well as any of the following effects.

---

[2]   Single doses within the therapeutic range, up to 60 mg per day in non-tolerant users.

[3]   Doses above the medically recommended level in non-tolerant users, or lower doses in particularly sensitive individuals.

CNS, behavioral, subjective: exhilaration, excitation, agitation, muscle twitching, dilation of the pupils, confusion, hallucinations and paranoid thinking.

Cardiovascular: flushing and increased blood pressure and pulse rate.

Gastrointestinal: dryness of the mouth and other mucous membranes, and vomiting.

Other: fever and sweating.

Hazardous dose levels may result in delirium and possibly seizures, which may be followed by coma.

Effects of Long-Term Use

The principal favorable effects for children with attention deficits are reported to be decreased hyperactivity, decreased impulsiveness, increased attention span, and more directed and controlled motor activity. The principal unwanted effects that may occur are insomnia, decreased appetite, stomach-ache, headache and dizziness. Growth suppression is a concern of long-term use of methylphenidate although the issue is still controversial.

For adults, high doses taken daily by injection may result in a toxic state clinically identical to amphetamine psychosis, a disorder resembling acute paranoid schizophrenia. Cessation of use usually leads to a clearing of the syndrome. Characteristic lesions have been reported to occur at the sites of injection and in peripheral capillaries, which may be attributable to the filler present in tablets that are dissolved before injection.

Other effects of chronic abuse are similar to those produced by amphetamines (see the chapter on amphetamines in Section 3).

Lethality

Severe overdose can lead to seizures and coma.

Tolerance and Dependence

Children with ADHD and narcoleptics do not appear to develop tolerance to the therapeutic effects of methylphenidate. There is no evidence that use of stimulants in the treatment of ADHD in childhood leads to subsequent substance abuse. It has been suggested that the link between ADHD and later substance abuse may be the continued presence of psychiatric symptoms such as aggressivity or a conduct disorder.

Tolerance does develop to those desired effects sought by the abuser, and physical dependence can result from chronic heavy use. Withdrawal symptoms such as exhaustion and severe emotional depression have been observed. Psychological dependence may also occur, characterized by compulsive use of, and preoccupation with, the drug, and a craving for its psychological effects, which may be so intense that serious distress or feelings of panic may develop if it becomes temporarily unavailable.

Patterns of Use

Individuals who abuse methylphenidate are generally older and typically have long histories of polysubstance abuse. There are reports of abusers combining methylphenidate with pentazocine, although the incidence of this practice is unknown.

According to a survey of alcohol and drug use among Ontario students in Grades 7, 9, 11 and 13,[4] the medical use of stimulants in the past year increased significantly between the 1991 and 1993 survey (rising from 2.6 to 4.0 per cent of students) and remained at the higher level (4.1 per cent) in 1995. Despite this rise in use in the 1990s, the percentage of students reporting medical use of stimulants was lower than that reported prior to 1987.

---

[4]   The traditional "Grade 13" has been replaced by an Ontario Academic Credit (OAC) year in Ontario schools. However, the Ontario survey, and thus this text, continue to use the term "Grade 13" to facilitate comparison with surveys from previous years.

Potential for Abuse

Dependence Liability

While the dependence liability of methylphenidate is high, it is not as high as that of cocaine, amphetamine or methamphetamine. When injected, methylphenidate can produce intense euphoria and CNS stimulation, but these effects are reported to be less intense than those produced by those more powerful stimulants. As a result, methylphenidate is seldom the preferred drug for most stimulant abusers.

Inherent Harmfulness

When administered in low to moderate doses, the adverse effects produced by methylphenidate are usually mild. However, some experienced abusers administer methylphenidate intravenously in very high doses. These users generally appear to be aware of the heightened risks and willing to accept them.

Availability

Methylphenidate is available only by prescription and is considered a controlled drug.

Background Reading

Adlaf, E.M., Ivis, F.J., Smart, R.G. & Walsh, G.W. (1995). *The Ontario Student Drug Use Survey 1977-1995*. Toronto: Addiction Research Foundation.

Ahmann, P.A., Waltonen, S.J., Olson, K.A., Theye, F.W., VanErem, A.J. & LaPlant, R.J. (1993). Placebo-controlled evaluation of Ritalin side effects. *Pediatrics, 91 (6)*, 1101–1106.

Canadian Pediatric Society. (1990). Use of methylphenidate for attention-deficit hyperactivity disorder. *Canadian Medical Association Journal, 142 (8)*, 817-818.

Carter, H.S. & Watson, W.A. (1994). IV pentazocine/methylphenidate abuse — The clinical toxicity of another Ts and Blues combination. *Clinical Toxicology, 32 (5)*, 541-547.

Jaffe, S. (1991). Intranasal abuse of prescribed methylphenidate by an alcohol and drug abusing adolescent with ADHD. *Journal of the American Academy of Child and Adolescent Psychiatry, 30 (5)*, 773-775.

Keely, K.A. & Licht, A.L. (1985). Gradual vs. abrupt withdrawal of methylphenidate in two older dependent males. *Journal of Substance Abuse Treatment, 2,* 123-125.

Loney, J. (1988). Substance abuse in adolescents: Diagnostic issues derived from studies of attention deficit disorder with hyperactivity. Rockville, MD: National Institute of Drug Abuse Research Monograph, No. 77.

Vandoren Parran, T. & Jasinski, D.R. (1991). Intravenous methylphenidate abuse. *Archives of Internal Medicine, 151,* 781–783.

Morphine

Synopsis

Morphine, which occurs naturally in the opium poppy, *Papaver somniferum*, is a potent analgesic. Its primary clinical use is to manage moderately severe and severe pain. Next to heroin, morphine has the greatest dependence liability of the opioid analgesics in common use. Morphine may be administered by several routes (injection, smoking, sniffing or swallowing). When injected, particularly intravenously, morphine can produce intense euphoria and a general sense of well-being and relaxation. Regular use can result in the rapid development of tolerance to these effects. Physical and psychological dependence can also develop rapidly. The withdrawal syndrome that occurs when morphine use ceases suddenly is very similar to withdrawal from heroin, and many of the symptoms resemble those produced by a case of moderately severe flu.

Although morphine is infrequently encountered in the North American street drug culture, it is sometimes obtained through thefts from physicians' offices, pharmacies or hospitals. Given morphine's availability to health professionals, especially in hospitals, it is not surprising that morphine dependence has been reported more frequently in this population.

Drug Source

Morphine is isolated from crude opium, a resinous material that is collected from the capsule of the opium poppy.

Trade Names

Doloral®; M-Eslon®; Morphine HP®; Morphitec®-1,-5,-10,-20; M.O.S.®, M.O.S.-SR®; M.O.S.-Sulfate®; MS Contin®, MS•IR®; Oramorph SR®; Statex®.

Street Names

"M," morph, Miss Emma.

Combination Products

Use of morphine plus cocaine, as well as of morphine plus methamphetamine, has been reported. However, such combinations are not frequently encountered.

Medical Uses

Medical uses of morphine include:

- symptomatic relief of moderately severe to severe pain
- relief of certain types of difficult or labored breathing
- suppression of severe cough (rarely)
- treatment of severe diarrhea (e.g., that produced by cholera)
- reversal of naloxone-induced withdrawal.

Physical Appearance

Morphine is legally available as a pure substance only in the form of its water-soluble salts. Most common are morphine sulphate and morphine hydrochloride. Both are fine, white, bitter-tasting crystalline powders that are soluble in water and slightly soluble in alcohol.

Dosage[1]

Medical

For moderate to severe pain, the typical dose range by the intramuscular or subcutaneous route is 5 to 20 mg every four hours, depending on the severity of pain. The usual oral dose range is 10 to 30 mg every four hours. This higher oral dose reflects the fact that after oral administration a large portion of the morphine dose is destroyed as it passes through the liver immediately after absorption, so that only a small part of the dose reaches the central nervous system. With oral extended-release preparations for relief of chronic pain or pain in cancer patients, the dose must be individualized to the patient's situation. Intravenous injection is used primarily for severe post-operative pain or emergency situations, in which case the dose range is 2.5 to 10 mg every four hours.

Non-medical

Irregular or intermittent users (who are not substituting the drug for another opioid analgesic) may start with, and continue to use, doses within the therapeutic range (i.e., up to 20 mg). However, regular users who use morphine for its subjectively pleasurable effects frequently increase the dose as tolerance develops. To take several hundred milligrams per day is common, and there are reliable reports of daily use levels up to four or five grams (4,000 to 5,000 mg).

Routes of Administration

While morphine may be taken orally in tablet form, smoked, sniffed and injected subcutaneously, intramuscularly or intravenously, those who are dependent on morphine prefer the intravenous route.

---

[1]   All doses refer to adults

Effects of Short-Term Use: Low Doses[2]

CNS, behavioral, subjective: Effects of morphine use include suppression of the sensation of pain and emotional response to it, euphoria, drowsiness, lethargy, relaxation, difficulty in concentrating, decreased physical activity in some users and increased physical activity in others, mild anxiety or fear, pupillary constriction, blurred vision, impaired night vision and suppression of cough reflex.

Respiratory: slightly reduced respiratory rate.

Gastrointestinal: nausea and vomiting, constipation, loss of appetite, decreased gastric motility.

Other: slight drop in body temperature, sweating, reduced libido, prickling or tingling sensation on the skin (particularly after intravenous injection).

Effects of Short-Term Use: Higher Doses[3]

Intensification of morphine's low-dose effects may occur with administration of higher doses. Duration of effects also increases with increased dosage. As the dose increases, sensitivity and emotional response to painful stimuli decrease; probability of sleep increases; ability to concentrate is increasingly impaired; breathing becomes progressively slower and more shallow; heart rate gradually slows and blood pressure decreases.

The effect most desired by morphine abusers, referred to as a "rush," occurs almost immediately after intravenous injection. The experience is very similar to that reported for heroin at equivalent doses, although it is somewhat less intense. Users subjectively describe the experience as akin to an intense orgasmic-like sensation in the abdomen.

---

[2]   Single doses of 5 to 10 mg administered by subcutaneous or intramuscular injection in non-tolerant users; to a maximum of 40 mg in divided doses per day.

[3]   Single doses in excess of the therapeutic range (higher than 20 mg) administered by subcutaneous or intramuscular injection in non-tolerant users, or lower doses in particularly sensitive individuals.

In very high doses (i.e., overdose), morphine can produce deep sleep possibly progressing to stupor or coma, low blood pressure, slow and irregular heart rate, cyanosis, shallow and markedly reduced rate of breathing, low body temperature, flaccidity of skeletal muscles, cold and clammy skin, pinpoint pupils and sometimes pulmonary edema (rapid filling of the lungs with fluids).

Effects of Long-Term Use

When morphine has been provided to morphine-dependent patients in maintenance programs, there has been no indication of marked physiological deterioration or significant psychological impairment. Adverse consequences directly related to long-term morphine use include mood instability,[4] pupillary constriction (which impairs night vision), constipation, reduced libido, menstrual irregularity and certain types of respiratory impairment.

Lethality

Lethal overdose is characterized by profound coma, pinpoint pupils, cyanosis and severely depressed respiration, and death usually results from respiratory arrest. The lethal dose level by injection in non-tolerant persons is estimated to be between 120 and 250 mg but high-dose tolerant users have been known to survive 20 times that amount. In rare cases, acute withdrawal reaction has resulted in death.

Tolerance and Dependence

Tolerance
Marked tolerance to many of morphine's main effects can rapidly develop with regular (i.e., daily) heavy use,[5] particularly if the user administers the drug by intravenous

---

[4]   Mood instability is due to the relatively short duration of action of morphine and most other opioid analgesics; under controlled conditions the main effects of 10 mg of morphine are reported to last for approximately four to six hours.

[5]   Tolerance does not develop with infrequent or occasional use.

injection.[6] As a result, increasingly greater doses are required to produce the desired euphoric, analgesic and sedative effects. Tolerance to morphine's respiratory-depressant and nausea-producing effects also develops. Tolerance to its pupillary constricting effect has not been demonstrated, and tolerance develops only slightly to its constipating effect.

With long-term, continuing use of increasing daily dose to maintain the desired effects, the user reaches a dose plateau where no amount of the drug can produce the desired intensity of effects. At this point morphine may be administered with the same frequency (possibly as often as every six to eight hours) but without additional increases in dose. The main purpose of continued morphine use in this situation is to avert withdrawal sickness, which typically commences within 12 hours of the last dose.[7]

Physical Dependence/Withdrawal

Powerful physical dependence develops rapidly in the regular high-dose user. Withdrawal symptoms are virtually identical to those described for heroin (see the chapter on heroin in Section 3), and therefore will only be summarized here.[8]

Early symptoms of morphine withdrawal include watering eyes, nasal discharge, uncontrollable yawning and heavy sweating. This stage is characteristically followed by an agitated sleep, sometimes referred to as a "yen." Agitation upon awakening is accompanied by loss of appetite, depression, dilated pupils and tremor. At peak intensity (approximately 36 to 72 hours after morphine use has stopped) symptoms include alternations between chills and flushing; insomnia; continued loss of appetite; violent yawning and sneezing; "goose-flesh"; vomiting; nausea; abdominal cramps; elevated heart rate and blood pressure; pains in the bones, muscles and joints; muscle spasms and uncontrolled kicking movements.

The severity of the syndrome gradually declines, and most signs are no longer observable within seven to 10 days after the onset of withdrawal sickness.

---

6   Early experiments, under medical supervision, employing inpatients with a history of opioid analgesic dependence indicate that substantial tolerance develops as rapidly as within seven to 10 days.

7   Sensitivity to the desired effects of morphine can be restored after a period of abstinence from it, as well as from other opioid analgesics (there being a high degree of cross-tolerance among these drugs).

8   The duration of morphine withdrawal symptoms is slightly longer than that of symptoms associated with heroin.

Psychological Dependence

The serious impact of dependence on morphine-like drugs is often observable for prolonged periods following the classical phase of withdrawal sickness. Chronic depression, anxiety, insomnia, loss of appetite, periods of agitation and continued craving for the drug can persist for a very long time even among those who may be participating in a methadone maintenance program. Such symptoms are often considered indicative of psychological dependence. However, a purely psychological explanation may be an oversimplification. More research is needed into the complex physiological changes that occur in opioid dependence and the disruption of these adaptive changes when drug use is terminated.

Patterns of Use

During the period between the American Civil War and the early decades of the 20th century, morphine abuse was widespread.[9] Since then, heroin has largely replaced morphine as the drug of choice among street drug abusers who prefer to inject opioids intravenously.

In the past, when morphine was more freely available, physicians prescribed it not only for its analgesic properties but also to treat many conditions for which anxiolytics are now prescribed. At one time, physicians even recommended it as a recreational substitute for alcohol.

Today, heroin-dependent users may attempt to obtain morphine illegally when their drug of choice is unavailable, because morphine in sufficient quantities can rapidly and completely suppress heroin withdrawal symptoms. Because of its availability in medical settings, physicians, nurses and other health workers have been known to use morphine illegally. However, the few studies concerning opioid dependence among medical personnel report a higher rate of meperidine abuse.

Morphine has retained its clinical value as a potent analgesic, and in hospital settings it is among the most commonly used drugs in its class (along with meperidine) for relief of severe pain.

---

9   In fact, so many wounded Civil War soldiers developed physical dependence on morphine that the condition was commonly referred to as the "soldier's disease."

Potential for Abuse

Dependence Liability
The dependence liability of morphine exceeds that of all other opioids in common use except heroin. This reflects both its powerful euphoric and analgesic properties.

Inherent Harmfulness
In low to moderate doses, morphine does not usually produce hazardous effects. However, nausea and vomiting are common, and when they occur the user must be willing to continue use until tolerance to the unpleasant effects is developed.

Availability
Because morphine may be prescribed for chronically painful conditions, there is a risk to patients of iatrogenic[10] physical dependence. However, the great majority of physicians use morphine with caution, ordinarily reserving its extended use for patients suffering from severe pain, including those who are also terminally ill. For most other clinical indications, morphine is prescribed for relatively brief periods. Very strict regulations controlling production and distribution of morphine in Canada and in most other countries greatly reduce its potential for abuse.

Background Reading

Canadian Pharmaceutical Association. (1997). *Compendium of Pharmaceuticals and Specialties* (32nd edition). Ottawa: Canadian Pharmaceutical Association.

Martin, W. R. & Fraser, H. F. (1961). A comparative study of physiological and subjective effects of heroin and morphine administered intravenously in postaddicts. *Journal of Pharmacology and Experimental Therapeutics, 133,* 388–399.

Reisine, T. & Pasternak, G. (1996). Opioid analgesics and antagonists. (Chapter 23). In J.G. Hardman, L.E. Limbird, P.B. Molinoff, R.W. Rudden & A.G. Gilman (Eds.), *Goodman and Gilman's The Pharmacological Basis of Therapeutics.* (9th edition). New York/Toronto: McGraw-Hill Health Professions Division.

---

10   That is, accidentally or unavoidably produced by a course of medical treatment.

Naloxone

DRUG CLASS: Opioid Antagonist

Synopsis

Naloxone is an almost pure opioid antagonist. It reversibly blocks the pharmacological effects of opioids. When administered in a sufficient dose to someone who has taken an opioid analgesic, naloxone returns the person to a state in which opioid effects are not present. One important aspect of the antagonism of opioid effects is rapid reversal of overdose effects, including respiratory depression. However, if naloxone is administered to a person who is in a drug-free state, it exerts little or no pharmacological action. Naloxone and naltrexone (another opioid antagonist) are among the few antidotes that can successfully counteract the effects of hazardous overdose across an entire class of psychoactive drugs.

Because it blocks the effects of opioid analgesics, naloxone precipitates withdrawal when administered to an opioid-dependent individual. For this reason, it was once used by some methadone maintenance programs to verify physical dependence, as a requirement for admission to the program. Naloxone is effective only when administered by injection and has been included in some oral opioid preparations in an attempt to minimize intravenous abuse.

There is no evidence that extended use of naloxone can cause harmful physical or psychological effects or dependence. Tolerance to its antagonist actions does not appear to develop.

Drug Source

Naloxone is a semi-synthetic opioid antagonist derived from thebaine.

Trade Name

Narcan®.

Street Names

None in common use.

Combination Products

Naloxone, which is effective only by injection, has been included in some opioid preparations intended for oral use in an attempt to minimize intravenous abuse. The theory is that when these combination products are administered orally, the intended opioid effects will be obtained. However, if they are administered by injection, the antagonistic actions of naloxone predominate and block the desired euphoric effects of the opioid. Examples of such preparations are Talwin Nx® (pentazocine and naloxone) caplets, which are available in the United States, and Bu-Nx® (buprenorphine and naloxone) tablets, which are not commercially available in North America.

Medical Uses

Naloxone is used to rapidly reverse respiratory depression and other effects of opioid analgesics such as anileridine, codeine, fentanyl, heroin, hydromorphone, meperidine, methadone and morphine, as well as mixed agonist/antagonist opioids such as butorphanol and pentazocine. Its medical uses include:

- diagnosing respiratory depression induced by opioid analgesics

- treating patients experiencing opioid overdose effects

- treating asphyxia in newborn infants whose mothers were treated with opioid analgesics during labor

- verifying that candidates for naltrexone treatment programs are opioid-free

- precipitating withdrawal in individuals undergoing rapid opioid detoxification procedures. More research is needed on the safety, clinical effectiveness and costs of these techniques.

Using Naloxone to Diagnose Opioid Overdose

Respiratory depression is a principal feature not only of opioid (and mixed agonist/antagonist opioid) overdose but also of overdose of other substances such as sedative/hypnotics. Therefore, medical personnel need a quick and accurate method for determining whether opioids are the basis of this potentially life-threatening problem. This is the case particularly when a patient is stuporous or comatose and cannot provide information. Because naloxone exerts no direct respiratory-depressant action, it can be safely administered to a patient whose breathing is shallow, irregular and markedly slowed. If the patient quickly responds favorably to naloxone (i.e., breathing becomes deeper and more rapid), a diagnosis of opioid overdose is indicated. In such cases, and in the case of newborn infants experiencing respiratory depression, treatment with naloxone will be continued until normal breathing returns. Respiratory depression caused by overdose of sedative/hypnotics or other substances is not affected by naloxone in standard therapeutic doses.

Naloxone and Methadone Programs

Naloxone administered by injection precipitates symptoms of withdrawal in opioid-dependent individuals. Therefore, administration of this drug permits confirmation of dependence. While in the past some methadone maintenance clinics used naloxone (i.e., the so-called "naloxone challenge test") for this purpose, this practice has been discontinued. Today, opioid-dependent individuals are admitted to methadone maintenance programs on the basis of positive urine tests for opioids and physical evidence of injection behavior (i.e., "track marks").

Oral preparations combining methadone and naloxone have been used in methadone maintenance programs to prevent patients or others from injecting their methadone. Naloxone exerts little or no pharmacological activity when taken orally, because it is metabolized very rapidly to inactive breakdown products immediately after absorption, as it passes through the liver. However, if the patient attempts to inject such methadone-naloxone combinations, the naloxone can completely block the desired effects of methadone and precipitate mild withdrawal symptoms.

Physical Appearance

Naloxone is a slightly off-white, odorless crystalline substance soluble in water and slightly soluble in alcohol.

Dosage

Medical

For adults between 0.1 and 2.0 mg, repeated if necessary at two to three minute intervals.

Non-medical

Naloxone is not subject to abuse.

Routes of Administration

Usually by intravenous, intramuscular or subcutaneous injection, or intravenous infusion.

Effects of Short-Term Use: Low Doses[1,2]

Naloxone has an onset of action of one to two minutes when given intravenously, or two to five minutes if given subcutaneously or intramuscularly. The duration of action depends on the dose and route of administration.

In individuals who are opioid-dependent, naloxone precipitates a withdrawal syndrome that is very similar to that following abrupt cessation of opioid use, except that symptoms appear within minutes and last about two hours.

An "overshoot" phenomenon can occur when naloxone is administered in cases involving either overdose or dependence. Not only is the overdosed patient's depressed respiratory rate reversed by naloxone, but for a while the patient's breathing may actually become more rapid than before the overdose. This "overshoot" may be related to the unmasking of acute physical dependence.

---

[1]   All doses refer to adults.

[2]   Up to 1 mg by injection.

In the absence of opioids in the body, administration of naloxone results in little or no pharmacological effect. If an opioid is administered a short time after naloxone has been taken, the effects of the opioid on the non-tolerant person will be blocked either partially or totally (depending on the relative size of the doses). For example, 1 mg of naloxone has been demonstrated to completely block the effects of 25 mg of heroin.

Individuals treated with this antagonist must be carefully monitored. Since the duration of action of some opioids exceeds that of naloxone, additional doses of naloxone may be required until a substantial portion of the opioid has been metabolized.

High and low blood pressure, rapid and irregular heartbeat, and fluid in the lungs have been reported in some individuals who received naloxone after surgery, but these effects may be unrelated to naloxone. Cardiac effects have occurred in those who had pre-existing heart disease or received other medication with effects on the heart.

Effects of Short-Term Use: Higher Doses[3]

There have been rare instances of nausea and vomiting, rapid heartbeat, sweating and excitement in post-operative patients when higher-than-recommended doses have been inadvertently administered. However, a causal relationship to naloxone has not been established.

High oral doses have resulted in apathy, depression, difficulty with concentration, irritability, sleepiness, anorexia, nausea and vomiting. These effects subsided with continued therapy or a reduction in dose. In rare cases, seizures have occurred after administration but may be unrelated to naloxone. One case of *erythema multiforme* resolved after naloxone was discontinued. There have been no reported instances of naloxone overdose.

---

3   Doses above the medically recommended level, administered by injection.

Effects of Long-Term Use

Long-term use does not appear to produce any harmful consequences.

Lethality

No reported deaths have been attributed to naloxone overdose.

Tolerance and Dependence

There is no evidence that naloxone produces tolerance or physical dependence. However, long-term administration of opioid antagonists such as naloxone increases the density of opioid receptors in the brain and causes temporary exaggeration of responses to subsequent administration of opioid analgesics.

Patterns of Use

Naloxone is used only under medical supervision and is virtually never taken knowingly by street drug users.

Potential for Abuse

Naloxone does not produce dependence and has no potential for abuse.

Background Reading

Canadian Pharmaceutical Association. (1997). *Compendium of Pharmaceuticals and Specialties* (32nd edition). Ottawa: Canadian Pharmaceutical Association.

Heishman, S. J., Stitzer, M.L., Bigelow, G.E. & Liebson, I.A. (1989). Acute opioid physical dependence in postaddict humans: Naloxone dose effects after a brief morphine exposure. *Journal of Pharmacology and Experimental Therapeutics, 248,* 127–134.

McEvoy, G. (Ed.), (1997). Naltrexone hydrochloride. *American Hospital Formulary Service (AHFS) Drug Information.* Bethesda MD: American Society of Health-System Pharmacists.

O'Connor, P.G. & Kosten, T.R. (1998). Rapid and ultrarapid opioid detoxification techniques. *Journal of the American Medical Association, 279 (3),* 229-234.

Reed, D.A. & Schnoll, S.H. (1986). Abuse of pentazocine-naloxone combination. *Journal of the American Medical Association, 256,* 2562–2564.

Robinson, G.M., Dukes, P.D., Robinson, B.J., Cooke, R.R. & Mahoney, G.N. (1993). The misuse of buprenorphine and a buprenorphine-naloxone combination in Wellington, New Zealand. *Drug and Alcohol Dependence, 33,* 81–86.

Naltrexone

DRUG CLASS: Opioid Antagonist

Synopsis

Naltrexone is essentially a pure opioid antagonist with little or no agonist activity. It reversibly blocks the pharmacological effects of opioids. Naltrexone is administered orally and is both more potent and longer acting than naloxone, which is ineffective when administered orally. Acute opioid withdrawal symptoms may result if naltrexone is administered to individuals who are physically dependent on opioids.

Naltrexone is a useful continuing treatment for individuals formerly physically dependent on opioids who have already been successfully detoxified and are attempting to maintain abstinence. It is believed that naltrexone minimizes opioid-seeking behavior by blocking the euphoric effects of opioids. Individuals taking naltrexone soon realize that any opioid administered will be ineffective and therefore money spent on opioids will be wasted. Since naltrexone lacks opioid-agonist activity, many opioid-dependent clients do not accept this treatment well, and retention rates in naltrexone treatment programs tend to be poor. Naltrexone treatment of opioid dependence appears to be most beneficial in more highly motivated and psychologically healthier populations (e.g., health care professionals; other employed, socially functioning individuals detoxified from methadone maintenance; or individuals leaving prison or residential treatment facilities). Naltrexone treatment is more effective when combined with behavioral therapy.

Naltrexone is also used to treat alcohol dependence because it has been shown to have a beneficial effect on abstinence and relapse rates. Although the exact mechanism by which these effects are achieved is not known, it is thought that naltrexone may block the rewarding or pleasurable effects associated with alcohol use. This treatment has been shown to be more effective when combined with behavioral therapy.

Naltrexone does not produce physical or psychological dependence. Tolerance to the opioid antagonist properties of this compound has not been demonstrated.

Drug Source

Naltrexone is a semi-synthetic opioid antagonist derived from thebaine.

Trade Names

ReVia® (formerly Trexan®).

Street Names

None.

Combination Products

None.

Medical Uses

Medical applications of naltrexone include its use:

- as an adjunct in the treatment of opioid dependence, to maintain abstinence following detoxification from opioids
- as an adjunct in the treatment of alcohol dependence.

Naltrexone has also been investigated for:

- accelerating the withdrawal process for individuals undergoing
- detoxification from opioids
- treating obesity.

Physical Appearance

Naltrexone hydrochloride is a white, bitter-tasting crystalline compound.

Dosage

Opioid Dependence

The following doses are recommended to block the pharmacological effects of opioids, in order to assist formerly dependent individuals to maintain an opioid-free state.

1. Starting Therapy

The patient should be opioid-free for seven to 10 days (up to 14 days if the patient was maintained on methadone). Opioid-free status should be confirmed by a negative urine screen. No withdrawal symptoms should be present.

A naloxone challenge test[1] should then be administered. The patient should show no signs of opioid withdrawal.

The patient may then be given a 25-mg test dose of naltrexone and observed for one hour. If no signs of withdrawal are present, the patient may be given another 25-mg dose.

2. Continuing Treatment

The length of treatment must be individualized. Several months may be required — some consider six months to be a minimum treatment period. The maintenance dose is 50 mg daily (50 mg will block or significantly attenuate the effects of 25 mg of intravenous heroin for 24 hours). Less than daily dosing can be used; for example, 100 mg on alternate days or 150 mg every three days.

3. Sporadic Treatment

Naltrexone is sometimes prescribed intermittently after a course of treatment has been completed, e.g., during periods of stress when risk of relapse may be great. The dose administered would be the same as the dose recommended for maintenance therapy.

NOTE: Patients should be counselled against attempting to override the blockade effect with large doses of opioids, since this could result in fatal opioid intoxication. Patients should carry a medical identification card while undergoing naltrexone therapy.

---

[1]   See the chapter on naloxone in Section 3.

Depending on the patient, it may be important that a family member, employer or health worker observe and confirm that the patient takes the dose of naltrexone. The continuing presence of the naltrexone metabolite 6-beta-naltrexol in urine may be used as an indicator that the naltrexone is being taken regularly.

To maximize its effectiveness, naltrexone treatment should be accompanied by behavioral therapy.

Alcohol Dependence

Prior to initiating naltrexone therapy for the treatment of alcohol dependence, the physician should verify that the patient has not taken opioids in the past five to seven days. An initial dose of 25 mg has been suggested because patients frequently complain of gastrointestinal upset. A once-daily dose of 50 mg has been recommended for the maintenance phase. Naltrexone treatment for alcohol dependence should also be accompanied by behavioral treatment.

Routes of Administration

Naltrexone is administered orally. A "depot injectable" form of naltrexone has been investigated. Depot injection involves injecting a small amount of a naltrexone-containing liquid formulation intramuscularly to provide a "reservoir" of the drug that would gradually diffuse into the bloodstream to maintain the opioid antagonist effects over a long period (e.g., several weeks). This method would eliminate the risk of patients skipping their oral doses — and the need to supervise oral dosing.

Effects of Short-Term Use: Low Doses[2]

While naltrexone is generally well tolerated, the following adverse effects have been reported.

CNS, behavioral, subjective: dysphoria, loss of energy, decreased mental acuity, depression, anxiety, nervousness, headache and sleep disturbances.

---

[2]   All doses refer to adults.

Gastrointestinal: nausea, vomiting, abdominal pain/cramps,[3] loss of appetite and constipation.

Other: possible liver toxicity (particularly in those with pre-existing, or potential, impairment of liver function). Joint and muscle pain, thirst, dizziness, changing hormone levels, neuroendocrine effects, rash and chills have also been reported.

Effects of Short-Term Use: Higher Doses

At higher doses, effects of the short-term use of naltrexone include the following.

CNS, *behavioral, subjective:* One anecdotal case of euphoria has been reported.

Liver: Injury to liver cells has been reported in a substantial number of obese patients who used naltrexone 300 mg per day.[4]

Effects of Long-Term Use

The optimal duration of naltrexone therapy has not been established. The length of treatment should be based on the individual patient's needs. Generally, patients who were formerly opioid-dependent require at least six months to make the necessary behavioral changes, and naltrexone may be appropriate throughout this period. Additional naltrexone therapy may be useful in some patients on an intermittent basis, during a crisis or during episodes of intense craving, for example.

Lethality

There is little experience with overdose of naltrexone in humans. In overdose situations, patients should be treated symptomatically in a hospital setting.

---

[3]   These may be minimized by taking naltrexone with food or antacids, or after meals.

[4]   That is the toxic dose appears to be no more than five times the size of the apparently safe dose.

Lethality is more of a concern in cases in which patients taking naltrexone attempt to override its opioid-blocking effects by taking high doses of opioids. These individuals are at risk of serious consequences including respiratory depression, coma and death due to opioid intoxication. This issue is of concern when an analgesic is required in patients on naltrexone therapy. Non-opioid analgesics should be used whenever possible. If opioids are required, they should be administered cautiously, bearing in mind that higher-than-usual doses may be required and that deeper, more prolonged respiratory depression may result. Such patients may experience what appear to be non-opioid receptor-induced effects such as swelling of the face, pruritus and erythema due to such mechanisms as opioid-induced histamine release.

Tolerance and Dependence

Naltrexone does not produce either physical or psychological dependence. Tolerance does not appear to develop to naltrexone's opioid-antagonist activity.

Naltrexone will produce withdrawal symptoms if given to someone who is physically dependent on opioids.

Patterns of Use

Naltrexone treatment has a very high early dropout rate and has been poorly accepted by street addicts, partly due to the drug's lack of reinforcing properties. Naltrexone works best in highly motivated and psychologically healthier individuals. Strong family support improves the beneficial results of this medication. Health professionals and white-collar workers appear to benefit more from naltrexone than those from lower socioeconomic groups. Potential candidates for naltrexone therapy may also include those with recent employment and a good educational background, probationers, parolees and those recently detoxified from, or waiting for admission to, methadone maintenance programs.

Potential for Abuse

Dependence Liability

It is generally thought that naltrexone does not produce dependence and that it is not abused. However, in one anecdotal case, four former addicts claimed to have abused naltrexone. They reported euphoric effects, increased their dosage of naltrexone beyond that prescribed and had difficulty stopping use of the medication.

Inherent Harmfulness

In recommended doses, the incidence of adverse effects due to naltrexone is low. When adverse effects do occur, they are generally mild to moderate in severity and usually subside in a few days. Naltrexone may cause dose-related injury to liver cells.

Patients should be warned of the serious consequences of attempting to overcome the opioid-blocking effects of naltrexone by using large doses of opioids. Such overdoses may produce potentially lethal intoxication, respiratory depression and circulatory collapse.

Availability

In Canada and the United States, naltrexone is available by prescription.

Background Reading

Berg, B.J., Pettinati, H.M. & Volpicelli, J.R. (1996). A risk-benefit assessment of naltrexone in the treatment of alcohol dependence. *Drug Safety, 15 (4),* 274–282.

Galloway, G. & Hayner, G. (1993). Haight-Ashbury free clinics; Drug detoxification protocols; Part 2: Opioid blockade. *Journal of Psychoactive Drugs, 25 (3),* 251–252.

Greenstein, R.A., Fudala, P.J. & O'Brien, C.P. (1997). Alternative pharmacotherapies for opiate addiction. In J.H. Lowinson et al. (Eds.), *Substance Abuse, A Comprehensive Textbook.* (3rd edition) Baltimore: Williams and Wilkins.

Lerner, A.G., Sigal, M., Bacalu, A. & Gelkopf, M. (1992). Naltrexone abuse potential. *Journal of Nervous and Mental Disease, 180,* 734–735.

McEvoy, G. (Ed.), (1997). Naltrexone hydrochloride. *American Hospital Formulary Service (AHFS) Drug Information.* Bethesda MD: American Society of Health-System Pharmacists.

Volpicelli, J.R., Alterman, A.I., Hayashida, M. & O'Brien, C.P. (1992). Naltrexone in the treatment of alcohol dependence. *Archives of General Psychiatry, 49,* 876–880.

Nicotine

DRUG CLASS:	CNS Stimulant

Synopsis

Nicotine is a potent drug with complex biological actions, classified by pharmacologists as a ganglionic stimulant. In usual doses, it produces a variety of physiological and psychological effects. The nature and intensity of these effects are related to the amount of nicotine used, and the duration and recency of use. Tobacco,[1] the almost-exclusive natural source of nicotine, is native to the Western Hemisphere and may have been used by the ancient Maya. North American Indians are believed to have used tobacco in cigarettes, cigars, chewing tobacco and pipes. Columbus introduced tobacco into Europe at the end of the 15th century, and since then nicotine has become one of the world's most widely used psychoactive drugs. The term "nicotine" derives from the surname of a 16th-century French diplomat, Jean Nicot (1530-1600), who extolled the virtues and beneficial effects of tobacco smoking.

Nicotine, as it occurs naturally in tobacco, has no present medical or therapeutic use, but pure nicotine delivered in small doses has been used to treat nicotine addiction (see below). Compounds derived from or related to nicotine may prove to have therapeutic applications in the future. The physiological effects of nicotine include small increases in heart rate, blood pressure, respiration and motor activity. Depending on the dose and circumstances of present use, nicotine may produce a range of behavioral effects, from mild stimulation and euphoria to relaxation, anxiety reduction and sedation.

---

[1]   Oviedoy y Valdus first used the term "tobaco" in his *Historia* published in 1535. The term was used to refer to a "a long bifurcated tube" used to snuff tobacco in Hispaniola (Haiti), the act of smoking, the tobacco plant or a narcotic state induced from inhaling the powdered plant (Brooks, 1952).

Nicotine is most commonly ingested through tobacco cigarette smoking. When the smoker draws in air through the lit cigarette, temperatures as high as about 1000 C are produced at its tip. High-temperature combustion produces smoke (an aerosol), which is composed of extremely fine particles (less than one micron in average diameter) suspended in hot gases (including carbon monoxide). Nicotine molecules are attached to these particles[2] and, because of the particles' extremely small size, easily reach the lungs' alveoli[3] during each smoke inhalation. From here they are rapidly absorbed into the bloodstream and carried to the brain and other parts of the body. By design, cigarette smoke is mildly acidic, and this, coupled with the very fine particle size, facilitates the comfortable inhalation for which cigarettes are known.

Nicotine may also be obtained by smoking cigars or pipes. These produce an alkaline smoke that is more irritating to the respiratory system when inhaled. The smoke's alkalinity, however, facilitates absorption of nicotine directly through the (mucous) membranes lining the mouth and throat. Nicotine is also readily absorbed from forms of tobacco that are chewed (chewing tobacco), held against the lining of the mouth (wet snuff), or sniffed into the nasal passages (dry snuff).

Drug Source

Nicotine is isolated mainly from the tobacco plants *Nicotiana tabacum* and *Nicotiana rustica*. Significant quantities of nicotine occur naturally only in tobacco plants. The leaves of the two varieties contain between one to six per cent nicotine. Very small quantities of nicotine have been isolated from other members of the *Solanaceae* (nightshade) family,[4] but these are not of toxicological significance.

The combustion of tobacco produces smoke that is composed of a gas and a particulate phase. The particulate phase is the solid component of tobacco smoke that is trapped in the filters of smoking machines. The gas phase passes through these filters. Since 1973, tar has been defined as the portion of the particulate phase plus water minus nicotine. Tar is formed during the combustion of tobacco products. It is not present in unburned tobacco. When a cigarette is puffed, the smoker inhales the

---

2   In aggregate these particles plus moisture make the dark brown substance known as "tar."

3   Tiny air sacs in the lungs from which small molecules are transferred to and from the bloodstream.

4   Tomato, eggplant and others.

"mainstream" smoke that passes through the cigarette. This is the main source of nicotine and other compounds for the smoker. "Sidestream" smoke is emitted from the end of the burning cigarette. Environmental smoke is composed of sidestream smoke and exhaled smoke.

Tobacco, when combusted during smoking, yields more than 4,000 compounds in addition to nicotine. Carbon monoxide has negative effects on cardiac function, and appears to be involved in reducing the birth weight of children born to smoking mothers. Many of the compounds found in tobacco smoke have been shown to be cancer-causing (carcinogenic) and others have been shown to affect the metabolism of other drugs.

Trade Names

There are hundreds of cigarette brand names. Many brands and styles of cigarettes are made by a small number of large corporations to meet the needs of various markets, as well as to acquire a market share from their competitors. Chewing tobacco, roll-your-own tobacco, and various forms of wet and dry snuff are also available, under a variety of trade names. Concentrated solutions of nicotine salts (e.g., nicotine sulphate) were used in the past as garden insecticides (Black Leaf 40®). Pure nicotine for human therapeutic use is discussed below in the section on medical uses.

Since the 1980s, nicotine resin (gum) containing 2 to 4 mg of nicotine per piece, has been marketed in Canada and the United States under trade names such as Nicorette® and Nicorette Plus® for use by smokers who are attempting to quit or cut down. More recently transdermal patches containing nicotine have been marketed for the same purpose under trade names such as Habitrol®, Nicoderm®, Nicotrol® and Prostep®.

Street Names

Various colloquial terms exist for tobacco, but few are currently used. Of those that are (e.g., smokes, butts, cigs, cancer sticks, tumor candy, coffin nails), most refer to cigarettes.

Combination Products

Street drug users sometimes mix tobacco with other drugs such as cannabis, phency-clidine (PCP), heroin or cocaine. Some combinations are smoked after being combined and hand-rolled into a cigarette. Others are vaporized (or aerosolized) at the tip of the cigarette and inhaled as the tobacco smoke is drawn into the lungs. In a third method, a track of the non-tobacco substance is laid along the length of the cigarette using a thin needle. Heroin, which was often cheap and easily available to American soldiers in Vietnam, was smoked with tobacco. With falling street prices and increasing purity of heroin in North America, this practice appears to be re-emerging. Finally, "blunts" are cigars that are hollowed out and then refilled with a mixture of tobacco and cannabis or other drugs.

Medical Uses

Pure nicotine (for therapeutic purposes) has been available in Canada for more than 10 years in the form of a chewable polacrilex resin or "gum," and comes in forms containing 2 mg and 4 mg of nicotine. The 2-mg formulation is now available "over the counter." For a given strength, the amount absorbed into the body depends on the pattern and duration of chewing. The manufacturer has specified the appropriate technique.

Since the early 1990s, transdermal *nicotine patches* have become available from several manufacturers. These patches, while differing somewhat physiochemically and structurally, are designed to allow small amounts of nicotine to be absorbed through intact skin. The stated "dose" of a nicotine patch is the amount of nicotine normally absorbed into the bloodstream during a single application of 16 or 24 hours, depending on the brand.

All the above forms of therapeutic nicotine replacement are most effective as an aid to smoking cessation in clients who are motivated to quit, and when ongoing behavioral support is also provided. For some years, nicotine aerosols and sprays have also been used both experimentally and therapeutically as aids to quitting. The comfort of use depends on a number of factors including the particle size and physiochemical properties of the solution being aerosolized. Different methods of aerosol generation have been used with particle sizes ranging from 0.1 to 5 microns. While nicotine aerosols and sprays are not currently available for treatment in Canada, the speed with which they achieve the desired blood nicotine concentrations makes these pro-ducts possible nicotine therapies.

Physical Appearance

Nicotine is a volatile oily liquid varying in appearance from colorless, through pale yellow, to brown (depending on its state of oxidation). Chemically, it exists as a number of stereoisomers, of which S-nicotine is the dominant form found in tobacco. R-nicotine, which is less pharmacologically active, may comprise some 10 per cent of the nicotine found in tobacco. Nicotine is a weak base, and in the presence of acids forms salts such as nicotine sulphate, which are white or colorless in their pure form.

Smoking tobacco is tobacco leaf that has been prepared and cured in a number of ways, depending on its intended use and on local consumer preferences. The fresh leaf is medium to dark green, while the air-cured and flu-dried leaf is a golden color. Various proprietary ingredients may be added to flavor shredded tobacco for cigarettes and pipes. Cigarette and pipe tobacco is medium to dark brown in color. Tobacco leaves that are used to make cigars are brown but may have different green hues. Chewing tobacco is generally a dark brown, moist, compressed mass of plant-leaf material. Dry snuff is a powdered plant material, and is usually a lighter brown to ginger color, while wet snuff tends to be darker brown.

Dosage

Medical

The medical (or therapeutic) use of nicotine should be associated with a program that incorporates behavioral support components (individual and/or group). The recom-mended maximum dose for the 4-mg gum is 20 pieces per day, but most patients can be stabilized on 10 to 16 pieces during their first month of treatment. Treatment may be continued for up to six months, and the manufacturer recommends that users carry the product for up to three months after they have quit smoking, to help deal with "overwhelming" urges to smoke. The 2-mg formulation is recommended for people who are "less tolerant" as indicated by a score of six or less on the Fagerström Tolerance Questionnaire (FTQ). An updated version of the FTQ, called the Fagerström Test for Nicotine Dependence (FTND), has been developed.

Non-medical

A typical cigarette contains approximately 10 to 15 mg of nicotine. However, when a cigarette is smoked in the usual manner, about 1 mg reaches the bloodstream. Yields of nicotine for Canadian brands of cigarettes reported by manufacturers range from less than 0.1 to as much as 1.46 mg per cigarette.[5] Tar yields per cigarette, which correlate very highly with nicotine yields, are reported to vary from 0.7 to 19.0 mg per cigarette. Different cigarettes also produce between 0.7 and 17 mg of carbon monoxide, a poisonous gas that impairs the oxygen-carrying capacity of the blood. "Tar" contributes to debilitating lung disease when chronically inhaled, and contains a large number of compounds known to cause cancer in a variety of organs (see below).

The actual amounts of these substances reaching the bloodstream may differ considerably from the figures reported and depend on the following factors:

- whether there is a filter
- the filter's type and effectiveness
- the type of tobacco
- the number of puffs per cigarette and the depth of inhalation
- the proportion of the cigarette smoked prior to its being extinguished
- the way in which the cigarette is smoked.[6]

A smoker who uses one pack of 20 Canadian cigarettes per day will typically take in between 1.8 to 29.2 mg of nicotine, between 14 and 380 mg of tar and between 14 and 340 mg of carbon monoxide.

Routes of Administration

The usual route of administration for non-medical use is by smoking. When acidic tobacco cigarette smoke is inhaled, nicotine is absorbed rapidly across the membranes of the alveoli in the lungs. However, because of the more alkaline pH of cigar and

---

[5]   Constituent yields are determined under highly regulated conditions of machine smoking, using standards defined by the Tobacco Control Regulation (Schedule 1).

[6]   For example, with low-tar/low-nicotine cigarettes, if smokers cover the small air holes in the filter with their fingers, the nicotine yield increases to a level approaching that of a regular cigarette.

pipe smoke, nicotine from these sources is also absorbed through the membranes of the mouth and upper respiratory tract. The drug can also be absorbed through the membranes of the mouth from chewing tobacco or wet snuff, and through the lining of the nose from dry snuff. As a smoking cessation treatment, nicotine may be administered through the buccal mucosa (lining of the mouth) from nicotine gum, or through the skin using a transdermal nicotine patch.

Effects of Short-Term Use

For the non-smoker, a few inhaled puffs may result in dizziness, headache, nausea, abdominal cramps and possibly vomiting or weakness. The smoke itself may produce coughing or gagging. In regular smokers, these symptoms abate with continued use as tolerance develops to the autonomic effects of the drug, such as heart rate and certain subjective effects.

In the regular user, nicotine produces mild euphoria (or a feeling of well-being), increased arousal, enhanced ability to concentrate, relaxation and a temporary reduction in the urge to smoke. The exact mechanisms underlying nicotine's effects on mood are not yet known, but activation (by direct or indirect means) of norepinephrine[7] and mesolimbic[8] dopamine may be involved. Even in established users, nicotine causes a mild increase in heart rate and blood pressure and constriction of peripheral blood vessels, lowering skin temperature. Nicotine is also reported to decrease appetite, increase metabolic rate and lower the body-weight set point (the weight at which individuals feel comfortable). These effects are sometimes sought by users for weight control and may explain part of the (often transient) weight gain experienced by many smokers after quitting.

Effects of Long-Term Use

Cigarette smoking is recognized as the major preventable cause of premature death and disability in developed and developing countries. When tobacco smoke is

---

[7]   Norepinephrine (noradrenaline) and dopamine are substances in the brain (neurotransmitters) that act to chemically regulate brain activity.

[8]   The mesolimbic part of the brain is believed to be involved in the regulation of appetitive behavior.

inhaled chronically, the nicotine, carbon monoxide and thousands of constituents of tar damage the cardiovascular and respiratory systems. As a result, smoking greatly increases the incidence of heart attack, stroke, lung cancer and chronic lung disease in smokers as compared with non-smokers. Good evidence of harmful effects on a host of other human systems also exists. Passive smoke[9] has also been shown to be a major risk factor in the development of disease in non-smokers.

Of every 1,000 Canadians age 20 who smoke, about half (500) will die from smoking, if they continue; 250 will die before the age of 70.[10] In Canada about 40,000 deaths, or 21 per cent of deaths from all causes, were attributable to smoking in 1991. This number is expected to increase. More than 400,000 deaths per year in the United States are attributable to smoking. On average, 15 years of a smoker's expected life are lost through smoking.

In Canada, smoking causes more than 11,000 deaths from cardiovascular disease (a third of all deaths from heart disease, stroke and diseases of blood vessels) and accounts for more than 30 per cent of all deaths from cancer. Smoking also accounts for almost 90 per cent of deaths from lung cancer, which has replaced breast cancer as the leading cause of cancer death in Canadian women. There is a strong link between smoking and cancers of the pancreas, kidney and urinary bladder. About 75 per cent of deaths from chronic obstructive lung disease (chronic bronchitis and emphysema) are attributable to smoking.

Estimates of the social and economic costs of tobacco use in Canada range from $9.5 billion to $12.3 billion per year, including the costs of premature death, lost productivity and increased health care.

The economic cost of tobacco is more than that of alcohol or any other substance of abuse, although a portion of this cost is offset by tobacco taxes collected by government, reduced health care costs to the elderly (due to premature death) and reduced pension payments.

---

9   Active smoke is that inhaled directly by a smoker from the lit cigarette; passive smoke (sometimes called environmental tobacco smoke) is that exhaled by an active smoker plus that which enters the atmosphere directly from the lit cigarette.

10   In contrast, nine will die in traffic accidents and one will be murdered.

Smoking and Pregnancy

Smoking regularly during pregnancy increases a woman's risk of having problems during the pregnancy, delivering a low birth weight baby and having problems associated with breast feeding.

The risk of having a baby weighing less than 2,500 grams is more than twice as high in mothers who smoke compared to non-smoking mothers, and the risk is higher for heavy smokers than for lighter smokers. On average, smoking during pregnancy reduces the baby's birth weight by 150 to 300 grams. Low birth weight babies are more likely to be premature, to be stillborn, to require special neonatal care and to have a higher rate of infant mortality. Women who quit smoking during pregnancy are less likely to have low birth weight babies than those who smoke throughout pregnancy.

Smoking during pregnancy also increases the risk of bleeding, spontaneous abortion and abnormalities of the placenta. After delivery, women who smoked during pregnancy are likely to produce less breast milk, and it may be necessary to wean the baby early because of changed quality of the breast milk.

Environmental Tobacco Smoke

In 1992, the United States Environmental Protection Agency declared environmental tobacco smoke (ETS) a Group A carcinogen. ETS includes both the smoke exhaled by the smoker and the smoke that escapes directly from the burning cigarette ember. People in the immediate environment who inhale this smoke (sometimes called "passive smoking") are at increased risk of health problems. It is estimated that approximately 300 lung cancer deaths a year in non-smoking Canadians result from exposure to "second-hand" smoke. An even larger number of deaths likely result from ETS-related heart disease.[11] In children, ETS exposure increases the risks of bronchitis and pneumonia, asthma, middle ear infection, sudden infant death syndrome and other problems.

Lethality

Nicotine and the many other constituents of tobacco are known to be harmful to health, and chronic use of tobacco has been shown conclusively to be linked to numerous fatal diseases. Death directly attributable to nicotine overdose (especially from nicotine in tobacco) has been reported in the past. Infants, young children and adults have been known to suffer toxic doses of nicotine through the ingestion of

---

[11]   In the United States, ETS is estimated to cause at least 10 times more deaths from heart disease than from lung cancer. A similar ratio in Canada would be equivalent to 3,000 deaths among non-smokers from environmental tobacco smoke.

cigarettes and other sources of nicotine. The absorption of nicotine through the skin leading to toxic effects has also been documented. Gastric absorption is poor, acute ingestion induces vomiting through central mechanisms and nicotine absorbed from the intestinal tract is largely eliminated from the body by passage through the liver (high first-pass extraction).

The lethal dose in non-tolerant adults is estimated to be 60 mg, but much smaller amounts (2 to 5 mg) can cause nausea and vomiting. As little as a few drops (200 to 300 mcL) of pure nicotine may be lethal to humans. Fatal overdose is associated with nausea, salivation, abdominal pain, sweating, headache and dizziness. Blood pressure falls, and breathing becomes difficult. Death is from respiratory paralysis and may be associated with seizures. Treatment involves gastric lavage and the infusion of activated charcoal, with support of respiration and management of shock.

Tolerance and Dependence

In 1989, the Royal Society of Canada outlined its rationale for considering cigarette smoking to be an addiction as follows.

> *Cigarette smoking can, and frequently does, meet all the criteria for the proposed definition of addiction:*
>
> i. *It is used regularly (usually many times a day) by the majority of users, and most of those who experiment with cigarette smoking become regular daily smokers.*
>
> ii. *The amounts and patterns of use by regular smokers are in most cases sufficient to maintain pharmacologically significant blood levels of nicotine throughout most of the day.*
>
> iii. *Such nicotine levels have been shown to produce a variety of effects on the brain, altering chemical and electrophysiological aspects of brain function, and producing subjective effects that the smoker recognizes, differentiates from those of other drugs, and usually finds pleasurable.*
>
> iv. *Sudden cessation of smoking gives rise to a withdrawal syndrome which can be alleviated by the administration of nicotine. Other drugs which act on nicotine receptors in the brain also modify smoking patterns.*

v.   *In experimental studies, both laboratory animals and humans will expend considerable effort to self-inject nicotine intravenously, in a manner similar to that shown in studies of heroin, cocaine and other drugs that are generally regarded as addicting, i.e., the effects of nicotine are clearly reinforcing.*

vi. *Regular cigarette smokers have great difficulty in giving up smoking, even when motivated to do so by the occurrence of respiratory, cardiovascular or other diseases caused or aggravated by smoking. Relapse rates among those who do stop smoking are high. The urge to smoke, among those who are also heavy users of alcohol or other drugs, is, in over 50 per cent of cases, as strong as, or stronger than the urge to use these other substances.*

vii. *Although much less evidence is available for other forms of tobacco use, including cigars and pipes, snuffs, and chewing tobacco, they are capable of giving rise to plasma nicotine concentrations as high as, or higher than, those achieved by cigarette smokers, though somewhat more slowly. The risk of addiction to these forms of tobacco use therefore warrants further study.[12]*

The Society recommends that patterns of cigarette use that meet these criteria be regarded as nicotine addiction. Their analysis of tobacco smoking clearly puts it in the realm of a complex biopsychosocial phenomenon in which genetics, psychology, pharmacology and environment all interact to produce a tenacious pattern of drug use, associated with which there are proven and serious health consequences, and that extracts a heavy personal and social cost.

Withdrawal from regular tobacco use involves a myriad of sometimes very unpleasant symptoms, which may intensify for three to four days and persist for a week, or sometimes much longer. The first symptoms to appear include irritability, restlessness, anxiety, insomnia, fatigue, lack of ability to concentrate and strong urges to smoke (cravings). The latter two may persist for weeks or months. People are more likely to quit smoking successfully when they have a strong personal motivation to quit; a clear strategy for quitting, including behavioral and, where appropriate, pharmacological support; and when they avoid former smoking situations or relationships.

---

12   Reprinted with permission from Tobacco Nicotine and Addiction: A committee report prepared by the Royal Society of Canada for the Health Protection Branch, Health and Welfare Canada. Copyright 1989 Royal Society of Canada.

Patterns of Use

A daily smoker uses an average of 17.7 cigarettes per day, which corresponds to an average yearly consumption of about 6,500 cigarettes each. Canadians are among the heaviest per-capita tobacco consumers in the world. In 1990, 1,700 manufactured cigarettes were consumed yearly per capita. In 1994, there were 6.5 million smokers in Canada.

In Canada, the proportion of men over 15 years of age who smoked cigarettes regularly declined steadily from 61 per cent in 1965 to 29 per cent in 1995. Among women over 15 the proportion who smoked regularly declined from 38 per cent in 1965 to 25 per cent in 1995, with the decrease's having begun in the late 1970s. In 1995, the proportion of adults of both sexes who smoked was 27 per cent.

Socioeconomic factors such as education and employment are also related to rates of smoking. The more education individuals have and the higher their occupational level, the less likely they are to smoke.

Major smoking-related concerns include:

- the rise in female mortality from lung cancer, which overtook breast cancer as a cause death among Canadian women in 1994[13]

- the young age at which both boys and girls begin smoking

- the difficulty that teenage smokers have in quitting once they have become established smokers

- the evidence of an increase in smoking, particularly among high school students, following a reduction in tobacco taxes in several Canadian provinces in 1994.

---

[13] Recent evidence suggests that females may be more susceptible to the pulmonary effects of tobacco smoke.

Potential for Abuse

Nicotine is a powerful drug of addiction with a high degree of abuse liability. A significant number of those who start smoking cigarettes during their teenage years become regular, often lifelong, users. Many factors promote the initiation of smoking, including smoking by friends and family, the urge to experiment, attitudes toward smoking, academic expectations, rejection of established authority, risk-taking and peer pressure. The development of tolerance to the initial negative physical effects, the early experience of positively reinforcing effects (e.g., euphoria, stimulation, relaxation, stress reduction) and, finally, the experiencing of withdrawal during attempts to quit all act to ensure continued use.

Other factors that promote smoking, especially among young people, include the rapid effects produced by inhalation (faster than by intravenous injection of comparable doses of nicotine), the time lag and uncertainty of harmful physical consequences for each smoker, and the availability of less expensive tobacco products. Nevertheless, social opinion is generally strongly against smoking, and there is a high level of public awareness of the serious consequences associated with prolonged and regular use of tobacco.

Attempts to quit smoking are characterized by relapse. A practical and humane treatment approach is to view relapse as a learning opportunity, in which the predisposing factors may be identified and dealt with proactively in subsequent attempts to quit. Feelings of guilt have no useful role in treating nicotine addiction, while positive reinforcement for incremental improvement and transient success are associated with positive outcomes.

Established smokers are most often successful in quitting when they have clear and personal reasons for quitting and a supportive work and home environment, coupled with the availability of individual or group treatment. Reasons associated with successful attempts to quit often include concerns about the risk to personal health, or to that of family members — including fetuses, infants and young children — posed by smoking. Success in quitting may also be associated with the adoption of a generally healthier lifestyle, the use of coping skills, the desire to take control (that is, to no longer view oneself as "an addict" or "controlled" by smoking), the wish to save the after-tax dollars spent on tobacco, and feelings of confidence and motivation with respect to quitting.

Background Reading

American Heart Association, Committee on Atherosclerosis and Hypertension in Children, Council on Cardiovascular Disease in the Young. (1994). Active and passive tobacco exposure: A serious pediatric health problem. *Circulation, 94*, 2581-2590.

Brooks, J.E. (1952). *The Mighty Leaf: Tobacco through the Centuries*. Boston: Little Brown.

Chilmonczyk, B.A., Salmun, L.M., Megathlin, K. N., Neveux, L.M., Palomaki G.E., Knight, G.J., Pulkkinen, A.J. & Haddow, J.E. (1993). Association between exposure to environmental tobacco smoke and exacerbations of asthma in children. *New England Journal of Medicine, 328*, 1665-1669.

Cohen- Klonoff, H.S., Edelstein, S.L., Schneider Lefkowtiz, E., Srinivasan, I.P., Kaegi, D., Chang, J.C. & Wiley, K.J. (1995). The effect of passive smoking and tobacco exposure through breast milk on sudden infant death syndrome. *Journal of the American Medical Association, 273*, 795-798.

Fiore, M.C., ed. (1992). The Medical Clinics of North America. *Cigarette Smoking: A Clinical Guide to Assessment and Treatment*. Toronto: W.B. Saunders.

Fredricsson, B. & Gilljam, H. (1992). Smoking and reproduction: Short and long term effects and benefits of smoking cessation. *Acta Obstetrics Gynecol Scandinavia, 71*, 580-592.

Heatherton, T.F., Kozlowski, L.T., Frecker, R.C. & Fagerström, K-O. (1991). The Fagerström test for nicotine dependence: A revision of the Fagerström Tolerance Questionnaire. *British Journal of Addiction, 86*, 1119-1127.

Hughes, J.R., Gust, S.W., Skoog, K., Keenan, R.M. & Fenwick, J.W. (1991). Symptoms of tobacco withdrawal. *Archives of General Psychiatry, 48*, 42-59.

Le Houezec, J. & Benowitz, N.L. (1991). Basic and clinical psychopharmacology of nicotine. In J.M. Samet & D.B. Coultas (Eds.), *Clinics in Chest Medicine: Smoking Cessation*. Toronto: W.B. Saunders.

Makomaski Illing, E.M. & Kaiserman, M.J. (1995). Mortality attributable to tobacco use in Canada and its regions, 1991. *Canadian Journal of Public Health, 86*, 257-265.

McKenzie, D., Williams, B. & Single, E. (1997). *Canadian Profile: Alcohol, Tobacco and Other Drugs, 1997*. Toronto: Canadian Centre on Substance Abuse/Addiction Research Foundation.

Muscati, S.K., Gray-Donald, K. & Newson, E.E. (1994). Interaction of smoking and maternal weight status in influencing infant size. *Canadian Journal of Public Health, 85*, 407-412.

National Cancer Institute of Canada. (1996). *Canadian Cancer Statistics 1996*. Toronto: National Cancer Institute of Canada.

Peto, R., Lopez, A.D., Boreham, J., Thun, M. & Heath, C. Jr. (1994). *Mortality From Smoking in Developed Countries 1950-2000: Indirect Estimates From National Vital Statistics.* New York: University Press.

Pomerleau, O.F., Flessland, K.A., Pomerleau, C.S. & Hariharan, M. (1992). Controlled dosing of nicotine via an intranasal nicotine aerosol delivery device (INADD). *Psychopharmacology, 108,* 519-526.

Rickert, W.S. (1995). *A Historical Study of Nicotine Yields of Canadian Cigarettes in Relation to the Composition and Nicotine Content of Cigarette Tobacco (1968-1995).* Ottawa: Government of Canada.

Royal Society of Canada (1989). *Tobacco, Nicotine and Addiction.* Ottawa: Royal Society of Canada.

Silagy, C., Mant, D., Fowler, G. & Lodge, M. (1994). Meta-analysis on efficacy of nicotine replacement therapies in smoking cessation. *The Lancet, 343,* 139-142.

Single, E., Robson, L., Xie, X. & Rehm, J. (1996). *The Costs of Substance Abuse in Canada, Highlights of a Major Study of the Health, Social and Economic Costs Associated With the Use of Alcohol, Tobacco and Illicit Drugs.* Ottawa: Canadian Centre on Substance Abuse.

U.S. Department of Health and Human Services. (1988). *The Health Consequences of Smoking: Nicotine Addiction.* A Report of the Surgeon General. Rockville, MD: U.S. Department of Health and Human Services, Public Health Service, Office on Smoking and Health. DHHS Publication No. (PHS) 88-8406.

U.S. Department of Health and Human Services. (1993). *Respiratory Health Effects of Passive Smoking: Lung Cancer and Other Disorders. The Report of the U.S. Environmental Protection Agency.* Public Health Service, National Institutes of Health, National Cancer Institute. Smoking and Tobacco Control, Monograph 4. NIH Publication No. 93-3605.

Wigle, D.T., Mao, Y., Wong, T. & Lane, R. (1991). Economic burden of illness in Canada, 1986. *Chronic Diseases in Canada, 12 (3),* supplement.

Wright, A.L., Holberg, C., Martinez, F.D., Taussig, L.M. & Group Health Medical Associates. (1991). Relationship of parental smoking to wheezing and nonwheezing lower respiratory tract illnesses in infancy. *Journal of Pediatrics, 118,* 207-214.

Oxycodone

DRUG CLASS: Opioid

Synopsis

Oxycodone is a semi-synthetic opioid derived from the chemical modification of codeine. It produces potent euphoric, analgesic and sedative effects and has a dependence liability similar to that of morphine. Its main clinical use is in the management of moderate to severe pain. One of the principal advantages of oxycodone over some other opioid analgesics is its substantial potency when administered orally. For this reason it is widely used for pain relief for patients functioning in the community and, for the same reason, has become a popular drug of abuse. Chronic high-dose abuse of oxycodone can produce powerful physical dependence. The withdrawal syndrome that develops upon abrupt termination of use is similar to that produced upon termination of morphine. When used for medicinal purposes for extended periods, at even low doses, it can produce physical dependence. Tolerance to its euphoric, pain-relieving and sedative effects can develop rapidly, particularly when the drug is abused at high dose levels.

Oxycodone has a very high potential for abuse, not only because it is highly effective when taken orally, but also because its extensive medicinal use makes it relatively easily available in dosage forms of high purity at relatively low cost.

Drug Source

Oxycodone is produced by the pharmaceutical industry through the chemical modification of codeine.

Alternative Non-Proprietary/Generic Name

Dihydrohydroxycodeinone

Trade Names

Oxycontin®, Supeudol®.

Street Name

Percs.

Combination Products

- Percocet® (oxycodone hydrochloride, acetaminophen)

- Percocet-Demi® (oxycodone hydrochloride, acetaminophen)

- Percodan® (oxycodone hydrochloride, ASA)

- Percodan-Demi® (oxycodone hydrochloride, ASA)

- Endocet® (oxycodone hydrochloride, acetaminophen)

- Endodan® (oxycodone, ASA)

- Oxycocet® (oxycodone hydrochloride, acetaminophen)

- Oxycodan® (oxycodone hydrochloride, ASA)

- Roxicet® (acetaminophen, oxycodone hydrochloride).

Medical Uses

Relief of moderate to severe pain.

Physical Appearance

Oxycodone in pure form occurs as a white, odorless crystalline powder that is slightly soluble in water and soluble in alcohol. Its salts are freely soluble in water and only slightly soluble in alcohol.

Dosage[1, 2]

Medical

Oxycodone is used medically to treat moderate to severe pain in the following formulations and doses:

- with oral tablets, 5 to 10 mg up to four times daily as necessary for adequate pain relief

- with oral controlled-release formulations, initially 10 mg every 12 hours, with subsequent adjustment based on patient's response, or the dose level of oxycodone equivalent to one-half the patient's previous daily dose of opioid analgesic

- with suppositories, 10 to 40 mg up to four times daily as necessary for adequate pain relief

- with oral products containing ASA 325 mg or acetaminophen 325 mg, combined with oxycodone hydrochloride 5 mg, usually one tablet up to four times per day.

Non-medical

Daily doses of up to 100 mg or more have been reported. Dosage is progressively increased as tolerance develops to the desired effects.

---

[1] All doses refer to adults.

[2] Oxycodone hydrochloride 5 to 10 mg administered parenterally or 10 to 15 mg administered orally is approximately equal in analgesic potency to 10 mg of morphine injected intramuscularly.

Routes of Administration

Orally[3] or by suppository. Dependent users have occasionally been reported to inject the drug.

Effects of Short-Term Use: Low Doses[4]

CNS, behavioral, subjective: suppression of the sensation of pain and of emotional response to it; euphoria; relaxation; sedation; lightheadedness; dizziness; drowsiness; some clouding of mental function; in some people, mild depression and anxiety; pupillary constriction (which can impair night vision); and blurred vision.

Respiratory: reduction in respiratory rate.

Gastrointestinal: dry mouth, nausea and vomiting, loss of appetite and constipation.

Other: blurred vision, sweating, reduced libido, and itching.

Effects of Short-Term Use: Higher Doses[5]

Intensification of oxycodone's low-dose effects may occur with administration of higher doses. The duration of effects also increases with the size of the dose, including reduced awareness of and response to pain, increasing inability to concentrate and greater likelihood of sleep. Breathing tends to become progressively slower and more shallow; the heart rate and blood pressure tend to decrease.

In very high doses (i.e., overdose), oxycodone can produce deep sleep that may progress to stupor or coma; low blood pressure; slowed heart rate; cyanosis; shallow,

---

[3]   One of the principal advantages of this drug is that it is much more potent than an equal weight of codeine taken orally and retains at least half of its analgesic potency when administered orally.

[4]   Single doses within the therapeutic range administered orally to non-tolerant users, up to approximately 20 mg per day.

[5]   Single doses in excess of the therapeutic range administered orally in non-tolerant users, or lower doses in particularly sensitive individuals.

slowed breathing; reduced body temperature; flaccidity of skeletal muscles; and cold and clammy skin.

Effects of Long-Term Use

There have been no indications of marked physiological deterioration or significant psychological impairment among long-term oxycodone abusers. Adverse effects that can be directly attributed to chronic abuse of this drug include mood instability,[6] pupillary constriction, blurred vision, impaired night vision, constipation, menstrual irregularity and certain types of respiratory impairment.

Lethality

Severe overdose may result in respiratory arrest, circulatory collapse, cardiac arrest and death. The estimated lethal dose for a non-tolerant adult is approximately 500 mg. Overdose of the combination products produces additional effects:

- Ingestion of large quantities of products containing a combination of ASA and oxycodone may result in acute salicylate poisoning.

- Ingestion of large quantities of products containing a combination of acetaminophen and oxycodone may result in acute acetaminophen poisoning.

Tolerance and Dependence

Tolerance

Tolerance to many of the main effects produced by oxycodone can develop rapidly with regular use. These effects include the euphoric, analgesic, sedative and, to some extent, respiratory-depressant and nausea-producing actions. Tolerance does not appear to develop to oxycodone's pupillary constricting effect, and it develops only partially to the constipating effect.

---

6   This is due to the relatively short duration of the effects of oxycodone, i.e., four to five hours.

As tolerance develops to the desired effects, the daily dose of the drug must be increased to compensate for decreased sensitivity. After several such increases, the user may reach a dose plateau where no further increase in the size of the dose can produce the intensity of effects desired. If users do not then switch to a more potent opioid analgesic, they are likely to self-administer the drug with the same frequency and dose, but primarily to prevent the onset of withdrawal symptoms.

Physical Dependence/Withdrawal

Powerful physical dependence on oxycodone can result for the regular heavy user, and abrupt abstinence results in a withdrawal syndrome as severe as that produced upon abstinence from morphine.[7] Early symptoms may be present approximately eight hours after the last dose. These include watering eyes, nasal discharge, uncontrollable yawning and heavy sweating, often followed by agitated sleep. At peak intensity (approximately 36 to 72 hours after use has stopped), these symptoms are intensified and may be accompanied by severe agitation, alternations between chills and flushing, tremor, severe yawning and sneezing, loss of appetite, insomnia, "goose-flesh," vomiting, nausea, abdominal cramps, elevated heart rate and blood pressure, pains in the muscles and joints, muscle spasms and uncontrolled kicking movements. Intensity of the syndrome gradually declines and most signs persist no longer than one week.

Psychological Dependence

The impact of long-term dependence on oxycodone (and other opioids) is often observable for a long time after the classic signs of withdrawal have disappeared. Chronic depression, anxiety, insomnia, loss of appetite, periods of agitation and continued craving for the drug can persist for months (or in some cases even years). Although such symptoms have often been interpreted as indications of psychological dependence, they are likely associated with complex physiological adjustments after withdrawal.

---

[7]   At any time during withdrawal, administration of a suitable dose of oxycodone (or many other opioids) can either partially or completely suppress the syndrome.

Patterns of Use

Several decades have passed since oxycodone was introduced into medicine as a powerful orally effective analgesic, with the hope that it would be a safe alternative to morphine. Because of its oral effectiveness and greater analgesic potency than morphine, oxycodone became widely used in the management of moderate to severe pain among patients in community settings.[8] Further, because it can produce a potent euphoric effect, oxycodone also rapidly became an important drug of abuse. Street abusers obtain oxycodone-containing medications by stealing from pharmacies, by forging prescriptions on stolen prescription blanks and by faking painful conditions that are difficult for a physician to confirm objectively (e.g., back pain). It is not unusual for an oxycodone abuser to obtain several prescriptions per week from different doctors ("double doctoring"). Oxycodone-containing products obtained by such methods are sometimes diverted to the illicit drug market, where they are prized for the consistency of their dose level and effects.

Potential for Abuse

Dependence Liability

Currently available oxycodone preparations contain fillers that make injection both difficult and painful. Therefore, abusers generally take the drug orally. When the drug is administered in this way, its euphoric effect, although still powerful, is experienced less rapidly and in lower intensity than is the case when oxycodone or other powerful opioids are injected.

Oxycodone hydrochloride in pure form is soluble and can be injected in large quantities directly into the bloodstream. Under these conditions, both the immediacy and potency of its effects are approximately equal to those that would result from injection of a similar dose (by weight) of morphine. Thus, its inherent dependence liability is as great as that of morphine. However, pure oxycodone is not generally available on the street.

---

[8]   The estimated per-capita quantity of oxycodone used in Canada for medical and scientific purposes more than tripled during the 1970s.

Inherent Harmfulness

In low to moderate doses, oxycodone usually does not produce hazardous effects. However, nausea and vomiting are common early side effects, and the user must be willing to continue taking the drug regularly in order to acquire tolerance to these effects.

Availability

Because oxycodone is frequently prescribed for painful chronic conditions, there is a risk of patients, developing iatrogenic (medically induced) physical dependence. Some physicians mistakenly believe that the risk of physical dependence on oxy-codone is greatly reduced because it is administered orally. As a result, they tend to prescribe oxycodone less prudently than they would prescribe other powerful opioid analgesics. Nevertheless, chronic use of oxycodone, even if administered orally at low doses, can still produce physical dependence.

The main issues related to the current popularity of oxycodone among opioid abusers appear to be its relatively easy availability, relatively low cost and high degree of relatively consistent purity. For these reasons, regular abusers of oxycodone are willing to forgo the more immediate and intense effects of injected opioids.

Background Reading

Canadian Pharmaceutical Association. (1997). *Compendium of Pharmaceuticals and Specialties* (32nd edition). Ottawa: Canadian Pharmaceutical Association.

Reisine, T. & Pasternak, G. (1996). Opioid analgesics and antagonists. (Chapter 23). In J.G. Hardman, L.E. Limbird, P.B. Molinoff, R.W. Rudden & A.G. Gilman (Eds.), *Goodman and Gilman's The Pharmacological Basis of Therapeutics*. (9th edition). New York/Toronto: McGraw-Hill Health Professions Division.

PCP
(Phencyclidine)

DRUG CLASS: Dissociative Anesthetic, Hallucinogen

Synopsis

Phencyclidine is a dissociative anesthetic[1] originally used in human anesthesia but later limited to veterinary medicine because of the delirium with hallucinations that occurred post-operatively in some patients. However, these hallucinogenic effects are what make PCP so attractive to street drug users. The drug possesses both stimulant and depressant properties and can produce hallucinations, relaxation, feelings of dissociation from the environment and sometimes intense euphoria. Further, it can cause changes in perception and thought processes that are similar to those produced by LSD. Users commonly experience distortions in their perceptions of time, space and body image, as well as visual and auditory distortions.

PCP can also produce very severe traumatic psychic effects even at low doses and in those who have had previous favorable experiences with the drug. Users commonly report agitation, disorganization of thinking and intense feelings of alienation accompanied by paranoia while under PCP's influence. This last experience has sometimes provoked violent and bizarre behavior. Large doses can produce convulsions and respiratory arrest.

Drug Source

Phencyclidine was formerly produced through chemical synthesis by the veterinary pharmaceutical industry, but now originates almost exclusively in illicit laboratories.

---

[1]   Like ketamine it is a member of the cycloalkylarylamine family of psychoactive drugs and has an anesthetic effect without overt loss of consciousness. Patients who receive these drugs as anesthetics remain conscious, with a staring gaze and rigid muscles.

Trade Names

No products containing PCP are legally marketed for human use.

Street Names

Among the many street names for PCP, a few of the more widely used are amoeba, angel dust, animal tranquillizer, cadillac, CJ, crystal, crystal joint, cyclones, DOA (dead on arrival), dust, elephant tranquillizer, goon, hog, horse tranquillizer, KJ, lovely, lovely high, mist, peace pill, peace, rocket fuel, synthetic THC, scuffle, seams, sheet, snorts, super rods, surfer and synthetic marijuana. The abbreviation PCP is derived from the drug's chemical name, *l*-(*l*-phenylcyclohexyl)-piperidine.

Drug Combinations

PCP is sometimes taken with LSD. It is also sprinkled on marijuana and smoked. This combination is sometimes marketed as "peace weed," "supergrass," "superweed" or "killer weed."

Medical Uses

PCP has no current uses in human medicine. It was initially investigated as an anesthetic for human use, but was not marketed for this purpose. It was used by veterinarians and researchers to anesthetize and tranquillize large animals, particularly primates.

Physical Appearance

Although, in its pure form, phencyclidine occurs as a white crystalline powder that dissolves rapidly in water or alcohol, PCP is encountered on the street in variously colored tablets, capsules or powders. It is quite often misrepresented to the street buyer as methamphetamine ("speed"), mescaline, LSD or other psychoactive substances such as THC (tetrahydrocannabinol, the active ingredient in cannabis). When it is mixed with marijuana (i.e., in products such as supergrass) or other leaf material such as parsley, tobacco or mint, it may not be visible to the user.[2]

Dosage[3]

Medical
Phencyclidine is no longer used in clinical medicine. When it was used by veterinarians, the dose varied in proportion to the type of animal and the purpose for which it was used (tranquillization or anesthesia).

Non-medical
The typical dose is 5 to 10 mg. There have been reports that chronic users may take single doses of up to 80 to 100 mg, two to three times per day continuously over a period of a few days, in the form of PCP "joints," made of a leaf substance such as parsley sprinkled with the drug and smoked. There have been unsubstantiated reports of users consuming 0.5 to 1.0 gram (500 to 1,000 mg) over a 24-hour period.

Routes of Administration

PCP may be taken orally in the form of a liquid, tablet or capsule; "snorted" (sniffed); smoked sprinkled on marijuana, parsley, tobacco, mint or other smokable substance; or injected (usually intravenously).

---

[2]   Such products are typically prepared by adding a solution of PCP to leaf material and then drying the product so that a film of PCP remains on the leaf material.

[3]   All doses refer to adults.

Effects of Short-Term Use: Low Doses[4]

The effects of the short-term use of low doses of PCP include the following.

CNS, *behavioral, subjective:* There is a fairly wide variation among users in their perceptual, cognitive and emotional experiences resulting from PCP use. In addition to the size of the dose, drug effects are influenced by the setting, as well as the user's expectations,[5] past drug experiences and personality. It is not unusual for a user to experience differing reactions to PCP during different drug-taking episodes. CNS effects may include the following:

- mild to intense euphoria

- relaxation, drowsiness or pleasant stimulation

- feelings of dissociation from the environment and of unreality

- distortion of the user's perception of his or her body, including sensations of weightlessness and floating

- distortion in perception of time (minutes may seem to pass as slowly as hours)

- distortion in perception of space

- numbness of the extremities

- visual and auditory distortions (true hallucinations can occur, but are much more likely to be experienced at higher doses) and possibly distortions involving any of the other senses

- difficulties in concentrating, thinking or maintaining attention

- a "body trip," related to a schizophrenic-like state.

Primarily physical CNS effects can include speech disturbances such as difficulty in articulating, impairment of motor co-ordination, impairment of fine dexterity, pupillary constriction, blurred vision and sometimes dizziness.

---

4   Five milligrams or less, taken orally by non-tolerant users.

5   The user's subjective expectations are particularly important in the case of PCP because this drug is so frequently misrepresented to be other substances. Severe agitation or panic may ensue for the unsuspecting user who is anticipating the very different effects of another drug.

Adverse effects may range from mild to severe and may include any of the following symptoms: anxiety (quite common), agitation, paranoid thinking, panic or even terror; confusion and thought disorganization; precipitation of previously latent psychosis; blank staring, stupor and catatonic rigidity; mutism (inability to speak); intense feelings of alienation; depression, sometimes severe enough to precipitate a suicide attempt; hostile and possibly violent and bizarre behavior; amnesia for events occurring during the drug-taking episode; and a painful reaction to sounds.

At moderately higher doses (e.g., 10 mg), the anesthetic and analgesic properties of PCP are likely to be evident. Sensitivity to pain decreases and probability of sleep increases. There may be a psychic experience similar to sensory isolation.

Cardiovascular: increased blood pressure and heart rate.

Respiratory: increased breathing rate, but with breathing tending to be more shallow.

Other: increased urinary output, sweating, nausea and vomiting.

The effects of relatively pure PCP when smoked are perceptible within a few minutes and peak in approximately 30 minutes. The "high" lasts between four and six hours, with a gradual decline of effects ("coming down") usually completed within 24 hours.

Effects of Short-Term Use: Higher Doses[6]

Intensification of low-dose effects of PCP may occur at higher doses, as well as any of the following effects.

CNS, behavioral, subjective:[7] erratic and bizarre behavior and compulsive repetitive movements; severe psychological disorganization and acute toxic psychosis, often evident in a clinical picture that can include confusion, incoherent speech, disorientation, paranoia, possibly hostile or violent behavior, agitation and restlessness,

---

[6]   In excess of 10 mg in non-tolerant users, and lower doses in particularly sensitive individuals.

[7]   As with low doses, perceptual, cognitive and emotional experiences may vary considerably among users.

autism, preoccupation or obsession with what would otherwise be trivial matters, hallucinations and grandiose delusions. States of panic, terror, and overwhelming fear of imminent death have been observed. This state frequently lasts for several days.

Other physical CNS effects can include involuntary rapid movement of the eyes, especially rolling movements (nystagmus), which can be used to distinguish PCP intoxication from a naturally occurring psychotic state; dilated pupils; muscular rigidity; decreased awareness of the sensations of pain, touch and position; absence of or decreased gag and corneal reflexes; posture spasms in which the body arches from head to heel; stupor or coma.

Cardiovascular: irregular heartbeat, alternation between abnormally high and abnormally low blood pressure.

Respiratory: slow, shallow and irregular breathing.

Gastrointestinal: severe nausea and vomiting and persistent heavy salivation.

Other: decreased urinary output, deterioration of muscle tissue (rhabdomyolysis). Increased body temperature and heavy sweating may alternate with chills and shivering.

At very high doses (i.e., severe overdose), coma, convulsions and death (usually attributed to respiratory arrest) can occur. Treatment of phencyclidine intoxication/overdose has typically included attempts to decrease absorption of the drug from the gastrointestinal tract (e.g., by administering activated charcoal) and increase the rate of excretion of absorbed drug from the body (e.g., by administering ammonium chloride or ascorbic acid to make the urine more acidic).[8] Results of recent animal studies also suggest the potential effectiveness of anti-PCP antibody therapy in treating phencyclidine overdose. When anti-PCP antibodies were administered after PCP absorption, PCP levels in the brain were reduced.

---

8   The mechanism of increased excretion is explained in Section 1.

Effects of Long-Term Use

What is known about the effects of chronic use of PCP is based largely on clinical case reports. Although some of these reports appear to provide no more than users' perceptions, the symptoms described by regular users are consistent.

Like methamphetamine ("speed") users, chronic PCP users often engage in "runs," using the drug repeatedly over an uninterrupted period of two to three days without sleeping and with little or no eating. The "run" is followed by a protracted period of sleep from which the user often awakens feeling disoriented and depressed. "Runs" may be repeated as frequently as two to four times per month.

Chronic high-dose users report impaired thinking and memory, particularly recent memory, but in most users, these functions recover within a period of several months after PCP use has stopped. As well, some users report unpleasant "flashbacks" similar to those experienced by LSD users. Persistent speech problems (including stuttering, the inability to articulate and the inability to speak at all) have been observed, which may also continue for extended periods after the PCP use has been terminated. Chronic and possibly severe anxiety and depression are common, and some regular users become sufficiently depressed to attempt suicide.

Although early experiences with PCP usually occur in the company of others, there is often gradual social withdrawal and isolation. Many users report marriage breakdown, lost employment and disrupted education. Since most regular users of PCP also use alcohol, marijuana and/or other drugs, these other substances may contribute to this spectrum of symptoms.

PCP-influenced behavior is frequently unpredictable and sometimes includes extreme violence against other people. Toxic psychosis, similar to amphetamine psychosis or acute schizophrenia, has been observed in some chronic users who had no known psychiatric disturbances prior to their regular use of PCP. Symptoms of this syndrome include aggressive or violent behavior towards others, paranoia, delusional thinking and (mainly auditory) hallucinations. However, research studies indicate that higher levels of violence are reported by PCP users with a history of psychiatric treatment. As a study conducted in hospital emergency rooms showed, intoxicated users with acute psychiatric problems are often extremely difficult to manage.

Most chronic users acknowledge having experienced at least one "bad trip," but in most cases the unpleasant experience did not result in their terminating use of PCP. Apparently the possibility of the extraordinary "high" and feelings of euphoria is enough to encourage further use. Psychological dependence does seem to develop for many high-dose users (see Tolerance and Dependence, below).

PCP and Pregnancy

Exposure to phencyclidine in the uterus has been found to have serious effects on fetal growth, although these effects were less pronounced than those produced by exposure to cocaine. Similarly, phencyclidine is less likely than cocaine to be associated with infants with small head circumference. Although PCP-exposed newborns may exhibit signs and symptoms that suggest a withdrawal syndrome somewhat like that experienced by opioid-exposed newborns (including poor attention and increased muscle tone), it has been suggested that these are effects of PCP itself, not evidence of withdrawal symptoms.

Lethality

Deaths from acute overdose of PCP have occurred after use of (estimated) amounts of 150 and 200 mg.[9] While the usual clinical picture is seizures, coma and respiratory arrest, acute hypertensive crisis, hemorrhage of the blood vessels in the brain and kidney failure have also been reported to result from extremely high doses of PCP. The overdose profile may also be complicated by the presence of other drugs in the body. For example, high doses of CNS-depressant drugs (e.g., sedative/hypnotics or opioids) substantially increase the risk of respiratory arrest.

Many PCP-related deaths have also resulted from the psychological impact of the drug. Some PCP users, for example, have reported trying to swim in an effort to enhance the sensations of weightlessness and floating, but depressed sensory and muscle control has led to several accidental drownings. Other deaths have resulted from leaps from high places and motor vehicle accidents. Suicides, homicides (sometimes bizarre), self-mutilations and other results of extremely violent behavior have also been reported to be associated with use of this drug.

---

9   It is likely that lower doses could prove fatal to some.

Tolerance and Dependence

Tolerance to the effects of PCP has yet to be clearly demonstrated. However, preliminary observations and subjective reports suggest that tolerance can develop with long-term, regular use. Two separate investigations of chronic users of PCP, conducted in widely separated geographic areas, have resulted in similar findings. Initially, only a few puffs (a few milligrams) of a PCP "joint" were required to produce the euphoric "high" in users. Most of the subjects indicated a consistent need to increase their intake in order to maintain the "high," and within two to six weeks many were smoking one or two "joints" at a time. (It was estimated that each "joint" contained between 50 and 80 mg of PCP.) Some users reported taking even higher doses at one sitting. Although their reports were unsubstantiated, some also claimed to use up to one gram (1,000 mg) within a 24-hour period.

Reports of physical dependence in humans are rare, and none have been objectively confirmed. Although withdrawal symptoms upon abrupt termination of use have been reported for some animal species,[10] PCP abusers in drug treatment do not report a physiological withdrawal syndrome when stopping PCP use. Psychological dependence has been reported in several chronic users in the form of a craving for the effects of PCP when it was temporarily unavailable and difficulty stopping use despite adverse consequences.

Patterns of Use

Phencyclidine was initially introduced into clinical medicine as an anesthetic in the 1950s. Disturbing reports regarding convulsions during surgery and such postoperative effects as agitation, confusion, disorientation and hallucinations quickly ended its medical use for humans. It was again marketed in the 1960s exclusively as an animal anesthetic under the trade name Sernylan®. It also appeared on the streets in San Francisco at the same time, and was referred to in the drug subculture as the "peace pill," adapted from the name PCP which, in turn, is an abbreviation for the chemical name, *l*-(*l*-phenylcyclohexyl)-piperidine.

---

[10]   Experiments designed to study withdrawal symptoms in humans have not been performed. Such experiments were necessary, for example, to establish that humans could become physically dependent on cannabis.

Because of the variety of the drug's psychoactive properties, it has been sold on the street not only as PCP but also, falsely, as a host of other drugs, most commonly THC, methamphetamine, mescaline and LSD. Large profits have been made by such misrepresentation, particularly in areas where the desired drugs are scarce and expensive, since the chemicals needed to synthesize PCP cost relatively little.

Although caution should be exercised in interpreting the statistics, the number of PCP-related deaths and hospital emergency department admissions due to PCP overdose appeared to increase consistently during the 1970s and 1980s. Although PCP is currently used across North America, its use appears to be most common among males aged 18 and older in some major cities. A 1997 survey of Ontario students in Grades 7 to 13[11] found that two per cent of the students reported having used PCP in the previous 12 months, and that more males than females had used the drug.

A trend toward increased incidence of PCP abuse seems to have continued in the 1990s despite the substantial negative publicity the drug has received.

In recent years, a number of substances structurally related to PCP have been synthesized by "basement" chemists, particularly in California. Many of these congeners produce effects that are similar to those of PCP. One key reason for their current popularity is that they are less readily detected in routine urine screenings for PCP, which are commonly required by drug abuse treatment and parole services.

Potential for Abuse

Dependence Liability
Physical dependence on PCP has not yet been demonstrated, and the incidence of psychological dependence is not known. However, intense euphoria appears to be one common reaction to PCP and accounts at least in part for its appeal for those who use it regularly.

---

11   The traditional "Grade 13" has now been replaced by an Ontario Academic Credit (OAC) year in Ontario schools. However, the Ontario survey, and therefore this text, has kept the term "Grade 13" to facilitate comparisons with surveys from previous years.

Inherent Harmfulness

The effects of PCP vary considerably among users and from one drug episode to another. As a result it is not possible to predict with any certainty how a given user will react to this drug on any given occasion. Even in low doses, PCP can produce very harmful psychological effects, and at higher doses the effects may be life-threatening.

The drug is currently widely abused. No doubt abuse would be even more widespread if it were not for the dangers attendant on its use, the unpredictability of these dangers and the drug's consequent reputation in the street-drug subculture.

Availability

PCP is currently widely available on the illicit North American drug market.

Background Reading

Adlaf, E.M., Ivis, F.J. & Smart, R.G. (1997). *Ontario Student Drug Use Survey, 1977-1997.* Toronto: Addiction Research Foundation.

Carroll, M. (1985). PCP. *The Dangerous Angel.* The Encyclopedia of Psychoactive Drugs Series. New York: Chelsea House Publishers.

Caroll, M. (1990) PCP and hallucinogens. *Advances in Alcohol and Substance Abuse, 9 (1-2),* 167-190.

Gorelick, D.A. & Wilkins, J.N. (1989). Inpatient treatment of PCP abusers and users. *American Journal of Drug and Alcohol Abuse, 15 (1),* 1–12.

Gorelick, D.A., Wilkins, J.N. & Wong, C. (1989). Outpatient treatment of PCP abusers. *American Journal of Drug and Alcohol Abuse, 15 (4),* 367–374.

McCardle, L. & Fishbein, D.H. (1989). The self-reported effects of PCP on human aggression. *Addictive Behaviors, 14 (4),* 465–472.

Poklis, A., Graham, M., Maginn, D., Branch, C.A. & Gantner, G.E. (1990). Phencyclidine in violent deaths in St. Louis, Missouri: A survey of medical examiners' cases from 1977 through 1986. *American Journal of Drug and Alcohol Abuse, 16 (3-4),* 265–274.

Rahbar, F., Fomufod, A., White, A. & Westney, L.S. (1993). Impact of intrauterine exposure to phencyclidine (PCP) and cocaine in neonates. *Journal of the National Medical Association, 85 (5),* 349–352.

Tabor, B.L., Smith-Wallace, T. & Yonekura, M.L. (1990). Perinatal outcome associated with PCP versus cocaine use. *Journal of Drug and Alcohol Abuse, 16 (3-4)*, 337–348.

Thombs, D.L. (1989). A review of PCP abuse trends and perceptions. *Public Health Reports, 104 (4)*, 325–328.

Pentazocine

DRUG CLASS:	Opioid Agonist/Antagonist

Synopsis

Pentazocine was synthesized as part of a continuing effort to find a drug sufficiently potent to relieve moderately severe to severe pain without the danger of abuse associated with opioid analgesics such as morphine. In fact, while pentazocine has opioid analgesic properties, it is also a weak opioid antagonist. As a result, it can precipitate mild withdrawal symptoms when administered to opioid-dependent users,[1] but does not block the respiratory depression caused by opioid agonists such as morphine.

When taken orally, pentazocine has an analgesic potency[2] greater than meperidine (e.g., Demerol®); when injected intramuscularly, its analgesic potency is approximately one-sixth that of morphine.

In the 1970s, pentazocine surfaced as a drug of abuse in its own right because it can produce the euphoria typical of opioids as well as pleasant sensations of floating. Some abusers have likened its effects to those produced by marijuana. At high doses, pentazocine can produce toxic psychosis. Furthermore, chronic injection of pentazocine can cause significant tissue damage at injection sites.

Studies have shown that physical dependence on pentazocine may result from chronic use at relatively low dose levels (e.g., 180 mg per day and higher). Distinctly unpleasant withdrawal symptoms following the abrupt cessation of chronic use include abdominal cramps, anxiety, restlessness, pallor, exaggerated breathing, nausea and vomiting, chills, elevated body temperature, sweating and watering eyes.

---

[1] See the chapter on opioid analgesics and antagonists in Section 2 for a discussion of agonists/antagonists.

[2] The analgesic effect of 50 mg of pentazocine has been reported to be approximately equivalent to that of 60 mg codeine.

In the late 1970s and early 1980s, a number of reports surfaced regarding widespread abuse of pentazocine in combination with an antihistamine, tripelennamine.[3] This combination, referred to as "Ts and Blues," produces a heroin-like effect when injected intravenously. The exceptionally rapid rise in popularity of Ts and Blues in many U.S. cities was related to a scarcity of heroin in the late 1970s, particularly in the midwestern states. Ts and Blues were cheap and easily available, and produced effects satisfactory to many opioid abusers. However, dangerous side effects, including seizures, respiratory impairment and psychotic symptoms, have been linked to abuse of this combination.

Drug Source

Pentazocine is produced through chemical synthesis by the pharmaceutical industry.

Trade Name

Talwin®.

Street Names

- Ts, big T, Tee, Tea

- for Talwin Nx® — butterballs; bananas; footballs.

Combination Products

Medical
- Talwin Nx® (pentazocine and naloxone[4]; not marketed in Canada)

- pentazocine in combination with ASA (not marketed in Canada)

- pentazocine in combination with acetaminophen (not marketed in Canada).

---

3   Tripelennamine is marketed under the trade name Pyribenzamine®.

4   Naloxone is an opioid antagonist. See the chapter on naloxone in Section 3.

Non-medical

- Ts and Blues, Ts and Bs (pentazocine and tripelennamine)

- One and Ones, Ts and Rs, Ts and Ritz, crackers (pentazocine and methylphenidate).

Medical Uses

Pentazocine is used medically for relief from moderate to severe pain.

Physical Appearance

Pentazocine hydrochloride occurs as a white crystalline powder that is soluble in water and alcohol.

Dosage[5]

Medical

Pentazocine is used medically in the following doses:

- oral — 50 to 100 mg every three to four hours

- by injection — 30 mg every three to four hours by the intramuscular, subcutaneous or intravenous route, usually not more than three doses daily, and not exceeding 360 mg daily.

Non-medical

Doses substantially in excess of 1 gram (1,000 mg) per day have been reported in tolerant users.

---

[5] All doses refer to adults.

Routes of Administration

Orally by tablet, and by subcutaneous, intramuscular and intravenous injection. Abusers may crush the tablets and prepare them in solution for injection, often in combination with tripelennamine.

Effects of Short-Term Use: Low Doses[6]

CNS, behavioral, subjective: Pentazocine's effects include relief from and reduced emotional response to moderate to severe pain,[7,8] euphoria in some and anxiety in others, sedation, lightheadedness, dizziness and blurred vision. Some users report sensations of floating. Less frequent effects include transient hallucinations (more often with injection than with oral use), confusion, nightmares, excitement and tremors.

Cardiovascular: infrequently, drop in blood pressure and increased heart rate.

Respiratory: slight to moderate respiratory depression.

Gastrointestinal: nausea and vomiting, constipation, abdominal distress and anorexia.

Other: sweating.

Because pentazocine is a weak opioid antagonist, individuals who are physically dependent on opioid analgesics may experience withdrawal signs and symptoms after use of pentazocine. Usually such signs and symptoms are not produced after a one- to two-day opioid-free period.

---

6   Single doses within the therapeutic range administered orally or by injection to non-tolerant persons. Symptoms tend to be similar to many of those produced by opioid analgesics.

7   The analgesic effects of pentazocine are thought to result from its action as an agonist at the κ (kappa) opioid receptors, while its antagonist properties are thought to be associated with its interaction with μ (mu) receptors.

8   Taken orally, 50 mg pentazocine has an analgesic potency approximately equivalent to 100 mg meperidine (e.g., Demerol®); by injection, 30 mg of pentazocine is approximately equivalent to 10 mg morphine.

Effects of Short-Term Use: Higher Doses[9]

Intensification of pentazocine's low-dose effects may occur at higher dose levels, as well as any of the following effects:

- abnormal increase in blood pressure and heart rate
- respiratory depression, usually more moderate than that which occurs with high doses of other opioids
- increasing impairment of ability to concentrate
- toxic psychotic states, characterized by hallucinations, delusions, disorientation and confusion.

With injection of doses above 60 mg, psychotomimetic effects similar to those produced by nalorphine (see Section 5) may occur. These effects may include strange or uncontrollable thoughts, anxiety, nightmares and hallucinations.

At very high doses (i.e., overdose), pentazocine can produce deep sleep, possibly progressing to stupor or coma. Blood pressure and heart rate may be abnormally high and heartbeat may be irregular. Seizures may occur.

Few cases of severe overdose of pentazocine have been reported. One such case involved ingestion of 1.5 grams of this drug. Symptoms included coma, continuous seizure activity, respiratory depression, acidosis, profoundly low blood pressure, irregular heartbeat and fixed pupils. Although the patient survived and regained consciousness, toxic psychotic symptoms persisted for four days.

Effects of Long-Term Use

In one study, normal volunteers received daily doses of 100 to 800 mg of pentazocine per day for 35 to 200 days. There were no significant effects on vital signs except in one case. However, there have been several clinical reports of pentazocine-induced emotional disturbances among medical patients on high-dose therapy. Most

---

9   Single doses in excess of the therapeutic range (or lower doses in particularly sensitive individuals) administered either orally or by injection to non-tolerant persons.

commonly occurring is depression, which can be quite severe. Acute toxic psychosis may persist until pentazocine use is discontinued. Nightmares, dizziness upon awakening, other sleep disturbances and concentration difficulties have also occasionally been associated with chronic use of this drug.

Chronic injection of pentazocine in the same area may result in hardening of the skin and subcutaneous and muscle tissue near the injection sites. The resulting ulcers may be deep and surrounded by a halo of discoloration, but may not be painful despite the tissue damage.

"Ts and Blues": Chronic Injection of Pentazocine and Tripelennamine

During the late 1970s and early 1980s, the abuse of pentazocine in combination with the antihistamine tripelennamine (and less frequently in combination with other drugs[10]) reached epidemic proportions in a number of U.S. cities. The popular street name "Ts and Blues" derives from the trade name, Talwin, and from the light-blue color of tripelennamine tablets marketed under the trade name Pyribenzamine®.

The size of individual doses taken by users varied greatly. It was not unusual for 150 to 200 mg (or more) of pentazocine to be injected along with half as much of tripelennamine. The tablets of each were crushed and dissolved as much as possible (but not completely) in a small quantity of water. The crude solution was then filtered through cotton (or a similar substance), drawn into a syringe and injected intravenously or subcutaneously. The subjective experience immediately following intravenous injection is reputed to be similar to the typical heroin "rush" — an intense orgasm-like sensation in the abdomen, lasting for five to 10 minutes. Dysphoric feelings, such as irritability and restlessness, often follow the rush, and this discomfort may prompt a second or even third injection. A satisfactory "high" may then be maintained for four to six hours.

It is not yet understood why these drugs combine to produce a highly potent euphoric effect. Taken alone, tripelennamine appears to produce little or no euphoria (although there are a few reported cases of intravenous abuse for a pleasant "high"). Furthermore, the intensity of euphoria produced by pentazocine, whether taken orally or by injection, is mild when compared with that of the opioids most prized by users. It would therefore seem that the antihistamine potentiates the effects of pentazocine.[11]

---

10   For example, methylphenidate, diphenhydramine.

11   Potentiation is a phenomenon that occurs with many drug combinations, in which the effect created by their combined actions is greater than one would expect from the simple addition of their separate effects. See Section 1 for a discussion of this effect.

In addition to irritability and tension, common adverse effects that may follow injection of Ts and Blues include pain and burning sensations at the site of injection, nausea, vomiting, headache, blurred vision, chest pain or tightness, palpitations, chills, profuse sweating, dizziness, rapid heartbeat, anxiety, fearfulness and short-term memory loss.

Several major health problems have been linked to the use of Ts and Blues. Most frequently reported is significant damage to veins and other tissue at the injection sites. Lung impairment is also common in regular users, and can be much more harmful. The damage is caused mainly by insoluble particles such as talc (magnesium silicate) contained in the tablets used to prepare the injected mixture. These particles can cause blood clots and other obstructions of the arterioles and capillaries of the lungs. This can result in impairment of oxygen transfer across the alveolar/capillary membrane, pulmonary hypotension or other abnormalities of respiratory function. In comparison with users of heroin and other intravenous drugs, users of Ts and Blues develop respiratory abnormalities more rapidly, and the abnormalities are more severe.

Excessive doses of either tripelennamine or pentazocine taken alone present a substantial risk of seizures. Taken together, smaller doses of each can result in seizures. It is thought that tripelennamine is the more toxic with respect to the induction of intense CNS stimulation, and reports by users seem to confirm this. It is not unusual for users to gradually increase the amount of tripelennamine from one injection to another, until stimulation becomes too unpleasant or until a seizure occurs; thereafter, they take less tripelennamine. Even so, seizures can recur, and this unpredictability is one important reason users give for taking Ts and Blues in the company of others. Other potential CNS complications linked to injecting Ts and Blues include stroke and infection, either of which can result in permanent brain damage or death. As with all other injected drugs of abuse, the use of non-sterile needles and syringes increases the user's risk of contracting diseases such as hepatitis and AIDS.

Extreme psychological symptoms seem to occur much more frequently among users of Ts and Blues than among users of other opioids. The appearance of these symptoms — which include moderate to severe depression, suicidal thoughts, severe anxiety and panic states, paranoid thinking, disorientation, hallucinations and violent behavior — often coincides with the onset of use. The intensity of these symptoms appears variable.

Agitation and other unpleasant symptoms of CNS stimulation are often cited by users as reasons for their frequent use of alcohol, diazepam or other non-opioid depressants.

Lethality

Deaths due exclusively to overdose of pentazocine are rare. Respiratory depression is usually much less severe than that which occurs with other opioid analgesics. A minimum lethal dose in humans has not been established, although blood concentrations in a few fatalities have ranged between 1 and 5 mg/L.

A number of deaths have been associated with Ts and Blues, although most were not attributable to fatal intoxication. In one report, for example, 63 deaths involving Ts and Blues were investigated by the St. Louis City Medical Examiner's Office. Only six were believed to result from fatal intoxication associated with intravenous injection; the remainder were homicides in which the presence of Ts and Blues in the body was determined by post-mortem examination.

Ts and Blues users are frequent visitors to hospital emergency departments for treatment of a variety of acute and chronic drug effects. However, life-threatening situations linked to the pharmacological effects of Ts and Blues account for a relatively small number of these visits. Nevertheless, many users have experienced at least one seizure; it is generally agreed that seizures are the principal life-threatening effect of this drug combination, although kidney failure and respiratory arrest were recorded in one patient who died in hospital.

Tolerance and Dependence

With frequent repeated use of pentazocine, tolerance develops to both its analgesic and euphoric properties.

When pentazocine was originally marketed, it was considered a non-addictive drug with low potential for abuse. However, it is clear that this early optimism was not justified. Indeed, studies have shown that physical dependence can occur even at moderate therapeutic doses (i.e., 180 mg per day and higher) when the drug is administered daily for at least one month. Underestimation of pentazocine's dependence liability has led to accidental dependence among users. In most cases, the dependence resulted from needle administration, but in a few cases it has resulted from exclusively oral use.

The withdrawal syndrome that occurs after abrupt termination of chronic high-dose use of pentazocine is not as intense as withdrawal from morphine. It is, however, sufficiently unpleasant to cause dependent users to strongly resist discontinuing its use. Commonly observed withdrawal symptoms include abdominal cramps, anxiety, chills alternating with elevated temperature, nausea and vomiting, sweating and watering eyes. Agitation, insomnia and depression have also been reported.

In most cases, withdrawal from Ts and Blues is mild and very similar to pentazocine withdrawal. However, a few users have experienced hallucinations and other manifestations of psychosis.

Like methadone, heroin and other opioids, pentazocine crosses the placental barrier. Withdrawal signs have been observed in a number of neonates whose mothers were regular users of Ts and Blues.

Patterns of Use

Pentazocine taken by itself is much less popular with street drug users than are Ts and Blues. Furthermore, because pentazocine also possesses opioid antagonist properties, dependent users of other opioids cannot substitute this drug to postpone withdrawal sickness when their preferred drug is unavailable.

In the late 1970s, abuse of Ts and Blues had become a major social, medical and legal problem in many large U.S. cities (and in some areas in Western Canada). For example, among drug cases handled by the city police laboratory in St. Louis between 1979 and 1981, the number involving Ts and Blues was exceeded only by those involving cannabis. In Dayton, Ohio, intravenous use of Ts and Blues "for several years represented the most common form of street drug abuse (excepting alcohol) presenting in [the] inner city Emergency Department." In 1980, researchers suggested that in Chicago "if widespread availability continues, the pentazocine and tripelennamine combination could conceivably replace heroin as the drug of choice among addicts."

The principal consumers of Ts and Blues were among the urban poor, a disproportionately high percentage of whom were young (under 30), male and black. (In New Orleans, however, one-third of Ts and Blues users presenting for treatment were female.) Many Ts and Blues users of both sexes had a history of heroin or other opioid abuse. In fact, some returned to heroin, citing as their reason the high incidence of adverse effects associated with Ts and Blues.

Several reasons have been advanced for the sudden rise in popularity of Ts and Blues. Researchers in the midwestern United States — where the epidemic began — observed that the quality and availability of heroin in the Midwest declined in the mid-1970s, while prices increased. Virtually all observers agreed that the T's and Blues combination (rather than other opioids) was the preferred substitute for heroin: in many respects, it produced a similar "high"; Ts and Blues were cheap and easily available from legal sources; controls over pentazocine were not strict (i.e., most legal and medical authorities did not recognize the high potential for abuse of pentazocine); and quality was assured (both drugs were manufactured by the legal pharmaceutical industry).

The origins of this combination are obscure and subject to speculation. There were reports in the 1950s of users of heroin, morphine and paregoric taking tripelennamine in combination with their drug of choice to enhance and prolong the "high" they achieved; these combinations, referred to as "blue velvet," have been mentioned in a number of volumes devoted to drug abuse. A report was also published in the 1940s by a physician who claimed that tripelennamine substantially relieved the symptoms of morphine withdrawal.

In response to concern over widespread abuse, stricter regulatory controls were placed on pentazocine in both the United States and Canada; the purposes of this action were to reduce the availability of pentazocine and to increase penalties for illicit possession and distribution. In 1983, the manufacturers of Talwin in the United States voluntarily introduced Talwin Nx, a combination of pentazocine and naloxone. When this product is taken orally, the naloxone has virtually no effect. However, when it is injected, not only are the effects of pentazocine blocked, but withdrawal is also precipitated in physically dependent users of pentazocine or any other opioid. It appears that these measures (along with reports of adverse effects and increased availability of heroin) resulted in a decrease of Ts and Blues abuse.

Potential for Abuse

Dependence Liability

When it is taken orally at therapeutic doses, pentazocine's dependence liability appears to be relatively low among the opioid analgesic family. When administered intravenously or orally at somewhat higher doses, this drug can produce pleasant sensations of floating and moderately intense euphoria in some users who therefore find repeated use attractive; in other users, however, it may produce decidedly unpleasant effects. Nonetheless, some researchers believe that, irrespective of the route of administration, the dependence liability of pentazocine remains similar to that of the weak opioid analgesics.

There is little disagreement over the dependence liability of the combination of pentazocine and tripelennamine. The intense euphoria reputed to accompany intravenous injection of this combination is similar to that produced by heroin. In fact, even when the availability of heroin returned to customary levels in the midwestern United States, some users continued taking Ts and Blues.

Inherent Harmfulness

Pentazocine does not produce significant toxic effects in most users when taken orally at therapeutic dose levels, although chronic use may result in mild physical and/or psychological dependence. Some users also experience disturbing psychological effects, more often when pentazocine is administered by injection rather than orally. Chronic injection often results in tissue damage at injection sites. Very high doses can produce seizures; however, fatalities involving pentazocine are rare.

A high rate of serious adverse effects accompanies chronic intravenous abuse of Ts and Blues; these include seizures, lung damage and severe psychological reactions, as well as significant tissue damage associated with chronic injection and a variety of diseases related to the use of non-sterile equipment. Most users have persisted despite these hazards. However, it is likely that the epidemic of Ts and Blues abuse in the late 1970s and early 1980s would have been greater had it not been for the serious risks associated with injecting this combination.

Availability

The Ts and Blues epidemic is a striking example of the rapidity with which drug abuse trends can shift dramatically. The principal reasons for the sudden popularity of Ts and Blues seem quite straightforward: a drop in the availability of street heroin and the easy availability of a substitute that produced heroin-like effects. No doubt pentazocine's low cost enhanced its attractiveness, particularly among the urban poor.

The more recent decline in Ts and Blues abuse also seems to have resulted from specific policy actions: a change in regulatory controls on pentazocine, with the imposition of more severe penalties for illicit possession and distribution and, in the United States, a reformulation of the oral product (i.e., the addition of naloxone). The impact of these policy actions on the use of Ts and Blues was complemented by increased availability of heroin.

Background Reading

Canadian Pharmaceutical Association. (1997). *Compendium of Pharmaceuticals and Specialties.* (32nd edition). Ottawa: Canadian Pharmaceutical Association.

De Bard, M.L. & Jagger, J.A. (1981). "T's and B's" — midwestern heroin substitute, *Clinical Toxicology, 18,* 1117–1123.

Garey, R.E., Daul, C.C., Samuels, M.S. & Egan, R.R. (1982-1983). Medical and sociological aspects of T's and Blues abuse in New Orleans. *American Journal of Drug and Alcohol Abuse, 9,* 171–182.

Lahmeyer, H.W. & Steingold, R.C. (1980). Pentazocine and tripelennamine: A drug abuse epidemic? *International Journal of the Addictions, 15,* 1219–1232.

McEvoy, G. (Ed.) (1997). *American Hospital Formulary Service (AHFS) Drug Information.* Bethesda, MD: American Society of Health-System Pharmacists.

Reisine, T. & Pasternak, G. (1996). Opioid analgesics and antagonists. (Chapter 23). In J.G. Hardman, L.E. Limbird, P.B. Molinoff, R.W. Rudden & A.G. Gilman (Eds.), *Goodman and Gilman's The Pharmacological Basis of Therapeutics* (9th edition). New York/Toronto: McGraw-Hill Health Professions Division.

Propoxyphene

DRUG CLASS: Opioid

Synopsis

Propoxyphene is a wholly synthetic opioid that binds primarily to μ (mu) receptors to produce its analgesic effects. It is among the least potent of the commonly used opioid drugs in terms of analgesia and euphoria, and is used medically for relief of mild to moderate pain. Estimates of propoxyphene's analgesic potency compared with codeine are inconsistent: some sources indicate that oral administration of propoxyphene is one-half to two-thirds as potent as codeine, while others indicate that, at some dose levels, it is somewhat more potent than codeine. Combinations of propoxyphene with ASA have been reported to produce greater pain relief than either drug alone.

Abusers report that they can achieve a pleasant state of euphoria (including a heroin-like "rush") when propoxyphene is injected intravenously, but chronic injection of this drug can cause severe damage to veins and to local tissue at the injection sites. In very high abusive doses (e.g., 800 mg daily) in chronic users, its principal toxic effects are respiratory depression, psychosis and seizures. For these reasons, it is rarely the exclusive drug of choice for abusers of opioid analgesics. Because of its easy availability, however, propoxyphene is frequently used with other drugs in order to produce a more pleasurable "high."

When propoxyphene is administered chronically in higher-than-recommended oral doses, tolerance to its mild analgesic and euphoric effects develops gradually. While chronic high-dose oral abuse can result in physical and psychological dependence, withdrawal symptoms after chronic oral use at 800 mg daily may be milder than those that occur in withdrawal from other opioid analgesics. Propoxyphene will only partially suppress withdrawal in individuals dependent upon other opioids.

In recent years, the prescribing of propoxyphene has declined markedly, probably largely because of a greater awareness among health professionals of its potential for abuse and its toxicity when taken at high doses or in combination with other CNS depressants.

Drug Source

Propoxyphene is produced through chemical synthesis by the pharmaceutical industry.

Trade Names

- propoxyphene napsylate — Darvon-N®

- propoxyphene hydrochloride — Darvon® (not marketed in Canada), Novo-Propoxyn®, 642®

Street Names

"Yellow footballs" (propoxyphene napsylate).

Combination Products

Propoxyphene is included in the following combination products:

- Darvon-N® with ASA (propoxyphene napsylate and ASA)

- Darvon-N® Compound (propoxyphene napsylate, ASA and caffeine)

- 692® (propoxyphene hydrochloride, ASA and caffeine)

- Novo-Propoxyn® Compound (propoxyphene hydrochloride, ASA and caffeine).

Medical Uses

Propoxyphene is used medically for treating mild to moderate pain that is not adequately relieved by ASA. In the United States, the use of propoxyphene napsylate maintenance in heroin-dependent persons has been investigated.

Physical Appearance

Propoxyphene hydrochloride in pure form is a white, bitter-tasting crystalline powder that is freely soluble in water and in alcohol. Propoxyphene napsylate is an odorless, bitter-tasting, white crystalline solid that is only slightly soluble in water and soluble in alcohol.

Dosage[1,2]

Medical

For mild to moderate pain — 65 mg propoxyphene hydrochloride or 100 mg propoxyphene napsylate three to four times per day.

Non-medical

Daily doses of propoxyphene hydrochloride in excess of 600 to 800 mg have been commonly reported. In rare instances, some highly tolerant abusers have been known to take as much as 3,000 mg per day.

Routes of Administration

Orally: by tablet, by capsule, or, rarely, in liquid suspension. Preparations specifically for injection are no longer marketed, and currently available oral preparations are difficult to dissolve for needle administration. Propoxyphene napsylate is particularly difficult to inject because it is practically insoluble. Injection may result in severe tissue damage at injection sites.

---

1   All doses refer to adults.

2   Sixty-five mg of propoxyphene hydrochloride contains the same amount of propoxyphene and has approximately the same analgesic potency as 100 mg of propoxyphene napsylate.

Effects of Short-Term Use: Low Doses[3]

CNS, *behavioral, subjective*: Effects of propoxyphene use include suppression of the sensation of mild to moderate pain,[4] occasionally mild euphoria or in some cases mild emotional depression, anxiety, dizziness, headache (infrequently), sedation, drowsiness or in some cases excitement and insomnia, pupillary constriction (which can impair night vision) and blurred vision.

Gastrointestinal: nausea, vomiting, abdominal pain, constipation (occurring less frequently than with other opioid analgesics).

Other: sweating, itching, skin rash.

Effects of Short-Term Use: Higher Doses[5]

Intensification of propoxyphene's low-dose effects may occur at higher doses, with the duration of effects increasing with the size of the dose. Other effects may include:

- increasing impairment of ability to concentrate

- sleepiness, progressing to stupor or coma

- decrease in blood pressure and heart rate, cardiac arrhythmias

- respiratory depression, usually more moderate than for high doses of other opioids, and at overdose levels, pulmonary edema

- in contrast with some other opioids, muscle twitches and tremors, and at overdose levels, generalized seizures.

---

3   Single doses within the therapeutic range administered orally to non-tolerant persons to a maximum of approximately 250 to 300 mg propoxyphene hydrochloride or 400 mg propoxyphene napsylate per day in divided doses.

4   The analgesic potency of propoxyphene has recently been a subject of controversy among researchers. Some sources indicate that its analgesic potency is approximately one-half to two-thirds that of codeine (Goodman and Gilman, 1996), while other sources indicate that its potency exceeds that of codeine (CPS 1997). While there has been debate about whether propoxyphene hydrochloride alone at a dose of 65 mg is more effective in relieving pain than ASA 650 mg, it has been shown that combinations of these two drugs are more effective than either drug alone (Goodman and Gilman, 1996).

5   Single doses in excess of the therapeutic range administered orally to non-tolerant persons, or lower doses in particularly sensitive individuals.

When administered intravenously to experienced users, higher doses of propoxyphene can produce a state of moderately intense euphoria and the typical "rush" associated with opioid analgesics. This is described as an intense orgasmic-like sensation in the abdomen, experienced almost immediately after injection. (Because of its severely irritating properties, injection of propoxyphene is quite damaging and painful.)

At very high doses (i.e., overdose), propoxyphene can produce toxic psychosis in some users, characterized by disorientation, confusion, delusions and hallucinations. Documented cases of toxic psychosis have occurred after ingestion of 390 mg of propoxyphene hydrochloride (i.e., approximately six times greater than the usual analgesic dose). Other effects may include localized or generalized seizures or continuous seizure activity (i.e., *status epilepticus*), pinpoint pupils, disturbance of the acid-base balance in the body, deep sleep possibly progressing to stupor or coma, shallow breathing and markedly reduced rate of breathing, slow and irregular heartbeat, low blood pressure, severe lung congestion and cyanosis.

Toxic effects may occur within an hour of oral administration of propoxyphene hydrochloride, because it is rapidly absorbed from the gastrointestinal tract into the bloodstream.

It is important to recognize that when propoxyphene has been administered in combination with ASA or acetaminophen, the observed drug effects may be the combined effects of the two drugs.

Effects of Long-Term Use

Chronic injection of propoxyphene is more painful than injection of most other common opioid analgesics. Marked irritation and destruction of tissue at injection sites and severe damage to veins are common. These problems substantially limit continuous abuse by injection.

Very high-dose oral abuse is limited by potentially serious side effects. Users may experience a persistent toxic psychotic state that disappears only following a drastic reduction in daily dose or after abstinence. Marked agitation, tremors and startle responses (and sometimes seizures) are characteristic of chronic high-dose abuse. However, research studies of highly tolerant users of opioid analgesics such as heroin have found that many users can be maintained on daily doses of 800 to 1,200 mg of propoxyphene napsylate without harmful effects. (See Physical Dependence/Withdrawal below.)

Lethality

Severe overdose can result in coma, seizures, severe congestion of the lungs, cardiac arrest and death. Seizures are particularly common in fatal overdoses. The lowest reported quantity of propoxyphene resulting in death is 800 mg, although it has been estimated that 500 mg can be lethal. In most deaths, propoxyphene blood levels exceed 0.1 mg/100 mL. In cases where propoxyphene-ASA combination products have been used at overdose levels, the resulting effects may include toxic effects of both drugs.

Because propoxyphene hydrochloride is so readily absorbed, death may occur very rapidly after overdose, much more rapidly than with overdose of propoxyphene napsylate. In one well-documented report of several accidental (i.e., abuse-related) fatalities, death occurred as early as 30 to 45 minutes after ingestion.

Although a large number of fatalities have been attributed exclusively to propoxyphene and propoxyphene compound products, deaths from multiple-drug overdose are more common. For example, in two large-scale surveys of postmortem findings in almost 3,000 propoxyphene-related fatalities, only 20 per cent involved no other drug. In most cases, alcohol, anxiolytics and/or other sedative/hypnotics were also ingested.

The U.S. Food and Drug Administration (FDA) reported that during the 1970s, propoxyphene-related deaths ranked second in number only to the barbiturates among all prescription-drug-implicated fatalities. A substantial number of these deaths were suicides. The FDA urged physicians and other health professionals, such as dentists, to exercise caution in prescribing propoxyphene to patients who may be suicidal, abuse-prone or addiction-prone. Reports published in the 1980s indicate a substantial decline in the number of propoxyphene-related deaths since their peak in the late 1970s.

Tolerance and Dependence

Tolerance

Tolerance to the analgesic and mild euphoric effects of propoxyphene occurs with regular use, but may develop more gradually than tolerance to the effects of other opioids when they are taken orally. With regular intravenous use of propoxyphene, tolerance develops rapidly (i.e., within a few weeks). The extent to which tolerance may develop to the CNS-stimulating effects of very high doses is uncertain. However, research evidence obtained from propoxyphene-maintained patients (who were formerly dependent on heroin) suggests that appreciable tolerance to these effects does not develop when single daily doses exceed 700 mg of propoxyphene napsylate.

Physical Dependence/Withdrawal

Propoxyphene, when chronically abused at doses substantially above the therapeutic range, can produce physical dependence. A withdrawal syndrome occurs after abrupt termination of long-term use. Propoxyphene's withdrawal symptoms are similar to those for other opioids, but are typically milder. Symptoms may include insomnia, agitation, profuse sweating and elevated blood pressure, pulse and temperature. There may also be abdominal and other muscular cramps, hyperactive deep-tendon reflexes, dizziness, "goose-flesh," nausea and vomiting. Seizures have been observed.

Administration of sufficient doses of propoxyphene or other opioid analgesic drugs can completely suppress propoxyphene withdrawal sickness.

Although relatively few in number, documented cases do exist of medically induced accidental acquisition of physical dependence on propoxyphene among patients suffering from chronic pain. In one study, while none of the patients had a history of either psychiatric illness or previous drug abuse,[6] the daily dose reached as high as 2 grams (2,000 mg) in some cases. Upon abrupt cessation of use, all patients experienced withdrawal symptoms.

---

[6]   In fact, some of these patients had become physically dependent on propoxyphene without experiencing the typical euphoria associated with opioid analgesics.

Propoxyphene Napsylate (PN) Maintenance

Beginning in the mid-1970s, several experimental studies were performed to determine the efficacy of propoxyphene napsylate (PN) as an alternative to methadone in drug maintenance programs. Several reasons were advanced for giving serious consideration to PN maintenance, including the following:

- PN is extremely difficult to inject and produces much less euphoria than methadone, limiting its potential for abuse.

- High doses of propoxyphene produce decidedly unpleasant effects. As a result, patients maintained on this drug would be less likely than methadone-maintained patients to demand (or seek) higher doses.

- Withdrawal symptoms associated with abstinence from propoxyphene are less unpleasant and less protracted than those associated with methadone withdrawal.

- Both constipation and male impotence occur less frequently with propoxyphene than with methadone.

- It was thought that propoxyphene would be more attractive to patients with relatively moderate dependence problems who objected to taking a drug as potent as methadone.

- One early study found that many patients who attempted to use heroin while maintained on high doses of propoxyphene experienced either unpleasant effects or none at all.

It has generally been found that patients dependent on heroin and other opioid analgesics can tolerate two daily doses of PN (taken orally) in the range of 400 to 600 mg (i.e., 800 to 1,200 mg per day) without experiencing disturbing side effects. At such dose levels, PN is as effective as (or more effective than) 10 mg of methadone in suppressing withdrawal activity, but less effective than 20 mg of methadone. Therefore, the usefulness of PN as a maintenance drug is likely to be limited to patients who are mildly dependent on opioid analgesics. However, because the purity of street heroin has increased in recent years, today's users generally consume larger quantities of heroin per day than in the past and are less likely to fit the criterion of mild dependence than were users two or three decades ago.

Psychological Dependence

Psychological dependence on propoxyphene can occur when it is regularly administered, even at low daily doses under medical supervision. Patients have been known to remain for years on the same small maintenance dose. In these cases, use persists even though tolerance to the analgesic effect of the regular daily dose has had ample time to develop and the drug no longer has any inherent pharmacological value.

These patients report a persistent craving for the psychological effects of propoxyphene, a preoccupation with securing an ample supply, and psychic distress when they are temporarily unable to obtain the drug. These symptoms can occur in the absence of physical dependence, when a consistent and clearly defined physiological withdrawal syndrome does not appear after abrupt abstinence.

Patterns of Use

Propoxyphene was introduced in the United States in 1957. It was marketed as a safe, apparently non-dependence-producing alternative to codeine and was widely prescribed in that country. This popularity continued until the late 1970s when the number of prescriptions reached a peak of more than 30 million each year. By then misuse and abuse were thought to be quite common, and a concerted effort was made to warn physicians and other health professionals about the drug's risks. Since the late 1970s, the prescribing of propoxyphene in the United States has declined sharply.

A similar pattern of declining propoxyphene use occurred in Canada. For example, the number of individual doses of propoxyphene and propoxyphene-compound products sold in Canada in 1977 was approximately 78 million; by 1981, the figure had dropped by more than 50 per cent to 38 million.

Propoxyphene continues to retain some value in the drug subculture, but it is rarely the drug of first choice among sophisticated users. Usually, it is taken with other drugs to heighten their effects. It is also used in large quantities by heroin-dependent users in order to (at least partially) suppress withdrawal sickness when other, more potent, opioid analgesics are unavailable.

Potential for Abuse

Dependence Liability
The dependence liability of propoxyphene is among the lowest of the commonly used opioid analgesics. Propoxyphene produces relatively mild euphoria when taken orally, even at high doses. Although more intense euphoria can occur when high doses are administered intravenously, the adverse effects of its administration by injection reduce the risk of its chronic abuse by this route.

Inherent Harmfulness

In addition to the negative consequences of protracted needle administration, the potentially hazardous effects of very high doses of propoxyphene greatly restrict the upper dose limits of abuse.

Availability

Since propoxyphene is still more easily available than many other opioid analgesics, with the exception of codeine, it has a relatively high potential for abuse. It is important to note that the intensity of its desired effects can be potentiated (although with considerable risk) by other easily available drugs such as alcohol.

Background Reading

Canadian Pharmaceutical Association. (1997). *Compendium of Pharmaceuticals and Specialties.* (32nd edition). Ottawa: Canadian Pharmaceutical Association.

Reisine, T. & Pasternak, G. (1996). Opioid analgesics and antagonists. (Chapter 23). In J.G. Hardman, L.E. Limbird, P.B. Molinoff, R.W. Rudden & A.G. Gilman (Eds.), *Goodman and Gilman's The Pharmacological Basis of Therapeutics* (9th edition). New York/Toronto: McGraw-Hill Health Professions Division.

Psilocybin

DRUG CLASS: Hallucinogen

Synopsis

Psilocybin and the closely related substance psilocin are hallucinogens found primarily in the *Psilocybe* and *Conocybe* mushrooms, which grow in many parts of the world. Psilocybin has been used ritually in Mexico and Central America for centuries to produce altered states of consciousness similar to those produced by mescaline and LSD. Among the psychoactive effects produced by psilocybin are vivid visual "pseudo-hallucinations" and distortions, which are known to the user to be unreal, synesthesias (the paradoxical melding of the senses in which, for example, the user seems to "see" music) and changes in the user's perceptions of time, space and his or her body.

In most instances, these effects are sought by the user and are the reason for taking the drug. Sometimes, however, the user may be frightened or even terrified by these same effects (i.e., experience a "bad trip"), particularly if their onset is rapid and the intensity greater than anticipated. Psilocybin is most highly valued for its ability to induce experiences that the user considers to be religious, cosmic or mystical in character.

Tolerance to the effects of psilocybin, and cross-tolerance to the effects of other hallucinogens such as LSD and mescaline, develop rapidly, and the user must periodically discontinue taking the drug to regain original sensitivity. There is no evidence that users develop physical or psychological dependence.

Drug Source

Psilocybin is chiefly derived from the mushroom *Psilocybe mexicana* and some other *Psilocybe* and *Conocybe* species. Psilocybin can be produced synthetically, but the process is relatively difficult and costly. Furthermore, the synthetic product deteriorates rapidly and is difficult to store. For these reasons, chemical synthesis of the drug is rare.

Trade Names

None. Psilocybin is not used for any medical purpose.

Street Names

Magic mushroom(s), mushroom(s), shroom(s).

Combination Products

None.

Medical Uses

None.

Physical Appearance

In its pure form, synthetic psilocybin is a white crystalline material that may be prepared in capsules, tablets or solution. Crude mushroom preparations containing psilocybin are sometimes distributed either as intact dried brown mushrooms (which remain potent for years with proper storage) or as powdered material in capsules.

Dosage[1]

Medical
Not applicable.

---

1   All doses refer to adults.

Non-medical

Non-medical doses range from 1 to 20 mg with typical doses between 4 and 10 mg. Approximately 15 to 20 mg of psilocybin produces the same psychoactive effects as 100 micrograms of LSD.

Routes of Administration

Synthetic psilocybin can be taken orally in tablets, capsules or solution. Psilocybin powder mixed with fruit juice — "fungus delight" — is a common form of preparation for oral ingestion. The mushroom itself may be eaten either fresh or dried. Psilocybin may also be sniffed, smoked or injected. However, injection of crude preparations can involve risk of medical complications resulting from the non-drug materials present.

Effects of Short-Term Use[2]

Short term use of psilocybin preparations produces the following effects.

CNS, *behavioral, subjective*: There is fairly wide variation among users in possible perceptual, cognitive and emotional experiences produced by psilocybin. In addition to the size of the dose, drug effects are also influenced by the setting and the user's expectations, past drug experiences and personality. Early effects[3] typically include facial numbness, tension and anxiety, rapid reflexes, muscle twitches and muscle weakness, dilation of the pupils and lightheadedness. Later effects can include the following:

- Users may experience vivid perceptual distortions, usually visual, such as "pseudohallucinations" and "pseudoillusions."

- The user's perception of time may be distorted (minutes may seem to pass as slowly as hours).

- Perception of space may be distorted.

---

[2] For doses of 4 to 10 mg taken orally by non-tolerant users. As with LSD, higher doses generally tend to produce quantitative (i. e., more intense) rather than qualitative changes in effects.

[3] Occurring 15 to 45 minutes after administration.

- Users' perceptions of their bodies may be distorted. They may experience sensations of heaviness or weightlessness and feelings of floating.

- Synesthesias (in which, for example users "see" music or "hear" colors) frequently occur.

- Users may experience a partial or complete loss of recognized boundaries between self and the environment, reactions to which may range from intense pleasure to terror.

- All sensory experiences tend to be heightened. The user perceives brighter colors, sharper definition of objects, increased hearing acuity, more sharply distinguished taste and so on. These heightened sensations may alternate with sensory impairment.

- Users often experience difficulties in concentrating, thinking and focusing attention.

- While memory may also be impaired, it is not unusual for past and possibly repressed experiences to be vividly recalled; these may meld with current experiences. The user's sense of the present reality (the "here and now") may be temporarily lost.

- Users may be intensely preoccupied with otherwise trivial thoughts, experiences or objects.

- Users may feel that they are undergoing a profound mystical, religious or "cosmic" experience. For many users this may be the most desired effect.

Some users may experience a highly adverse reaction to the above effects — a "bad trip" — characterized by the following symptoms: confusion, disorientation, fearfulness of non-existence or of disintegration of self, inability to distinguish between reality and unreality, paranoid thinking, true hallucinations, possibly severe agitation and/or depression, and panic or even terror.

Short-term use of psilocybin can also result in the following physical effects.

Cardiovascular: Increased blood pressure and heart rate are early effects.

Gastrointestinal: Early effects include nausea and vomiting, which are very common, and abdominal cramps.

Other: Early effects include elevated body temperature and sweating, which may be followed by chills and shivering.

The effects of psilocybin tend to wear off more rapidly than those of LSD, usually three to six hours after administration.

Effects of Long-Term Use

Because of the rapid development of tolerance to the effects of psilocybin, chronic daily use of psilocybin is unlikely to occur (see Tolerance and Dependence below).

Single episodes of psilocybin use have occasionally been known to precipitate a prolonged psychotic state similar to paranoid schizophrenia. Some observers have suggested that psychosis is likely only in those users who were latent psychotics prior to use of the drug.

Adverse effects directly attributable to chronic use of psilocybin have not been adequately researched.

Lethality

No reported deaths are known to have resulted from psilocybin overdose. However, severely adverse psychic effects of the drug on some individuals have been known to prompt hazardous or even life-threatening behavior. A recent report has associated magic mushrooms with end-stage renal failure.

Tolerance and Dependence

Users who take psilocybin for several days consecutively rapidly develop complete tolerance to the drug's subjective effects.[4] After tolerance has developed, no amount of this drug can then produce the desired psychic effects, and the user must abstain for several days to regain sensitivity to its effects. Nor is it of any use to take such

---

4   See the discussion of tolerance and tachyphylaxis in Section 1.

other hallucinogens as LSD or mescaline during the period of abstinence. Each of these drugs produces cross-tolerance to the effects of the other and once tolerance has developed, none can produce the desired effects until after the period of several days' complete abstinence. LSD produces tolerance to its effects even more rapidly than psilocybin.

Neither physical nor psychological dependence has been reported.

Patterns of Use

Mushrooms containing psilocybin and a closely related hallucinogen, psilocin, grow chiefly in Mexico, Central America and some areas of the southern United States.[5] Recently, psilocybin and psilocin have also been found in some related species of mushrooms indigenous to Australia, Great Britain, Europe, the northwestern United States, British Columbia and some other areas of Latin America.

Until the 1980s, psilocybin was very rarely encountered on the street drug market in most areas of North America. Most street samples presented for laboratory analysis that were alleged to be psilocybin in fact turned out to be low-dosage preparations of LSD added to ordinary mushrooms or other vegetable matter. However, beginning in the 1980s, police reports suggested that psilocybin is available at least occasionally in some areas of Canada. A 1997 survey of Ontario students found that reported use of hallucinogens such as mescaline and psilocybin had increased from the previous (1995) survey, especially among female students and those in Grades 9 and 13.[6] Use of hallucinogenic mushrooms has also been reported by Danish students in the 1990s. However, it is unclear whether these were actually psilocybin-containing mushrooms.

---

[5]   Use of these mushrooms among Indian tribes in Mexico on religious and other ceremonial occasions was common for centuries prior to the invasion of the Spanish conquistadors. They continue to be used to this day by Indians in some remote areas of southern Mexico.

[6]   Grade 13 has now been replaced by an Ontario Academic credit (OAC) year in Ontario schools. However, the Ontario survey, and thus this text, have continued to use "Grade 13" to designate this final year of high school, to facilitate comparison with earlier surveys.

Potential for Abuse

Because psilocybin is both infrequently available in most areas of North America and is not known to produce dependence, its abuse potential is low.

Background Reading

Adlaf, E.M., Ivis, F.J. & Smart, R.G. (1997). *Ontario Student Drug Use Survey 1977-1997*. Toronto: Addiction Research Foundation.

Franz, M., Regile, H., Kirchmair, M., Kletmayr, J., Sunder-Plassman, G., Horl, W.H. & Potianka, E. (1996). Magic mushrooms: A hope for a cheap high resulting in end-stage renal failure. *Nephrology, Dialysis, Transplantation, 11 (11)*, 2324–2327.

Lassen, J.F., Lassen, N.F. & Skov, J. (1993). Hallucinogenic mushroom use reported by Danish students: Patterns of consumption. *Journal of Internal Medicine, 233 (2)*, 111–112.

Lewis, W.H. & Elvin-Lewis, M.P.F. (1979). *Medical Botany: Plants Affecting Man's Health*. New York: John Wiley and Sons.

Schultes, R.E. & Hofmann, A. (1980). *The Botany and Chemistry of Hallucinogens*. (2nd edition). Springfield, IL: Charles C. Thomas.

Volatile Solvents
(Inhalants)

DRUG CLASS: Sedative/Hypnotic, Anesthetic

Synopsis

Almost all commonly abused inhalants are volatile hydrocarbon solvents produced from petroleum and natural gas.[1] The term "volatile" means that these substances evaporate when exposed to air, while "solvents" refers to their capacity, in liquid form, to dissolve many other substances. Volatile hydrocarbons have an enormous number of industrial, commercial and household uses. These include use as gasoline, cleaning fluids and paint thinners, and as ingredients in toiletries, adhesives, fillers and paints. Certain solvents have also been used as pressurized propellants in aerosols and as anesthetics. Frequently, two or more volatile hydrocarbon compounds are found in the same product.

Inhalants generally produce a number of dose-related CNS-depressant effects similar to those of other sedative/hypnotic substances. Inhalants produce alcohol-like intoxication, but with more perceptual distortions. This may give rise to bizarre behavior that can be injurious to the user and to others. At progressively higher dose levels, inhalants produce sleep and anesthesia.

Tolerance develops to the desired effects of inhalants with regular use, and psychological dependence can occur. Chronic abuse of these substances may result in physical dependence. Abrupt termination of inhalant use can produce a withdrawal syndrome. The symptoms of inhalant withdrawal are usually mild but in some cases severe symptoms have occurred.

---

[1]   Some principal exceptions are amyl nitrite, the related substance isobutyl nitrite and nitrous oxide.

A number of deaths have been associated with acute abuse of inhalants, most prominently "sudden sniffing deaths" and suffocations. "Sudden sniffing death" is caused by heart failure resulting from a severely irregular heartbeat, which is typically preceded by strenuous activity or sudden stress immediately following several deep inhalations. In the case of suffocation, death is a result of the person's falling asleep or otherwise becoming unconscious while a plastic bag containing the inhalant remains in place over the nose and mouth. Chronic abuse of inhalants can produce a spectrum of different harmful effects depending on the particular inhalant. These effects can range from relatively mild and reversible symptoms to severe damage to such vital organs as the kidneys and liver. Brain damage in some users has also been reported.

Table 1: Volatile Compounds That May Be Abused by Inhalation[2]

Aliphatic Hydrocarbons	iso-butane, n-butane, n-hexane, propane
Aromatic Hydrocarbons	toluene, xylene
Mixed Hydrocarbons	gasoline
Ketones	acetone, butanone, methyl iso-butyl ketone
Halogenated Compounds	bromochlorodifluoromethane, chlorodifluoromethane, chloroform, dichloroflduromethane, dichloromethane, enflurane, halothane, tetrachloroethylene, trichlorofluoromethane
Anesthetic Gases*	nitrous oxide
Room Odorizers*	(iso)amyl nitrite, (iso)butyl nitrite

* These substances are not discussed in this chapter. Please see the chapter on nitrous oxide in Section 4 and the notes on amyl nitrite and isobutyl nitrite in Section 5.

This article will be divided into two sections in order to distinguish important differences in effects of abuse (particularly in lethality) between commercial solvents used in products such as glues, paints and cleaning agents, and those solvents used as propellants in pressurized products such as hair sprays, deodorants and spray paints.

---

2   Adapted with permission from Ramsey, J., Anderson, H.R., Bloor, K. & Flanagan, R.J. (1989). An introduction to the practice, prevalence and chemical toxicity of volatile substance abuse. *Human Toxicology*, 8 (4), 261-269.

PART A: COMMERCIAL SOLVENTS

Drug Source

The most commonly abused commercial solvents are volatile hydrocarbon compounds produced from petroleum and natural gas through chemical synthesis by the chemical industry.

Trade Names

Not relevant for the individual solvents. They are found in a variety of commercial products in combination with other ingredients.

Street Names

Glue, gas and sniff. People who inhale solvents are said to be "sniffing" or "huffing."

Combination Products

Many commercial products contain volatile solvents in combination with other ingredients. The following table outlines the types of products commonly abused.

Table 2: Commercial Products Containing
Volatile Solvents That May Be Abused [3]

Adhesives

Airplane Glue	toluene, ethyl acetate
Rubber Cement	hexane, toluene, methyl chloride, acetone, methyl ethyl ketone, methyl butyl ketone
PVC Cement	trichloroethylene

Cleaning Agents

Dry Cleaning	tetrachloroethylene, trichloroethane
Spot Removers	tetrachloroethylene, trichloroethane, trichloroethylene
Degreasers	tetrachloroethylene, trichloroethane, trichloroethylen

Others

Polish Remover	acetone
Paint Remover	toluene, methylene chloride, methanol
Paint Thinners	toluene, methylene chloride, methanol
Correction Fluids	trichloroethylene, trichloroethane

Dosage

Medical

There are no medical uses for these commercial solvents.

Non-medical

Since many products contain volatile solvents, and because these substances vary in terms of concentration and combinations, it is not possible to accurately document the dosages necessary to produce intoxication. A single container of cleaning fluid or nail polish remover may be sufficient for a group of young abusers. A frequent and very heavy abuser of model cement (airplane glue) may use as many as a dozen tubes of glue in order to maintain intoxication for a period of several hours.

---

[3]   Adapted with permission from *Understanding Inhalant Users: An Overview for Parents, Educators, and Clinicians.* Copyright 1991, Texas Commission on Alcohol and Drug Abuse.

Routes of Administration

Volatile solvents are almost always inhaled. There are many methods of inhalation:

- One of the most common methods for inhaling semi-liquid solvents involves emptying the contents of the container into a plastic or paper bag, holding its opening tightly and firmly over the mouth and nose, and inhaling the vapors deeply.[4] The re-breathing of exhaled air causes an oxygen deficiency (anoxia), which can intensify the intoxicating effect of the solvent.

- When liquid solvents are used, they may be sniffed directly from the container.

- Liquid solvents may also be poured on to a rag or some other absorbent material. The saturated material is then held in the hands and cupped over the mouth or placed in a bag and then inhaled.

- Sometimes solvents are heated in order to achieve higher vapor concentrations. Because many solvents are highly flammable, this practice can be dangerous.

- Some other less common methods involve the use of such items as perfume atomizers. Solvents are also occasionally injected or mixed with alcoholic beverages.

Effects of Short-Term Use[5]

Effects of the short-term use of commercial solvents include the following.

CNS, behavioral, subjective: Users experience effects rapidly after the initial inhalations. Inexperienced users often feel drowsy and may fall asleep. Other early effects

---

4   The principal advantage of a paper bag, rather than a plastic one, is that it is not dissolved by the solvent. The use of a paper bag also reduces the probability of accidental suffocation.

5   The typical effects of these substances are generally dose-related, are similar to those of other sedative/hypnotic drugs, and at high doses, are similar to those of anesthetics. However, there is a wide variation among users with respect to the type and intensity of effects experienced. Little is known about the combined effects of the variety of solvents found in commonly used products. What is presented here is a composite picture of the observations of clinicians and researchers.

include euphoria and dizziness as well as sensations of numbness, and dissociation from the environment. Compared with alcohol, solvents produce a quicker, briefer intoxication with more perceptual distortions. Shortly after the onset of early effects, the following may also occur: giddiness, talkativeness, emotional disinhibition; impaired motor co-ordination and muscle weakness; slowed reflexes; slurred speech; impaired judgment; abnormal sensitivity to light; blurred vision and ringing in the ears.

Perceptual distortions may include distortions of the shape, size and color of objects and of time and space. Some users have suffered toxic psychosis manifested as delirium, disorientation, bizarre delusions and visual — and less commonly auditory — hallucinations. Users may experience exhilaration and temporary delusions of omnipotence and invincibility, which may encourage reckless behavior that can be harmful to the user and others. Users may deliberately or accidentally injure themselves or accidentally cause their own death by, for example, leaping from high places. Destruction of property is common.

While most users find solvent-induced intoxication to be pleasurable, some become depressed, occasionally so severely as to provoke suicide attempts.

Cardiovascular: increased heart rate, irregular heartbeat.

Respiratory: sneezing, coughing; nasal inflammation and nosebleed; respiratory depression.

Gastrointestinal: nausea, vomiting, diarrhea.

Other: irritation and/or watering of the eyes; diffuse pains in the muscles and joints; headache.

The duration of the euphoric effects is typically between 15 and 45 minutes, provided that the user does not attempt to prolong the effects with additional administrations. The euphoria is followed by a period of drowsiness or stupor. Once use has stopped, the CNS-depressant effects gradually decline in intensity and generally disappear within one to two hours, although some side effects can last much longer. Partial or total amnesia of the events of the solvent intoxication episode may occur.

The sophisticated solvent user can maintain a desired level of intoxication for prolonged periods of time by taking spaced inhalations over this period. However, prolonged concentrated and uninterrupted inhalation can result in a condition similar to severe alcohol or barbiturate intoxication. The user may even lapse into stupor or coma, which can be accompanied by depressed respiration, cardiovascular irregularities and sometimes seizures. Oxygen intake may also be significantly reduced with some methods of solvent inhalation, which can result in lack of sufficient oxygen to the brain, unconsciousness and brain damage, with possibly fatal results.

Effects of Long-Term Use

Several reports have provided evidence to support an association between solvent use and brain damage. The symptoms most frequently reported in long-term, heavy users of toluene-containing solvents include short-term memory loss, emotional instability, cognitive impairment, slurred speech, wide-based gait, staggering, nystagmus (uncontrollable eye movements) hearing loss and loss of sense of smell. In one study of heavy toluene users, neurological abnormalities included disorders of the sensory nerves and dysfunction of the cerebellum characterized by tremor upon attempting to move, poor co-ordination and difficulty walking. Brain scans of the impaired subjects demonstrated brain shrinkage (i.e., atrophy of the cerebellum and cerebral cortex) that was related to the severity of their neurological and performance deficits. The subjects showed very little evidence of recovery during a two-week drug-free period.

Observations of psychological impairment among chronic solvent users suggest that most have significant psychopathology. However, there is insufficient information to conclude that a direct cause and effect relationship exists between solvent abuse and psychological problems. Nonetheless, conduct disorders, personality disorders (e.g., antisocial personality disorder) and depressive disorders have been associated with solvent use.

It has not been possible to determine the incidence of permanent neuropsychological deficits from existing published reports. These reports do not distinguish between acute and chronic effects of abuse (for example, by allowing for a period of abstinence before testing) and they do not indicate the frequency of abuse. Moreover, they use different psychological testing techniques and lack adequate control groups for comparisons.

Other reported harmful effects that may occur in chronic solvent users include impairment of the liver, kidneys, lungs and heart, and blood abnormalities.

For some of the more common substances in chronically abused products, specific toxic effects include the following:[6]

- *N-Hexane* — Peripheral nerve damage, sometimes severe, has been reported to occur in some users after long-term abuse of this substance.

- *Toluene* — A broad range of toxic effects implicating chronic abuse of toluene has been reported, but none occurs invariably. Kidney damage (glomerulonephritis, distal renal tubular acidosis) may be reversible, but probably depends on the extent of the damage. Toluene has also been associated with peripheral neuropathy, respiratory damage, and liver, heart and blood toxicities.

- *Trichloroethylene and trichloroethane* — Severe and long-term liver and kidney toxicity has been reportedly caused by chronic abuse of both of these solvents. Peripheral nerve damage has also been observed including a slowly reversible trigeminal neuropathy.

- *Gasoline* — Chronic inhalation of leaded gasoline can result in such serious complications as the accumulation of toxic levels of lead in the body. The incidence of this problem has decreased with the introduction of unleaded gasolines.

- *Benzene*[7] — Benzene is one of the most toxic solvents of abuse. Chronic abuse can cause bone marrow deterioration as well as severe damage to the heart, liver and adrenal glands.

Lethality

The organ damage caused by long-term solvent abuse may result in death. Acute inhalation or ingestion of excessive amounts of any of the commonly abused solvents

---

[6] Similar effects, of course, are experienced by those who are accidentally exposed to high concentrations over extended periods in industrial settings.

[7] Benzene is now rarely available to Canadian abusers because of strict government controls over its commercial use.

can cause significant CNS depression including depression of the respiratory centre of the brain. Fortunately, fatalities directly arising from their toxic effects now occur only infrequently in abuse situations,[8] since the user normally lapses into sleep or sometimes stupor before quantities sufficient to cause death are inhaled. However, if the user is not awake and a receptacle such as a plastic bag remains firmly in place over the mouth and nose, there is a substantial risk of death from asphyxiation. This situation has caused a number of deaths, while other accidental deaths have resulted from the bizarre or impaired behavior induced by solvent intoxication.

Several substances in this group have been associated with the most common cause of death among solvent users — "sudden sniffing death." In these cases, death is gene-rally thought to result from heart failure brought about by a severely irregular heartbeat. In most instances the user had engaged in strenuous activity (e.g., running or wrestling) or was subjected to unexpected stress (e.g., being discovered), and often appeared to have been startled or become panicky. After stress or vigorous activity, collapse and death rapidly follow. The abnormal heartbeat is likely the result of the solvent sensitizing the heart to the effects of adrenaline, which is naturally produced and released during stressful periods.

Swallowing of solvents has sometimes resulted in poisoning. As little as 40 to 150 mL of trichloroethylene taken daily may produce unconsciousness in adults and be fatal in children.

Tolerance and Dependence

Tolerance
The development of tolerance to the intoxicating effects of solvents has been well documented. For example, within one year, a "glue sniffer" may be using eight to 10 tubes of toluene-containing plastic cement to achieve the desired intensity of effects initially produced by a single tube. With chronic and frequent abuse, tolerance is very likely to develop to other solvents.

---

8   Such highly toxic solvents as carbon tetrachloride and benzene accounted for several deaths in the past.

Psychological and Physical Dependence /Withdrawal

In general, adolescents use solvents experimentally and dependence on solvents is relatively rare by comparison with the total number who have tried them. However, among those who regularly abuse solvents, psychological dependence can develop. With frequent abuse, users begin to crave the psychological effects, and solvent use becomes an increasingly important part of their everyday life. These users rarely seek professional help on their own and almost all those in treatment have been compelled to participate by parents, the legal system or school authorities.

Physical dependence can result from chronic abuse of solvents. Withdrawal symptoms have been reported following abrupt termination of heavy use. However, such a response is not universal, and the symptoms experienced by chronic users who abruptly abstain are variable. In some cases the following symptoms have been reported after abrupt termination of use: anxiety, depression, loss of appetite, irritability, hostile outbursts, dizziness, tremors and nausea. Occasionally, toluene abusers have experienced severe symptoms similar to those occurring during alcoholic delirium tremens, although delusions (which accompany the alcoholic withdrawal syndrome) do not occur.

Patterns of Use

Solvent inhaling is frequently undertaken in groups, with each user usually inhaling from his or her own bag or saturated cloth until the desired degree of intoxication is achieved. Users may inhale solvents repeatedly over a period of several hours in order to maintain this level of intoxication. They typically stop inhaling either when their supply is exhausted or when they become too drowsy or tired to continue.

Surveys of Ontario students from Grades 7 to 13[9] have consistently confirmed that solvent use is inversely related to the age and grade of the students; that is, the lower the grade and age, the greater number of users. Data from a 1995 survey of drug use in Ontario indicated that 3.8 per cent of Grade 7 students acknowledged having sniffed glue at least once during the last 12 months, compared with 0.9 per cent of

---

[9]   The traditional "Grade 13" has now been replaced by an Ontario Academic Credit (OAC) year in Ontario schools. However, the Ontario survey, and thus this text, has continued to use the term "Grade 13" to facilitate comparisons with previous surveys.

students in Grade 13. These percentages are increased from the 1991 survey (1.1 per cent for Grade 7 and 0.4 per cent for Grade 13), but still considerably lower than in 1977 (6.5 per cent for Grade 7 and 1.8 per cent for Grade 13). The trends are similar for the use of solvents other than glue, with 3.8 per cent of Grade 7 students and 0.9 per cent of Grade 13 students, having used them in the 12 months prior to the 1995 survey. Of all the students who indicated the use of glue in the survey, 47 per cent report using it only once or twice in that 12-month period.

The large majority of young people who abuse solvents do so on an occasional or experimental basis. Those who more regularly abuse solvents are more likely to:

- come from economically disadvantaged homes

- perform less well in school

- have a substantially higher rate of truancy

- come from either unstable or broken homes, often with at least one alcoholic parent

- have shown a poorer personal adjustment prior to the onset of their solvent abuse.

Most young people outgrow solvent abuse, but others continue to abuse solvents into adulthood. What little valid research there is on solvent-abusing adults suggests that they tend to have significant adjustment problems, and most also frequently abuse alcohol or other substances.

One classification system for solvent abusers is shown in the following table. Some solvent abusers may progress from one stage to another.

Table 3: Clinical Classification of Inhalant Abuser[10]

Transient Social:	Transient Isolate:
• Short history of use	• Short history of use
• Use with friends	• Use alone
• Petty offences while intoxicated	• No legal system involvement
• Average intelligence	• Average/above-average intelligence
• Possible learning disabilities	• No learning disabilities
• 10 to 16 years of age	• 10 to 16 years of age

Chronic Social:	Chronic Isolate:
Long history of use (>5 years)	Long history of use (>5 years)
• Daily use with friends	• Daily use alone
• Legal system involvement — misdemeanors	• Legal system involvement — assaults common
• Poor social skills	• Poor social skills
• Grade 9 education	• Grade 9 education
• Brain damage	• Brain damage
• Mid-20s to early 30s	• Mid-20s
• Mental retardation prevalent	• Pre-use psychopathology prevalent

Potential for Abuse

Abuse Liability

When inhaled, solvents are rapidly absorbed into the bloodstream through the lungs, and the desired effects are then almost immediately perceptible. Most users claim to achieve a level of euphoria greater than that produced by alcohol. For these reasons, psychological dependence on this group of substances is common and the abuse liability of solvents is moderately high.

Inherent Harmfulness

Abuse of solvents can be harmful and even life-threatening. This knowledge is widespread among young people and probably deters a number of potential users. However, for some users the risk of harmful consequences can actually foster the desire to use the drugs. Sometimes, troubled younger adolescents feel a strong need to

---

10   Reprinted with permission from *Substance Abuse: A Comprehensive Textbook* (3rd edition). Copyright 1997 Williams and Wilkins.

increase their feelings of self-esteem and to achieve group acceptance by engaging in risk-taking behavior.

Availability

Few drugs of abuse are as cheap and as easily available to young adolescents as solvents. The low cost of and easy accessibility of most of these solvents contribute to their high potential for abuse.

PART B: AEROSOL SOLVENTS

Drug Source

Certain halogenated hydrocarbons that were used as aerosol propellants were formerly subject to widespread abuse as inhalants. These substances include the fluorinated hydrocarbons (also called freons) and, to a lesser extent, trichloroethane. The only fluorocarbon still in use in Canada for general aerosols is chlorodifluoromethane (FC22). Other propellants include gases such as nitrogen and carbon dioxide, and hydrocarbon propellants including butane.

Trade Names

Fluorinated hydrocarbons are given numerical designations based on their chemical structure. Chlorodifluoromethane is, therefore, referred to as FC22. One brand name for this propellant is Freon 22®.

Street Name

Gas.

Combination Products

Aerosol containers have one or more propellants in the form of pressurized liquids or gases that escape when the valve is released. The solid or liquid contents propelled by the gas vary from foodstuffs through antiseptics and cookware-coating agents to paints. These contents may also include other solvents that are liable to abuse, such as trichloroethane in cleaning fluids,[11] toluene in glues, and alcohol in hair sprays and disinfectants.

Table 4: Commercial Products Containing Gases That May Be Abused [12,13]

Aerosols

Paint Sprays	e.g., butane, propane, fluorocarbons
Hair Sprays	e.g., butane, propane, fluorocarbons
Deodorants, Air Fresheners	e.g., butane, propane, fluorocarbons
Analgesic Sprays	e.g., fluorocarbons
Asthma Sprays	e.g., fluorocarbons

Others

Fuel Gas	e.g., butane
Lighters	e.g., butane, isopropane
Fire Extinguisher	e.g., fluoromethane

Medical Uses

There are no directly medical applications of aerosol solvents themselves. However, aerosol-type packaging is used for a variety of products intended for medical use, including anti-asthma, antibacterial, antifungal, and local-anesthetic solutions and powders intended for application to skin or mucous membranes.

---

[11]   Trichloroethane was also used in the past as a low-pressure propellant in medicated vapor aerosols.

[12]   Adapted with permission from *Understanding Inhalant Users: An Overview for Parents, Educators, and Clinicians*. Copyright 1991, Texas Commission on Alcohol and Drug Abuse.

[13]   Because of regulations governing the composition of commercial aerosol products, some of the listed constituents may be prohibited in some jurisdictions.

Dosage

Since the composition and purpose of this class of products vary so widely, generalized statements regarding typical abusive doses are not possible.

Routes of Administration

Propellants may be separated from the other contents of a pressurized container by a variety of methods.

- The container may be held and the valve pressed in such a way as to permit only the gas to be released for direct inhalation.

- The contents may be filtered through a rag or cloth held firmly over the mouth and nose so that mainly the gas is inhaled.

- The propellants and other contents of the container may be sprayed into a plastic or paper bag, or sometimes into a balloon, and then inhaled directly (a method common among "glue sniffers").

- Some abusers spray the propellants and other contents directly into the mouth.

Effects of Short-Term Use[14]

These substances can produce a state of pleasurable intoxication, which can include sensations of weightlessness and numbness, emotional disinhibition, impaired motor co-ordination, impaired judgment, perceptual distortions, pseudohallucinations and sometimes true hallucinations, and delusions of grandeur. Bizarre behavior induced by these drugs can sometimes result in harm to the abuser and others and in the destruction of property.

---

[14] Most effects produced by aerosol solvents are similar to those arising from abuse of other solvents and, therefore, will be only briefly summarized here. However, aerosol solvents generally have a greater toxic effect on the heart.

Heartbeat can be abnormally rapid and irregular, blood pressure can quickly drop, respiration may be depressed, and temporary spasms in the bronchial tubes occasionally occur. Irritation of the eyes, throat, and nasal passages is frequent, as is minor gastrointestinal upset.

Concentrated, uninterrupted inhalation of aerosol solvents can result in a condition similar to severe alcohol intoxication, which may be accompanied by coma and potentially dangerous cardiac irregularities.

Effects of Long-Term Use

Kidney and liver damage may result from chronic abuse of (or accidental exposure to) aerosol solvents. Reversible damage to respiratory-tract tissue and mucous membranes can also occur. Sores on the nose and mouth ("glue sniffer's rash") are common. Aerosol solvent abusers may also suffer the following symptoms: chronic fatigue; nosebleeds; pallor; memory impairment; diminished ability to think clearly or logically; tremors; unsteady gait; constant thirst; loss of appetite accompanied by weight loss; and apathy, mood swings, emotional depression and paranoid thinking.

Lethality

There is evidence that among solvents of abuse, aerosol solvents are the most likely agents to cause "sudden sniffing death" and have accounted for more than half of all such deaths.[15]

Deaths involving aerosol propellants have also been attributed to other causes. These substances can produce "airway freezing" by the spraying of gases cooled by expansion into the mouth. This can lead to reflex inhibition of the heart (the heart may stop completely) by the vagal nerve. Death from suffocation can also occur if the user loses consciousness while a plastic bag containing the inhalant remains in place over the nose and mouth. Some substances propelled by the aerosol, such as paints, can themselves produce serious toxic effects. Finally, some deaths arise from the dangerous and bizarre behavior induced by inhalant intoxication.

---

[15]   A number of "sudden sniffing deaths" have also been caused by trichloroethane.

Tolerance and Dependence

With regular use, tolerance develops to the desired psychoactive effects of aerosol solvents, while psychological dependence can be as severe as that resulting from abuse of other solvents. It is unclear whether physical dependence develops.

Patterns of Use

Fluorocarbon propellants were the principal propellants used in aerosols until their replacement in Canadian aerosol products in 1980. This was due to concern over their environmental impact on the ozone layer, which filters the sun's harmful ultra-violet radiation. The replacement propellants (e.g., FC22) tend to be more water soluble, so there is less risk of the agents, reaching the upper atmosphere to cause damage. However the toxic effects of the replacement aerosols on humans are likely similar to those of the traditional propellants.

Potential for Abuse

Like other solvents of abuse, aerosol solvents have a moderately high abuse liability, although aerosol solvents are generally more toxic.

Background Reading

Adlaf, E.M., Ivis, F.J., Smart, R.G. & Walsh, G.W. (1995). *The Ontario Student Drug Use Survey 1977-1995*. Toronto: Addiction Research Foundation.

Chadwick, O.F.D. & Anderson, H.R. (1989). Neuropsychological consequences of volatile substance abuse: A review. *Human Toxicology, 8 (4)*, 307–312.

Crider, R.A. & Rouse, B.A. (Eds.). (1988). *Epidemiology of Inhalant Abuse: An Update*. Rockville, MD: National Institute on Drug Abuse, NIDA Research Monograph 85.

Edeh, J. (1989). Volatile substance abuse in relation to alcohol and illicit drugs: Psychosocial perspectives. *Human Toxicology, 8 (4)*, 313–318.

Fornazzari, L., Wilkinson, D.A., Kapur, B.M. & Carlen, P.L. (1983). Cerebellar, cortical and functional impairment in toluene abusers. *Acta Neurologica Scandinavica, 67*, 319–329.

Gosselin, R.E. Smith, R.P. & Hodge, H.C. (1984). *Clinical Toxicology of Commercial Products*. Baltimore: Williams and Wilkins.

Korman, M., Matthews, R.W. & Lovitt, R. (1981). Neuropsychological effects of abuse of inhalants. *Perceptual and Motor Skills, 53*, 547–553.

Novak, A. (1980). The deliberate inhalation of volatile substances. *Journal of Psychedelic Drugs, 12*, 105-122.

Ramsey, J., Anderson, H.R., Bloor, K. & Flanagan, R.J. (1989). An introduction to the practice, prevalence and chemical toxicity of volatile substance abuse. *Human Toxicology, 8 (4)*, 261-269.

Ron, M.A. (1986). Volatile substance abuse: A review of possible long-term neurological, intellectual, and psychiatric sequelae. *British Journal of Psychiatry, 148*, 235–246.

Sharp, C.W. & Rosenberg, N.L. (1997). Volatile Substances. In J.H. Lowinson, P. Ruiz, R.B. Millman & J.G. Langrod (Eds.), *Substance Abuse — A Comprehensive Textbook*. (3rd edition). (pp. 303-327). Baltimore: Williams and Wilkins.

Smart, R.G. (1986). Solvent use in North America: Aspects of epidemiology, prevention and treatment. *Journal of Psychoactive Drugs, 18 (2)*, 87-96.

Texas Commission on Alcohol and Drug Abuse. (1991). *Understanding Inhalant Users: An Overview for Parents, Educators, and Clinicians*. Austin, TX: Texas Commission on Alcohol and Drug Abuse.

Other Drugs in Brief

Amanita Muscaria

DRUG CLASS: Hallucinogen

Amanita muscaria (fly agaric) is a mushroom that is widespread in the temperate parts of Europe, Asia and North America. It is also known by the names fly agaric and fly amanita because of the presence of an insecticidal constituent that kills flies exposed to it. In Europe and parts of Asia, the mushroom has a bright red cap and is mottled with white warts. The North American variety has a yellow, orange-red or white cap, and is mottled with white, red or yellow warts.

The amanitas are well known for two aspects of their pharmacological activity. First, many of these mushrooms, including *Amanita phalloides* (also known as "deadly amanita," "destroying angel" and "avenging angel") and *Amanita verna*, are highly lethal, apparently because of the presence of certain potent toxins such as phalloin and amanitins. Amanita poisoning is characterized by a long delay (10 hours or longer) between ingestion of the mushrooms and the onset of symptoms. The large majority of mushroom poisonings in North America are due to the amanitas.

Second, *Amanita muscaria*, which has markedly lower toxicity than other members of this family, is capable of producing hallucinogenic experiences. Indeed, it has been suggested that this mushroom may be the fabled "Soma" mentioned in the ancient Vedic writings of India. Soma was regarded as a divine intoxicant by the priests, who valued its hallucinogenic properties as a vital part of their religious rituals.

Amanita muscaria has also been used ceremonially by native Americans in Michigan and in Siberia as an inebriant.

Amanita muscaria contains two psychoactive constituents, ibotenic acid and muscazone, together with the cholinergic alkaloid muscarine as a relatively minor component. When the mushroom is extracted, ibotenic acid is changed chemically to the psychoactive product muscimole. These components are thought to be responsible for the altered state of consciousness that usually begins within 30 minutes of ingesting the mushroom.[1]

Early pharmacological effects include dizziness, nervousness, dry mouth, rapid and deep respiration, diarrhea, nausea and vomiting, muscle twitches and numbness in the limbs. These are followed by a light and peaceful sleep accompanied by vividly colored imagery. Upon awakening, the user usually experiences a state of mescaline- or psilocybin-like altered perceptions, euphoria, exhilaration and intense involvement with self, as well as an increased ability to perform unusually demanding physical tasks. This period may last for three to four hours. Subsequently, muscle twitching may be noticeable, and CNS-depressant effects gradually develop to the point of ultimate loss of consciousness in the form of deep sleep.

Severe psychological consequences can occur for some users of *Amanita muscaria*, and may include paranoid thinking, violent and bizarre behavior and self-mutilation.

Deaths occasionally result from ingestion of *Amanita muscaria*, although much less frequently than with other amanitas, possibly because much of the mushroom is removed from the body through vomiting and diarrhea. A lethal overdose causes delirium, convulsions, deep coma and death from cardiac arrest.

It is important to note that amanita mushrooms vary greatly in appearance, and people who actively seek out *Amanita muscaria* for its mind-altering properties, or who come upon amanitas in their search for Psilocybe mushrooms, may inadvertently collect the more toxic — and potentially lethal — amanitas.

---

[1] The hallucinogenic components of this mushroom are eliminated in the urine without significant loss in potency. For this reason, users in some areas of Siberia have been known to recycle the active constituents several times through repeated consumption of their own urine.

Background Reading

Lewis, W.H. & Elvin-Lewis, M.P.F. (1977). *Medical Botany: Plants Affecting Man's Health.* New York, John Wiley and Sons.

Schultes, R.E. & Hoffman, A. (1980). *The Botany and Chemistry of Hallucinogens* (2nd edition). Springfield, IL: Charles C. Thomas.

Anileridine

DRUG CLASS: Opioid

Anileridine hydrochloride (Leritine®) is a synthetic opioid analgesic used for the relief of moderate to severe pain. It occurs as a white crystalline powder that is freely soluble in water and very soluble in alcohol. Anileridine is chemically similar to meperidine (e.g., Demerol®), but is approximately three times more potent as an analgesic (i.e., the same degree of pain relief is achieved using approximately one-third as many anileridine molecules as meperidine molecules). The usual oral dose is 25 to 50 mg, repeated every six hours as necessary. When administration by intra-muscular or subcutaneous injection is required to relieve severe pain, doses as high as 100 mg may be used at four- to six-hour intervals, to a limit of 200 mg in 24 hours. When anileridine is administered by these routes, the side effects are generally fewer and milder than those of other potent opioids. Although anileridine has been administered intravenously without problems, rapid intravenous injection of more than 10 mg can produce severe respiratory depression, a rapid drop in blood pressure, and cardiac arrest.[1] Such life-threatening consequences rarely occur with small doses of other medically used opioids given by intravenous injection.

While the dependence liability of anileridine is similar to that of morphine, anileridine is mainly used in hospital settings and is rarely found on the street drug market.

Background Reading

Canadian Pharmaceutical Association. (1997). *Compendium of Pharmaceuticals and Specialties.* (32nd edition). Ottawa: Canadian Pharmaceutical Association.

Reisine, T. & Pasternak, G. (1996). Opioid analgesics and antagonists. (Chapter 23). In J.G. Hardman, L.E. Limbird, P.B. Molinoff, R.W. Rudden & A.G. Gilman (Eds.), *Goodman and Gilman's The Pharmacological Basis of Therapeutics.* (9th edition). New York/Toronto: McGraw-Hill Health Professions Division.

---

[1]   These effects can be rapidly reversed by immediate administration of opioid antagonist drugs such as naloxone (see the chapter on naloxone in Section 3).

Anticholinergic Agents

DRUG CLASS: Anticholinergic Agent, Hallucinogen

A number of plants containing the naturally occurring alkaloids atropine and scopolamine are found in many areas throughout the world. Such plants belong to the *Solanaceae* (potato) family and include *Atropa belladonna* ("beautiful lady"), also known as "deadly nightshade," and *Datura stramonium* ("devil's weed," "locoweed"), also known as "jimsonweed." Atropinic alkaloids have long been used in medicine because they produce several effects resulting from the antagonism of the neurotransmitter substance acetylcholine. These effects are collectively referred to as anticholinergic effects. At lower doses (e.g., 1 to 2 mg of atropine) these effects include depression of stomach motility and gastric secretion, inhibition of glandular secretions (causing dry mouth), dilation of the pupils, paralysis of muscles in the eye causing blurring of near vision, relaxation of smooth muscle spasms, and increased heart rate.

Atropine (*dl*-hyoscyamine) is available in a number of medicinal preparations alone (e.g., eye drops, injection) or with other drugs for gastrointestinal disorders (e.g., Donnagel®, Lomotil® tablets). Scopolamine (hyoscine) is available in a transdermal patch for motion sickness (e.g., Transderm-V®) and, as the butylbromide salt as a treatment for gastrointestinal cramping (e.g., Buscopan®). At therapeutic doses, scopolamine is more likely than atropine to have CNS-depressant effects that may result in drowsiness, amnesia and fatigue. Synthetic anticholinergic agents have been developed that are useful in the treatment of Parkinson's disease and the extrapyramidal symptoms associated with traditional antipsychotic treatment (see the chapter on psychiatric medications in Section 2). These agents include benztropine (Cogentin®), trihexyphenidyl (Artane®), procyclidine (Kemadrin®) and biperiden (Akineton®).

Higher doses of anticholinergics (e.g., 5 to 10 mg of atropine) produce a number of CNS-stimulant effects, including hallucinations, mild euphoria, disorientation, confusion, memory loss, paranoid thinking, agitation, speech disturbances, impaired motor co-ordination, maximal dilation of the pupils and sometimes seizures. These effects are usually accompanied by abnormally rapid and irregular heart rate, abnormally high blood pressure, rapid and weak pulse, headache, high fever, dry and burning sensations in the mouth, flushing of the skin, nausea and vomiting. With even larger doses, CNS-stimulation is followed by depression in which paralysis results in circulatory and respiratory failure and coma. Children are especially susceptible to the toxic effects of anticholinergic agents.

Because anticholinergic agents also produce mild euphoria, hallucinations and disorientation, they have the potential to be abused. The medical literature has reported several cases of anticholinergic drug abuse. The first case, reported in 1960, involved a patient who overmedicated herself with trihexyphenidyl to achieve euphoria. While abuse has also been reported in schizophrenic patients receiving these drugs for therapeutic purposes, it is not limited to psychiatric patients. In general, trihexyphenidyl is the anticholinergic most frequently reported to be abused, in daily doses of 10 to 30 mg.

People who seek the drug for non-medical purposes have been known to feign symptoms to obtain the drug, buy drugs from several sources and request increased doses despite the absence of extrapyramidal symptoms. A history of abuse of other substances is common among those who abuse anticholinergics. There has been at least one report of prescription anticholinergic drugs being smoked.

Regular users develop tolerance to these drugs and may develop both psychological and physical dependence. It has been suggested that in some schizophrenic patients overuse may not be abuse, since the drug is described as helping them to "feel and function better." It has been suggested these patients may be treating the "negative symptoms" of schizophrenia, such as social withdrawal and affect blunting, rather than seeking the drugs' other psychoactive effects.

The abuse potential of anticholinergic agents is limited by the relative mildness of their euphoric effects and the number of unpleasant side effects associated with their use.

Background Reading

Brower, K.J. (1987). Smoking of prescription anticholinergic drugs. *American Journal of Psychiatry, 144 (3)*, 383.

Hidalgo, H.A. & Mowers, R.M. (1990). Anticholinergic drug abuse. *DICP The Annals of Pharmacotherapy, 24*, 40–41.

Kaminer, Y., Munitz, H. & Wusenbeek, H. (1982). Trihexyphenidyl (Artane) abuse: Euphoriant and anxiolytic. *British Journal of Psychiatry, 140*, 473–474.

Pullen, G.P., Best, N.R. & Maguire, J. (1984). Anticholinergic drug abuse: A common problem? *British Medical Journal, 289*, 612–613.

Wells, B.G., Marken, P.A., Rickman, L.A., Brown, C.S., Hamann, G. & Grimmig, J. (1989). Characterizing anticholinergic abuse in community mental health. *Journal of Clinical Psychopharmacology, 9 (6)*, 431–435.

Antipsychotics: Typical

DRUG CLASS: Antipsychotic

"Typical" antipsychotic agents, formerly referred to as "major tranquillizers," are effective for the treatment of acute and chronic psychotic states. These drugs are grouped together because they have a common set of therapeutic effects and side effects. In the past they were the only options for antipsychotic purposes. Since the late 1980s, however, "atypical" antipsychotic agents have become available that work in a different way and have a different set of effects (see the chapter on atypical antipsychotics in Section 4). There are many typical antipsychotic agents currently in use. Examples include haloperidol (e.g., Haldol®), chlorpromazine (e.g., Largactil®, Thorazine® in the United States), thioridazine (e.g., Mellaril®), trifluoperazine (e.g., Stelazine®), perphenazine (e.g., Trilafon®), methotrimeprazine (e.g., Nozinan®), loxapine (e.g., Loxapac®), fluphenazine (e.g., Moditen®, Modecate®), zuclopenthixol (e.g., Clopixol®), flupenthixol (e.g., Fluanxol®), thiothixene (e.g., Navane®) and the combination products Elavil Plus® and Etrafon® (perphenazine and amitriptyline).

Antipsychotics are used to manage the acute and chronic symptoms associated with schizophrenia (e.g., for controlling delusions, hallucinations and agitation); for calming mania and the psychotic manifestations of the manic phase of bipolar (manic-depressive) mood disorder; and for controlling the symptoms of psychoses of organic origin, including those produced by infection, by metabolic disorders and by some toxic substances. They are also used for controlling aggressiveness and agitation in patients with dementia.

The nature and intensity of effects produced by antipsychotics vary to some extent among patients and from one drug to another. Nonetheless, substantial overlap exists among drugs with respect to most of their effects. The intensity and frequency of hallucinations greatly declines, delusional thinking can be substantially suppressed, and agitation, mania and bizarre behavior may be eliminated. The user's orientation to reality can significantly improve. The overall results for patients can be fewer hospitalizations throughout their lifetime and, in some cases, lifelong maintenance in the community without hospitalization; briefer periods of hospitalization; improved quality of life (interpersonal and vocational functioning); and a greater capacity to care for themselves.

Prior to the introduction of the antipsychotics, most psychotic patients admitted to psychiatric hospitals remained there for most or all of their lives. While some chronic, severely psychotic patients who are maintained on antipsychotics do not improve sufficiently to function in the community, those who require permanent institutional care now represent a minority of patients.

Although the typical antipsychotics have proven highly beneficial to large numbers of psychotic patients, they can also produce a spectrum of undesired side effects. The severity and frequency of the symptoms vary both with the particular antipsychotic used and the size of the daily dose, and from one individual to another. These drugs may produce anticholinergic symptoms (e.g., dry mouth, constipation, urinary retention, or blurred vision) and may cause sedation. They may also produce acute involuntary painful muscle contractions, usually of the neck or eyes (called dystonias). Some patients undergoing antipsychotic therapy experience a compulsive need to move about constantly (called akathesia) and may become so restless that they are unable to sit or remain in one place except for short periods. It is important that this effect not be mistaken for anxiety or psychotic agitation, to avoid overmedicating. Typical antipsychotic agents may also cause muscle rigidity, fine tremors, "pin-rolling" movements of the fingers, drooling and shuffling gait (symptoms referred to as parkinsonism). As a group, these latter three effects (i.e., dystonias, akathesia and parkinsonism) are called extrapyramidal symptoms, or EPS. These effects can be partially or even fully controlled in many cases by reducing the patient's daily dose of antipsychotic or by introducing other medications. Benztropine (e.g., Cogentin®) is often used in combination to treat or prevent EPS (see the chapter on anticholinergic agents in Section 4).

Some patients experience a sudden drop in blood pressure when they attempt to stand up, and may feel faint and dizzy for a short period. Skin reactions to antipsychotic therapy sometimes occur and can include extreme sensitivity to sunlight (causing a reaction similar to severe sunburn). Occasionally, antipsychotics may cause seizures, particularly in patients who have a history of seizures. Some of these drugs also suppress nausea and vomiting.

A syndrome known as tardive dyskinesia may occur with chronic antipsychotic therapy. Tardive dyskinesia is characterized by rhythmic, involuntary movements of the jaw, face, tongue and/or mouth, sometimes accompanied by involuntary movements of the extremities. In some cases, these phenomena are irreversible.

Daily doses of the antipsychotics differ markedly from one drug to another, since these substances range widely in potency. For example, the daily oral dose of chlorpromazine is 25 to 1,000 mg. In contrast, the daily oral dose of haloperidol is 1 to 20 mg. Some drugs in this group (e.g., fluphenazine, flupenthixol, zuclopenthixol) can be administered by injection in a single dose once every two to four weeks, by virtue of the very slow speed at which they are absorbed into the body from the injection site.

Antipsychotics can potentiate the hazardous effects of other CNS depressant drugs such as barbiturates, alcohol and opioid analgesics, and such drug combinations have caused a number of fatalities. Deaths exclusively due to antipsychotic overdose occur infrequently. Overdose symptoms may include severe extrapyramidal effects, very low blood pressure, abnormal heart rhythms, respiratory depression and vasomotor collapse.

One of the most important features of these drugs is that they rarely produce physical or psychological dependence, even over an extended period of administration. Tolerance does not appear to develop, although some patients experience a mild withdrawal syndrome, characterized by muscular discomfort and sleeping difficulties, upon abrupt discontinuation. Street abuse of these drugs is extremely rare, since they are associated with many side effects and do not produce effects that drug abusers might desire.

Background Reading

Buckley, P., Cannon, M. & Larkin, C. (1991). Abuse of neuroleptic drugs (letter). *British Journal of Addiction, 86*, 789–790.

Canadian Pharmaceutical Association. (1997). *Compendium of Pharmaceuticals and Specialties* (32nd edition). Ottawa: Canadian Pharmaceutical Association.

Gillman, M.A. & Lichtigfeld, F.J. (1992). Abuse of neuroleptic drugs? (letter). *British Journal of Addiction, 87*, 937.

Antipsychotics: Atypical

DRUG CLASS: Antipsychotic

A new generation of antipsychotic agents has become available in North America since the late 1980s. Before this time, the many side effects associated with antipsychotic drugs were believed to be inherently linked with their antipsychotic actions (see the chapter on typical antipsychotics in Section 4). Through studies of the newer "atypical" agents, however, it was discovered that antipsychotic effects could be achieved through different types of action in the brain. These agents offer alternative choices for patients who do not respond well or fully to the typical antipsychotics, or who cannot tolerate their side effects. Significantly, they carry a much lower risk of extrapyramidal side effects, including involuntary movements, motor restlessness, rigidity.

Clozapine (Clozaril®) was the first atypical agent marketed. However, this drug has its own set of side effects. Because it presents an increased risk of a serious blood disorder (agranulocytosis), its use is restricted and must be carefully monitored by the physician, pharmacist and manufacturer. Also, seizures have occurred in some patients, especially those using higher doses and those with a history of seizures. It is used primarily to manage symptoms of treatment-resistant schizophrenia. The usual therapeutic dose is 300 to 600 mg daily in divided doses.

Risperidone (Risperdal®) offers another alternative to the typical antipsychotic agents. It has been shown to be effective for both the positive (e.g., hallucinations, delusions) and negative (e.g., social withdrawal, reduced emotional response) symptoms of schizophrenia. The most common side effects include insomnia, agitation, anxiety and headache. Extrapyramidal side effects may occur at higher doses (greater than 10 mg/day). The usual therapeutic dose is 4 to 8 mg daily.

Olanzapine (Zyprexa®), the third atypical agent marketed in Canada, is also indicated for both acute and maintenance treatment of schizophrenia. As with the other agents, it has been shown to be effective for both positive and negative symptoms. The most common side effects include drowsiness, dizziness, constipation, akathesia (inner restlessness) and weight gain. Doses range from 5 to 20 mg daily.

Antipsychotic medications are not considered to be substances of abuse.

Background Reading

Canadian Pharmaceutical Association. (1997). *Compendium of Pharmaceuticals and Specialties* (32nd edition). Ottawa: Canadian Pharmaceutical Association.

Buspirone

DRUG CLASS: Anxiolytic

Buspirone (e.g., Buspar®) is an anxiolytic agent that is very different from the other sedative/hypnotic-type drugs used to treat anxiety, including benzodiazepines, barbiturates. While buspirone has been shown to be as effective as benzodiazepines in treating generalized anxiety disorder, it has the major advantage of not causing general CNS-depressant effects. Buspirone does not cause the cognitive impairment and sedative effects that are generally thought to be necessarily linked to anti-anxiety effects, It does not impair motor co-ordination, enhance the effects of CNS-depressant drugs (e.g., alcohol) or demonstrate cross-tolerance with CNS depressants. Moreover, users do not appear to develop tolerance to the drug's effects, and no withdrawal syndrome occurs after long-term use is abruptly stopped. Buspirone may also help relieve symptoms of depression.

The most common side effects associated with buspirone include dizziness, nausea, headache, nervousness, lightheadedness and excitement. Another disadvantage of buspirone is that those who have taken benzodiazepines prior to buspirone therapy may not respond as well; they may have learned to expect the immediate sedating and muscle-relaxing effects associated with other anxiolytics. Buspirone has a relatively short half-life and therefore must be administered in two or three doses daily. The usual therapeutic dose is 20 to 30 mg daily. It is not effective in the treatment of all anxiety-related disorders; for example, it is not effective in treating panic disorder. Further research is required to fully evaluate the possible uses of buspirone in psychiatry.

Buspirone is not considered to be a drug of abuse.

Background Reading

Canadian Pharmaceutical Association. (1997). *Compendium of Pharmaceuticals and Specialties* (32nd edition). Ottawa: Canadian Pharmaceutical Association.

Gelenberg, A.J. (1994). Buspirone: Seven year update. *Journal of Clinical Psychiatry, 55* (5), 222–229.

Hardman, J.G., Limbird, L.E., Molinoff, P.B., Rudden, R.W. & Gilman, A.G. (Eds.) (1996). *Goodman & Gilman's The Pharmacological Basis of Therapeutics*. (9th edition). New York/Toronto: McGraw-Hill Health Professions Division.

Butorphanol

DRUG CLASS: Opioid Agonist/Antagonist

Butorphanol tartrate is a synthetic opioid with agonist and antagonist properties. It acts as an agonist at κ (kappa) receptors and as a mixed agonist-antagonist at μ (mu) receptors. It is structurally similar to morphine but has a pharmacological profile similar to those of other agonists/antagonists such as pentazocine and nalbuphine.

Butorphanol is used medically for the relief of moderate to severe pain. Its analgesic potency is about four to eight times that of morphine, 30 to 40 times that of meperidine and 16 to 24 times that of pentazocine. It has been available in the United States since 1978 for intramuscular or intravenous use, in 1 and 2 mg/mL strengths. More recently, butorphanol was made available in a nasal spray containing 1 mg per metered dose.[1] This preparation has been marketed for the treatment of migraine pain and it may be of particular use for those with severe headaches that are unresponsive to other treatments.

When administered orally, butorphanol undergoes extensive first-pass metabolism in the liver, but doses administered by nasal and parenteral routes are not subject to this type of metabolism. Butorphanol is, therefore, only administered by these latter routes. Studies suggest that a nasal spray dose resembles a parenteral dose in its pharmacokinetics. Effects with the nasal preparation have an onset of 15 minutes or less, and peak levels occur within 60 minutes. Approximately five per cent of butorphanol is excreted unchanged in the urine.

Principal adverse effects associated with butorphanol include confusion, sleepiness, dizziness, nausea and vomiting. Insomnia and nasal congestion may occur with use of the nasal spray. Some patients have reported hallucinations and dysphoria. These adverse effects may limit butorphanol's usefulness in chronic pain conditions, such as cancer pain. Butorphanol should only be used with caution in individuals with a history of heart problems.

---

1   This product has been marketed in Canada since 1994 under the trade name Stadol NS®.

Two mg of butorphanol can produce respiratory depression similar to that caused by 10 mg of morphine, but a "ceiling effect," in which increased dose levels are not accompanied by increased respiratory depression, appears to occur with higher doses. However, duration of respiratory depression appears to be dose-related. Naloxone is the recommended antagonist for treatment of butorphanol overdose, but repeated dosing with naloxone may be required since butorphanol's duration of action exceeds that of naloxone.

Butorphanol can induce withdrawal symptoms in opioid-dependent individuals, such as those maintained on methadone, because of its antagonist properties at μ (mu) receptors. Butorphanol will not suppress symptoms of withdrawal in individuals who are physically dependent on opioids.

Although mixed agonist-antagonist opioids such as butorphanol appear to have less potential for abuse than do pure opioid agonists such as morphine, some cases of dependence and withdrawal have been reported. Butorphanol has been abused by intravenous and intramuscular use, both alone and in combination with diphenhydramine,[2] in order to achieve heroin-like effects. The potential for abuse of nasal butorphanol appears to be the same as for the intramuscular route. However, the intramuscular formulation is primarily available only in institutional settings, while the nasal preparation is more widely available in community settings. During the first three years after the nasal formulation was marketed in the United States, reports of adverse effects increased from 60 to about 400 a year, with the percentage of dependence-addiction reactions, increasing from 6.5 to 24 per cent. Reports of suspected abuse, drug-seeking behavior and dependence associated with the nasal formulation have been received by the Canadian Adverse Drug Reaction Monitoring Program, and forged prescriptions and thefts have also been reported in Canada. Abrupt discontinuation of butorphanol after prolonged use can precipitate withdrawal symptoms similar to, but more intense than, those seen with pentazocine, including nausea, vomiting, cramping and diarrhea. In Canada, butorphanol is a controlled drug under Schedule I of the *Controlled Drugs and Substances Act*, and is available by prescription.

---

[2] This combination parallels the use of pentazocine and tripelennamine (i.e., "Ts and Blues"). For more information see the chapter on pentazocine in Section 3.

Background Reading

Canadian Pharmaceutical Association. (1997). *Compendium of Pharmaceuticals and Specialties* (32nd edition). Ottawa: Canadian Pharmaceutical Association.

Gillis, J.C., Benfield, P. & Goa, K.L. (1995). Transnasal butorphanol. A review of its pharmacodynamic and pharmacokinetic properties, and therapeutic potential in acute pain management. *Drugs, 50 (1)*, 157–175.

Homan, R.V. (1994). Transnasal butorphanol. *Clinical Pharmacology, 49*, 188–192.

Smith, S.G. & Davis, W.M. (1984). Butorphanol and diphenhydramine abuse. *Journal of the American Medical Association, 252*, 1010.

Springuel, P. (1997). Potential abuse of butorphanol nasal spray. *Canadian Adverse Drug Reaction Newsletter, 7 (2)*, April.

Chloral Hydrate

DRUG CLASS: Sedative/Hypnotic

Chloral hydrate is a synthetic sedative/hypnotic that occurs as colorless crystals with a pungent odor and a very bitter taste. Chloral hydrate (e.g., PMS-Chloral Hydrate®, Noctec® [U.S.]) is used both for sedation and to induce sleep, although its use on a regular basis has decreased since the introduction of benzodiazepines. It is commonly used prior to surgery or diagnostic procedures, including those involving children, to reduce anxiety or to produce sleep. The typical adult sedative dose is 250 mg, usually taken three times per day, and the typical sleep-inducing dose ranges from 0.5 to 1.5 grams (500 to 1,500 mg). Doses in excess of the therapeutic range can produce a state of pleasurable intoxication similar to that produced by alcohol or barbiturates. Some highly tolerant abusers reportedly take as much as 10 to 12 grams per day.

The principal drawbacks of this agent are its tendency to cause gastric distress (resulting in nausea and vomiting) and its disagreeable taste. The use of high doses on a regular basis can result in gastric hemorrhage. Therefore, chloral hydrate is not usually used in patients with a history of gastritis or ulcers. Other side effects include lightheadedness, impaired co-ordination and nightmares. Rarely, paradoxical reactions have occurred, producing hallucinations, unusual excitement and disorientation. "Hangover" effects may occur but are less likely than with barbiturates and longer-acting benzodiazepines.

The toxic effects of chloral hydrate are similar to those of the barbiturates. The main dangerous effects of very high doses (i.e., overdose) of this drug are respiratory depression and low blood pressure. Other effects may include abnormal heart rhythms, very low body temperature, severe damage to the stomach, and coma.

Chronic use or abuse of chloral hydrate results in tolerance to the desired effects. As a result, the user may resort to ever-higher daily doses to maintain the original intensity of effects. However, users do not develop appreciable tolerance to the respiratory-depressant effects produced by higher doses. Therefore, progressively higher daily doses increase the user's risk of respiratory arrest and death. The margin of safety can also be significantly reduced if high doses of chloral hydrate are taken with such other CNS depressants as alcohol or barbiturates.

Physical dependence on chloral hydrate can develop when daily doses are taken for prolonged periods. Users who abruptly stop taking the drug may experience a withdrawal reaction resembling alcoholic withdrawal, with symptoms including hallucinations and convulsions.

Background Reading

American Hospital Formulary Service (AHFS) *Drug Information 1991*. (1991). Bethesda, MD: American Society of Health-Service Pharmacists.

Canadian Pharmaceutical Association. (1997). *Compendium of Pharmaceuticals and Specialties* (32nd edition). Ottawa: Canadian Pharmaceutical Association.

Hardman, J.G., Limbird, L.E., Molinoff, P.B., Rudden, R.W. & Gilman, A.G. (Eds.) (1996). *Goodman & Gilman's The Pharmacological Basis of Therapeutics*. New York/Toronto: McGraw-Hill Health Professions Division.

Lichenstein, R., King, J.C. & Bice, D. (1993). Evaluation of chloral hydrate for pediatric sedation. *Clinical Pediatrics, 32 (10)*, 632–633.

Diethylpropion

DRUG CLASS: CNS Stimulant, Appetite Suppressant

Diethylpropion is a central nervous system (CNS) stimulant that produces effects similar to, but less intense than, those of the amphetamines. Diethylpropion (e.g., Tenuate®) is legally obtainable only by prescription, and it is used medically only in a short-term program of weight reduction. The usual dose is 25 mg taken three times daily, or one 75-mg controlled-release capsule taken each morning. Adverse effects are similar to those of other CNS stimulants — overstimulation, nervousness, restlessness, increased alertness and insomnia; dizziness; headache; psychotic episodes in rare instances; palpitations, increased heart rate, irregular heartbeat, elevated blood pressure and chest pain; dry mouth; nausea, vomiting, abdominal pain, diarrhea or constipation; and changes in libido.

Although it was initially believed to be a "safe" diet pill, diethylpropion is now recognized as having many of the same unfavorable attributes as the amphetamines. Chronic use of high doses may result in a toxic state that is clinically identical to amphetamine psychosis, characterized by hallucinations and paranoid delusions. Severe overdose can lead to seizures, coma and circulatory collapse.

Tolerance to the drug's effects, including its appetite-suppressant (anorectic) effects, develops fairly rapidly, and prolonged use can lead to both physical and psychological dependence. While withdrawal symptoms following abrupt cessation may include extreme fatigue, ravenous appetite, depression and marked agitation, these symptoms are not as severe as those associated with amphetamine withdrawal.

Diethylpropion was classified as a controlled drug in Canada in 1978. Its dependence liability is high, but not as high as that of cocaine, amphetamine and methamphetamine. When diethylpropion is injected, the euphoria and CNS stimulation it produces are less powerful than those produced by these other drugs. As a result, diethylpropion is not the drug of choice for most stimulant abusers. Reclassification of diethylpropion to its current status as a controlled drug has greatly reduced its previous widespread abuse.

Background Reading

Canadian Pharmaceutical Association. (1997). *Compendium of Pharmaceuticals and Specialties* (32nd edition). Ottawa: Canadian Pharmaceutical Association.

Dimenhydrinate

DRUG CLASS: Histamine Antagonist,
Anticholinergic Agent

Dimenhydrinate[1] (e.g., Gravol®, Dramamine® [U.S.]) is a non-prescription medication that is used primarily to prevent and treat nausea, vomiting or vertigo associated with motion sickness. The component of dimenhydrinate that is believed to give it its pharmacological activity is diphenhydramine. Therefore, many of its effects, including sedation and anticholinergic effects, are similar to those of other antihistamines (see the chapter on antihistamines in Section 3).

The adult therapeutic dose of dimenhydrinate is 50 to 100 mg every four to six hours to a maximum of 400 mg in 24 hours. Potential side effects at this dosage include drowsiness, dizziness, mild impairment of concentration and motor co-ordination, excitation and nervousness (more commonly in children than in adults), and dry mouth. Like other anticholinergic agents, dimenhydrinate in higher doses may have hallucinogenic, mood-elevating and stimulant effects (see the chapter on anticholinergic agents in Section 4). Taking dimenhydrinate with alcohol or other CNS-depressant drugs tends to intensify its effects.

There have been several reports of dimenhydrinate abuse by individuals who were unable to obtain their preferred substances and by adolescents using it for a "cheap high." Doses used by abusers range from 250 to 1,250 mg (5 to 25 tablets).[2] At higher doses, dimenhydrinate's effects include visual, auditory and tactile hallucinations; lethargy; paranoia; agitation; memory loss; increased blood pressure and heart rate; and difficulty swallowing and speaking. Fatal doses of dimenhydrinate are similar to those of other antihistamines, in the range of 25 to 250 mg per kilogram of body weight.

---

[1]   The 8-chlorotheophyllinate derivative of diphenhydramine.

[2]   All doses refer to adults.

Chronic use of dimenhydrinate has resulted in tolerance, dependence and withdrawal. In these cases, daily doses have escalated to 1,250 to 3,750 mg (25 to 75 tablets) per day and the users presented with complaints of depressed mood and loss of energy; confusion and inattentiveness; difficulty thinking; difficulty socializing; vomiting; and urinary retention. Such users who suddenly stop taking dimenhydrinate experience withdrawal symptoms such as increased excitability, extreme malaise, poor appetite, nausea and abdominal cramps.

Although dimenhydrinate may produce euphoria or feelings of well-being in some individuals, its side effects likely limit its widespread abuse. Dimenhydrinate's potential for abuse is moderate because of its easy availability.

Background Reading

Craig, D.F. & Mellor, C.S. (1990). Dimenhydrinate dependence and withdrawal. *Canadian Medical Association Journal, 142 (9)*, 970–973.

Gardner, D.M. & Kutcher, S. (1983). Dimenhydrinate abuse among adolescents. *Canadian Journal of Psychiatry, 38*, 113–116.

Malcolm, R. & Miller, W.C. (1972). Dimenhydrinate (Dramamine) abuse: Hallucinogenic experiences with a proprietary antihistamine. *American Journal of Psychiatry, 128 (8)*, 126–127.

Young, G.B., Boyd, D. & Kreeft, J. (1988). Dimenhydrinate: Evidence for dependence and tolerance. *Canadian Medical Association Journal, 138*, 437–438.

Diphenoxylate

DRUG CLASS: Opioid

Diphenoxylate (which is combined with atropine sulphate in the product Lomotil®) is a weak synthetic opioid that occurs in pure form as a white crystalline powder and is almost insoluble in water and slightly soluble in alcohol. For symptomatic relief of diarrhea, its only medical use, diphenoxylate is used in an oral dose of 5 mg, usually three to four times per day. At this dose level, diphenoxylate exerts little or no euphoric or analgesic effects. Nausea is the most common side effect of a therapeutic dose. Other reported effects include drowsiness, lethargy, restlessness, dizziness, respiratory depression and vomiting. However, at higher dose levels (e.g., 40 to 60 mg), this drug can produce typical opioid-like effects, including euphoria, and can partially suppress withdrawal symptoms produced by abrupt abstinence from other opioids.

Chronic use of diphenoxylate at the typical daily dose level does not appear to produce physical dependence, although regular high-dose abuse can result in a mild form of physical dependence. However, since diphenoxylate is much less potent than other opioids, and is combined with atropine in oral tablet products, it is unattractive to opioid abusers, who are likely to resort to it only when their preferred drugs are not available.

Severe overdose of diphenoxylate can produce symptoms similar to those that result from overdose of other opioids, including coma, severe respiratory depression and cardiac arrest. Young children may exhibit such symptoms after having consumed doses as small as 30 to 50 mg and are also at risk of the effects of atropine overdose.

Background Reading

Canadian Pharmaceutical Association. (1997). *Compendium of Pharmaceuticals and Specialties* (32nd edition). Ottawa: Canadian Pharmaceutical Association.

Reynolds, J.E.F. (1997). *Martindale's The Extra Pharmacopeia.* (30th edition). London: Royal Pharmaceutical Society.

Rubenstein, J.S. (1979). Deliberate use of diphenoxylate HCL a Schedule V narcotic. *Western Journal of Medicine, 131 (2),* 148–150.

DMT
(Dimethyltryptamine)

DRUG CLASS: Hallucinogen

DMT is structurally similar to psilocin, a hallucinogenic alkaloid found in the *Psilocybe* and *Conocybe* species of mushroom. As a pure substance, DMT is available as a white crystalline product of laboratory synthesis. However, together with a number of closely related chemicals, it is a naturally occurring component of several plants (e.g., *Piptadina peregrina*) found in the West Indies and South America. For centuries, South American Indians have used DMT in the form of snuff for its hallucinogenic effects. These effects were first noted by Europeans in 1496 during Columbus' second voyage to the West Indies.

The traditional use of these plant materials in the form of snuff is particularly interesting, because we know that DMT and closely related chemicals are far more active when inhaled or injected than when taken orally.[1] In North America, DMT has been found as an additive in some marijuana preparations in which the marijuana has been soaked in a solution of DMT and then dried. The smoking of this preparation takes advantage of DMT's high potency when inhaled.

Taken alone, doses of approximately 50 to 60 mg (injected or inhaled) can produce a spectrum of psychological and physical effects similar to those produced by other hallucinogens such as LSD and mescaline. The effects are consistent with DMT's similarity to LSD in its affinity for the 5-HT2 type of 5-hydroxytryptamine receptors. At low doses (0.05 to 0.1 mg/kg injected intravenously), DMT's primary effects include changes in mood and increased sensitivity to bodily sensations. At higher doses (0.2 to 4 mg/kg intravenously), it typically produces a "rush," visual (and less frequently, auditory) hallucinations, dissociation and euphoria. Other effects may include increased blood pressure and heart rate, dilation of the pupils and elevated rectal temperature. DMT's effects are perceived rapidly and, unlike other

---

[1]   Even large doses of DMT taken orally (e.g., 350 mg) fail to produce any significant effects.

hallucinogens, DMT's entire hallucinogenic episode is quite brief, lasting for 30 to 60 minutes (hence the drug's street name, "businessman's lunch"). Anxiety and non-psychotic panic states tend to be more frequent with DMT than with most other common hallucinogens. Some investigators have suggested that the anxiety may be due to the very rapid onset of this drug's potent effects, which does not allow the user time to acclimatize to the dramatic shift in subjective experience.

Repeated use of DMT appears to produce neither physical dependence nor tolerance to its subjective effects. The absence of tolerance appears to make DMT unique among classic hallucinogens. Evidence suggests that DMT does not produce cross-tolerance with LSD (although mescaline and psilocybin do). DMT may therefore have a somewhat different mechanism of action than these other hallucinogens.

Background Reading

Schultes, R.E. & Hoffman, A. (1980). *The Botany and Chemistry of Hallucinogens* (2nd edition). Springfield, IL: Charles C. Thomas.

Strassman, R.J. (1996). Human psychopharmacology of N,N-dimethyltryptamine. *Behavioural Brain Research, 73 (1–2)*, 121–124.

Strassman, R.J., Qualls, C.R. & Berg, L.M. (1996). Differential tolerance to biological and subjective effects of four closely spaced doses of N,N-dimethyltryptamine in humans. *Biological Psychiatry, 39 (9)*, 784–795.

Ephedrine

DRUG CLASS: CNS Stimulant, Decongestant

Ephedrine is a naturally occurring central nervous system (CNS) stimulant obtained from the plant *Ephedra equisetina*, also known as the Chinese herb *ma-huang*. *Ma-huang* has been used medicinally for several thousands of years, but it was not until 1887 that ephedrine was found to be the active ingredient in the herb. Ephedrine is now also produced by chemical synthesis and marketed in the form of its salt, ephedrine sulphate. In its pure form, ephedrine sulphate is as a white crystalline powder with a bitter taste, and is soluble in water and alcohol. Ephedrine is closely related in its chemical structure to methamphetamine, although its CNS actions are much less potent. Its peripheral stimulant actions are similar to but less powerful and longer-acting than those of epinephrine, also called adrenaline, a hormone produced in the body by the adrenal glands.

Ephedrine is a moderately potent relaxant of the bronchial muscles, and is used for symptomatic relief in asthma.[1] The typical adult dose ranges from 30 to 60 mg taken orally in the form of tablets, three to four times per day. Ephedrine in the form of nose drops has been used to relieve nasal congestion associated with upper respiratory-tract illnesses. It has also been used to treat low blood pressure, because it constricts blood vessels and stimulates certain actions of the heart.

Common side effects are qualitatively similar to those produced by amphetamines, and typically include dizziness, insomnia, tremor, rapid pulse, sweating, respiratory difficulties, confusion, hallucinations, delirium and (very infrequently) seizures. The most dangerous symptoms of overdose are abnormally high blood pressure and rapid, irregular heartbeat. Chronic use of ephedrine also has been associated with cardiac toxicity. Older adults are particularly sensitive to the effects of stimulant medications such as ephedrine. Finally, a number of instances of psychosis, clinically similar to amphetamine psychosis, have resulted from chronic high-dose use.

---

[1]   Newer agents (i.e., B2 [beta] agonists), which are more specific in their action, have largely replaced ephedrine for this purpose.

Regular users can develop tolerance to the main effects of ephedrine, but temporary abstinence restores sensitivity.

Pseudoephedrine (e.g., Sudafed®) is an isomer of ephedrine that is also used as a decongestant.

Because of their stimulant properties, both ephedrine and pseudoephedrine have been classified as banned substances by the International Olympic Committee and numerous other sports bodies. The presence of these drugs in the body can be readily detected in a urine test.

Because the stimulant effects of ephedrine may produce feelings of well-being, this drug has some potential for abuse.

Ephedrine and "Street Stimulants"

Prescription stimulants that were widely abused in the past — amphetamine, diethylpropion, methylphenidate, etc. — are now much more tightly restricted.[2] The result has been a proliferation since the 1970s of a group of legal stimulant products, collectively called "street stimulants" or "look-alikes."

Look-alike stimulant preparations normally contain mild (and legal) stimulants, such as ephedrine, caffeine and phenylpropanolamine (PPA) as single ingredients or in combination.[3] Look-alike stimulants are manufactured in capsule and tablet form and closely resemble (but do not exactly mimic) in appearance the more potent prescription stimulants. Even the registered trade names of some look-alikes closely resemble pharmaceutical trade names.

A 1985 laboratory study demonstrated that animals given certain combinations of ephedrine, caffeine and phenylpropanolamine (PPA) respond as if amphetamine had been administered. This finding suggests that the effects of this trio of drugs may be additive when taken simultaneously, possibly resulting in a state of stimulation sufficiently reinforcing to be a replacement for the less available, more potent CNS stimulants. Other factors, such as highly professional advertising (including advertisements in major magazines), low cost, ease of availability, and, to some extent, the naiveté of young users who have never experienced the "real thing," have also contributed to the widespread abuse of stimulant look-alikes.

---

[2]   See the chapters on amphetamines and methylphenidate in Section 3 and on diethylpropion in Section 4.

[3]   See the chapters on caffeine in Section 3 and phenylpropanolamine (PPA) in Section 4.

During the past 20 years, tens of millions of units of look-alike stimulants have been sold throughout North America, particularly to teenagers. One study of randomly selected tractor-trailer drivers detected ephedrine, pseudoephedrine or phenylpropanolamine in the blood and urine of 12 per cent of the sample. About half of those who tested positive for these stimulants had given no medical explanation for their use.

Serious toxic reactions to look-alikes containing low doses of these mild stimulants are uncommon and most reports of toxicity resulting from street stimulants involve combinations of these agents. All three ingredients adversely affect blood pressure, for example, and therefore can be particularly dangerous to those with high blood pressure or other cardiovascular problems. There have been reports of fatalities resulting from the ingestion of street stimulants.

While legislation has aimed at restricting the manufacture and marketing of street stimulants, they continue to be readily obtainable.

Background Reading

Canadian Centre for Drug Free Sport. (1993). *Drug Free Sport: Banned and Restricted Doping Classes and Methods*. Gloucester, Canada: Canadian Centre for Drug Free Sport.

Kalix, P. (1991). The pharmacology of psychoactive alkaloids from Ephedra and Catha. *Journal of Ethnopharmacology, 32*, 201–208.

Lund, A.K., Preusser, D.F., Blomberg, R.D. & Williams, A.F. (1988). Drug use by tractor-trailer drivers. *Journal of Forensic Sciences, 33 (3)*, 648–661.

Morgan, J.P., Wesson, D.R., Puder, K.S. & Smith, D.E. (1987). Duplicitous drugs: The history and recent status of look-alike drugs. *Journal of Psychoactive Drugs,19 (1)*, 21–31.

Pental, P. (1984). Toxicity of over-the-counter stimulants. *Journal of the American Medical Association, 252 (14)*, 1898-1903.

Theoharides, T.C. (1997). Sudden death of a health college student related to ephedrine toxicity from a ma huang-containing drink. *Journal of Clinical Psychopharmacology, 17 (5)*, 437–439.

Fenfluramine

DRUG CLASS: Anorexiant

Fenfluramine (e.g., Ponderal®, Pondimin®) is a pharmaceutically manufactured synthetic anorexiant (appetite suppressant). Dexfenfluramine (e.g., Redux®) is the more active *d*-isomer of fenfluramine. These agents were used clinically as diet pills for the short-term management of obesity until 1997. Although chemically related to amphetamines, fenfluramine and dexfenfluramine have pharmacological effects that are very different from those of amphetamines, likely due to their effects on the serotonin neurotransmitter system.

High doses of fenfluramine and dexfenfluramine can produce euphoria, hallucinogen-like perceptual changes and feelings of unreality. However their unique pharmacological profile compared with other anorexiant agents (e.g., diethylpropion, phentermine) reduced their potential for abuse.[1] Fenfluramine generally does not produce significant psychomotor stimulant actions, and indeed often produces drowsiness, sedation, lethargy and fatigue (although the more typical stimulant effects — anxiety and insomnia — sometimes occur). Other common side effects include dizziness, dry mouth, nausea and vomiting, diarrhea and increased urinary output. The principal hazards of very high doses (i.e., overdose) include very high fever, seizures and severe cardiovascular dysfunction. Fenfluramine overdose has caused a number of deaths.

Fenfluramine and dexfenfluramine were voluntarily withdrawn from the market in Canada and the United States in September 1997 due to concerns about a serious heart-valve disease observed in some patients taking these drugs. Although some reports involve patients taking the combination fenfluramine-phentermine ("fen-phen"), cases of valvular disease have not been associated with phentermine alone. This is an unusual type of drug reaction. Further study may clarify the risks and the extent of this adverse effect.

---

[1]   See the chapters on diethylpropion, phentermine in Section 4.

Background Reading

Canadian Pharmacists Association. (1997). Canadian Pharmacists Association drug alert: Fenfluramine and dexfenfluramine withdrawn from market. *Canadian Pharmaceutical Journal, 130 (8)*, 27–28.

Connolly, H.M., Crary, J.L., McGoon, M.D., Hensrud, D.D., Edwards, B.S., Edwards, W.D. & Schaff, H.V. (1997). Valvular heart disease associated with fenfluramine-phentermine. *New England Journal of Medicine, 337*, 581–588.

Harmaline and Harmine

DRUG CLASS: Hallucinogen with Stimulant Properties

Harmaline and a closely related alkaloid, harmine, are naturally occurring hallucinogens found in the bark of the South American vine *Banisteriopsis caapi* and other
members of the *Banisteriopsis* genus. They can also be obtained from the seeds of the
Middle Eastern shrub *Peganum harmala* (also known as Syrian rue). They are present
in the psychoactive drink *ayahuasca* (also known as *caapi, pinde, natéma or yajé*),
prepared from the bark of stems of the *Banisteriopsis* vine, and used in northern South
America as a magic hallucinogen. Both harmaline and harmine have central nervous
system (CNS) stimulant properties and are monoamine oxidase inhibitors.[1] The
hallucinogenic dose range for experienced users of harmaline is estimated to be
approximately 300 to 400 mg when taken orally and 70 to 100 mg when injected
intravenously. For harmine, the estimated dose ranges are twice as great.[2]

Early effects produced by these drugs include nausea and vomiting, sweating, weakness, dizziness, tremors, and numbness in the limbs. Users then become physically
relaxed and tend to lose interest completely in their surroundings. Eyes are usually
kept closed, and users experience long dreamlike sequences of vivid images and
fantasies, dominated by specific intense colors (usually blues, greens and purples).
Perceptions of the external environment are usually not as greatly affected as with
other hallucinogens, and delusions and feelings of unreality generally do not occur.
Unlike most other hallucinogens, harmaline and harmine do not appear to exert
significant effects on thought processes. The experience tends to be highly individualized and usually involves little social interaction. Hallucinogenic activity usually
lasts approximately six hours.

Preliminary psychiatric research on the content of the visual imagery induced
by harmaline suggests that, irrespective of the highly "personal" nature of the

---

1   See the chapter on monoamine oxidase inhibitors (MAOIs) in Section 4.

2   Higher doses can result in very distressing hallucinations and delirium.

hallucinogenic episode, certain archetypal and mythical images connoting aggression and sexuality seem to appear recurrently. These intense images are experienced by such divergent groups as South American Indians living in indigenous communities and middle-class South Americans.

Because harmaline and harmine are monoamine oxidase inhibitors, they have the potential to produce severe and even lethal increases in blood pressure when taken concurrently with foods containing tyramine (e.g., aged cheeses, chocolate, red wine). Also, some other drugs will, in the absence of MAO activity, produce more intense, long-lasting and sometimes dangerous effects.

It is not known whether harmaline and harmine produce tolerance and dependence with regular use. They have rarely been used in North America, although harmaline was experimentally employed for a short period as an adjunct to psychotherapy.

Background Reading

Schultes, R.E., and Hofmann, A. (1980). *The Botany and Chemistry of Hallucinogens*. (2nd edition). Springfield, IL: Charles C. Thomas.

Hydrocodone

DRUG CLASS: Opioid

Hydrocodone or dihydrocodeinone, is a synthetic opioid that occurs as a fine white crystalline powder and is insoluble in water but slightly soluble in alcohol. It is structurally similar to codeine, although it is much more potent. Traditionally, hydrocodone has been employed in clinical medicine only as a cough suppressant (antitussive; e.g., Hycodan®, Robidone®), even though it has powerful analgesic properties. Most hydrocodone preparations, commonly in liquid (cough syrup) form, contain additional medicinal ingredients such as a decongestant (e.g., Novahistine DH®), a decongestant and an expectorant (e.g., Novahistex DH Expectorant®) or a combination of decongestant, expectorant and antihistamine (e.g., Hycomine®; Dimetane Expectorant-DC®). These added drugs combat other symptoms that often accompany a severe cough due to a cold or other respiratory tract infection. A typical adult therapeutic dose is 5 mg of hydrocodone bitartrate administered orally once every four hours. However, some highly tolerant abusers claim to take as much as 250 to 300 mg of hydrocodone per day.

When taken orally in doses well in excess of the therapeutic level, hydrocodone produces relatively powerful euphoric and sedative effects, although these effects are not as intense as those produced by opioids of abuse administered by injection (e.g., heroin, morphine). Nonetheless, hydrocodone is popular among street drug abusers because it possesses several advantages over illicit injection drugs:

- Hydrocodone is more easily obtained, either by forged or legitimate prescription or by pharmacy theft.

- It is more consistently available, although almost always illegally.[1]

- The quality (purity) of hydrocodone products prepared by the legitimate pharmaceutical industry is highly consistent.

---

[1]   In Canada, it is a criminal offence for a patient to willfully omit reporting to a prescribing physician any other prescriptions obtained for an opioid analgesic during the past 30 days.

These advantages are particularly important to the physically dependent hydrocodone abuser who is constantly seeking to avoid experiencing withdrawal symptoms. Greater access to hydrocodone contrasts with the difficulties encountered by physically dependent heroin abusers, who must rely on street purchases. Street heroin addicts continuously risk being "burned" (cheated) or having their illicit sources completely dry up. Unlike the hydrocodone abuser, therefore, the heroin abuser cannot avoid periodic withdrawal symptoms.

Hydrocodone abusers also have a lower risk of detection by legal authorities, doctors and others because they do not have "track marks" and other evidence of superficial tissue damage associated with chronic needle administration. Moreover, hydrocodone abusers do not suffer the severe social stigma that is commonly attached to heroin abusers.

Given these advantages, it is not surprising that there is considerable abuse of hydrocodone and other potent opioids that retain much of their efficacy when taken orally, such as oxycodone (e.g., Percodan®) and hydromorphone (Dilaudid®).

Tolerance can rapidly develop to the desired effects of hydrocodone and other orally administered opioids when they are used regularly. The result is that ever-higher daily doses become necessary in order to maintain the original intensity of these effects. Powerful dependence can arise from long-term abuse, and abrupt abstinence can cause a morphine-like withdrawal, although it may be less severe than that produced by abrupt abstinence from morphine.

A life-threatening overdose of hydrocodone can produce coma, severe respiratory depression and cardiovascular collapse. The lethal overdose for adults is estimated to be between 0.5 and 1.0 grams (500 to 1,000 mg).

Background Reading

Canadian Pharmaceutical Association. (1997). *Compendium of Pharmaceuticals and Specialties.* (32nd edition). Ottawa: Canadian Pharmaceutical Association.

Reisine, T. & Pasternak, G. (1996). Opioid analgesics and antagonists. (Chapter 23). In J.G. Hardman, L.E. Limbird, P.B. Molinoff, R.W. Rudden & A.G. Gilman (Eds.), *Goodman and Gilman's The Pharmacological Basis of Therapeutics.* (9th edition). New York/Toronto: McGraw-Hill Health Professions Division.

Ketamine

DRUG CLASS: Dissociative Anesthetic

Ketamine (Ketalar®) is a synthetic drug, marketed initially as a dissociative anesthetic.[1] It also produces hallucinations, analgesia and amnesia similar to those produced by phencyclidine (PCP). In its hydrochloride salt form, ketamine occurs as a white crystalline powder that is freely soluble in water and soluble in alcohol. When the drug is injected intravenously over a period of one minute, patients rapidly experience dissociative feelings and unconsciousness may result almost immediately. The intravenous dose range for anesthesia is between 1 and 2 mg per kilogram of body weight (i.e., 70 to140 mg for a 70-kg adult). The dose range for intramuscular injection is approximately three times as great. An anesthetic dose causes increased heart rate and elevated blood pressure. Respiration is typically not affected, but spasm of the larynx and other forms of airway obstruction have been reported.

Unconsciousness lasts for only 10 to 15 minutes. As a result, ketamine is useful in short surgical procedures (especially procedures involving the head and neck where the use of an anesthetic mask is inconvenient) and for inducing anesthesia before switching to another anesthetic. It has also been widely used in children and in burn victims to avoid use of a mask. A number of problems associated with its use can further limit ketamine's therapeutic value. These include unsatisfactory muscle relaxation, increased muscle tone, unpredictable and sometimes violent jerking and twitching (which can be precipitated by otherwise relatively innocuous stimuli), vivid and unpleasant dreams during and after surgery, and slow recovery from anesthesia (taking up to several hours). During the recovery period, patients may experience an emergence reaction characterized by headache, nausea and vomiting, hallucinations, feelings of unreality, confusion and sensations of heaviness or floating. Irrational behavior may also occur. Hyperexcitability (and sometimes seizures) may be precipitated by even mild stimuli for up to several hours after surgery. Delayed psychological effects of ketamine have been reported to occur for some time after its

---

[1]   In this context, dissociative means producing in the user feelings of dissociation (or detachment) from the external environment.

clinical use. In children, this phenomenon may take the form of nightmares that persist for months or even years. In adults, the likelihood of a delayed psychological effect appears to be low, and in most cases the effect disappears within three weeks.

In recent years, ketamine has been used increasingly in sub-anesthetic doses to relieve pain and induce sedation. Research studies have indicated that as a non-opioid analgesic, ketamine acts as an antagonist at N-methyl-D-aspartate (NMDA) receptors. Although the drug has been used alone, especially for children in emergency department procedures, it has also been injected intramuscularly, intravenously and into the spinal column in combination with morphine or another opioid to relieve pain associated with terminal cancer, osteoporosis and post-surgical recovery.

As post-surgical medication, ketamine has been administered to children in a lollipop formulation. It has also been administered orally to adults for relief of pain that does not respond to other analgesics.

Ketamine has been subject to abuse in the United States, Canada and Europe. Typically, drug supplies were obtained by diversion from legitimate sources. Street preparations include powders, capsules, tablets, crystals and solutions. Non-medical users inject (estimated) doses of 50 mg or "snort" between 60 and 125 mg.[2] Such dose levels do not usually result in unconsciousness. The main desired effects are euphoria and "mystical" revelations, as well as hallucinations and pleasant sensations of both floating and stimulation. Although these effects are typically sought after by users, the intensity of the effects, which may continue for one hour, may be upsetting to novice users. Users generally experience impaired thought processes, confusion, dizziness, impaired motor co-ordination and slurred speech. Severe adverse episodes — or "bad trips" — sometimes occur and resemble the toxic psychotic state caused by PCP. The principal hazardous effect of high doses is respiratory depression.

Little research has focused on long-term non-medical use of ketamine, and it is not known whether tolerance or dependence develops with regular use. A number of regular users do experience "flashbacks" (recurrences of psychic events that originally occurred during a ketamine-taking episode).

---

2   All doses refer to adults.

Background Reading

Cherry, D.A., Plummer, J.L., Gourlay, G.K., Coates, K.R. & Odgers, C.L. (1995). Ketamine as an adjunct to morphine in the treatment of pain. *Pain, 62 (1)*, 119-121.

Cioaca, R. & Canavea, I. (1996). Oral transmucosal ketamine: An effective premedication in children. *Pediatric Anaesthesia, 6 (5)*, 361-365.

Dalgama, P.J. & Shewan, D. (1996). Illicit use of ketamine in Scotland. *Journal of Psychoactive Drugs, 28 (2)*, 191-199.

Haas, D.A. & Harper, D.G. (1992). Ketamine: A review of its pharmacologic properties and use in ambulatory anesthesia. *Anaesthesia Progress, 39 (3)*, 61-68.

Valentin, N. & Bech, B. (1996). Ketamine anaesthesia for electrocochleography in children, Are psychic side effects really rare? *Scandinavian Audiology, 25 (1)*, 39-43.

Khat

DRUG CLASS: CNS Stimulant

Khat (*Catha edulis*) is a plant found in Eastern Africa and the Arab Peninsula, where it is known by a variety of names, including *qat* (Yemen), *tschat* (Ethiopia) and *miraa* (Kenya). The leaves of the khat plant are chewed for their amphetamine-like stimulant effects. The active ingredient in khat is a compound called "cathinone," which is closely related to amphetamine and is found in higher concentrations in young leaves. Because cathinone becomes inactive when the leaves dry out, they must be chewed while still fresh to be effective. There may still be other, as yet unidentified, constituents in khat that contribute to its stimulant effects. However, it appears that cathinone is the most important chemical in the plant.

The effects of khat chewing are qualitatively similar to those of amphetamine use, and include feelings of elation, euphoria, increased energy and alertness. Systemic effects include dilated pupils, loss of appetite and increases in respiration, body temperature, blood pressure and heart rate. The likelihood of ingesting high doses of cathinone is limited somewhat by the bulkiness of the plant material containing the drug. However, excessive use of khat can cause psychosis and life-threatening events, including brain hemorrhage (bleeding), heart attack and pulmonary edema (lung congestion). Constipation is a common effect, and is believed to result from the high concentrations of tannin in khat. Long-term follow-up studies have not been conducted to determine the possible chronic effects of khat chewing. It is known that chronic khat use may be compulsive and that psychological dependence is possible. Withdrawal symptoms following prolonged use have been described as lethargy, mild depression, nightmares and tremor.

In general, khat is used by individuals as a recreational drug. In some countries, such as Yemen, khat has a long history of being used as part of formal social customs, to encourage group discussion of community issues, for example. Detailed studies of the psychosocial aspects of khat use are not available. However, the negative effects of its use on the individual and community are evident enough that countries in which its use is widespread have started to take steps to limit the availability of the drug. The United Nations Convention on Psychotropic Drugs has listed khat as a controlled substance.

With the availability of worldwide commercial air travel, it is not surprising that khat has been appearing in other regions of the world. Seizures of khat have occurred in Canada. It is questionable whether khat will ever become a drug of widespread abuse in North America because of the short-lived potency of the fresh leaves. A permit is required in order to import khat leaves into Canada.

Background Reading

Balint, G.A. & Balint, E.E. (1994). On the medico-social aspects of Khat *(Catha edulis)* chewing habit. *Human Psychopharmacology, 9,* 125–128.

Griffiths, P., Gossop, M., Wickenden, S., Dunworth, J., Harris, K. & Lloyd, C. (1997). A transcultural pattern of drug use: Qat (khat) in the UK. *British Journal of Psychiatry, 170,* 281–284.

Kalix, P. (1994). Khat, an amphetamine-like stimulant. *Journal of Psychoactive Drugs, 26 (1),* 69–74.

Widler, P., Mathys, K., Brenneisen, R., Kalix, P. & Fisch, H.U. (1994). Pharmacodynamics and pharmacokinetics of khat: A controlled study. *Clinical Pharmacology and Therapeutics, 55 (5),* 556–562.

LAAM
(Levo-alpha-acetylmethadol)

DRUG CLASS: Opioid

LAAM (levo-alpha-acetylmethadol) is a synthetic opioid agonist, chemically related to methadone, with properties qualitatively similar to those of morphine. It is a μ (mu) agonist that affects the central nervous system and smooth muscles (e.g., in the gastrointestinal tract). LAAM's effects include analgesia, sedation and respiratory depression.

Tolerance develops to LAAM's analgesic and sedating effects with repeated use. Abrupt discontinuation of this drug results in a withdrawal syndrome that is similar to that seen with other opioids, but with some differences: onset is slower, the course is more prolonged and the symptoms are less intense.

LAAM has the following properties that make it suitable for use in treating opioid-dependent individuals: 1) it effectively suppresses symptoms of withdrawal from heroin and other opioids, 2) chronic oral administration at appropriate doses produces cross-tolerance that blocks the euphoria and other subjective effects of administered opioids, and 3) it is effective when administered orally.

After oral administration, LAAM is well absorbed from the gastrointestinal tract. It is converted in the liver to two pharmacologically active metabolites: nor-LAAM and dinor-LAAM. Both of these metabolites are more potent agonists than the parent drug and have longer elimination half-lives. The long elimination half-lives of nor-LAAM and dinor-LAAM (48 and 96 hours respectively) are believed to be largely responsible for LAAM's long duration of action.

The onset of effects of a single oral dose of LAAM occurs two to four hours after the drug is taken, and the duration of action is 48 to 72 hours. Patients must be warned that the peak effects of LAAM do not develop immediately, and that effects continue for several days after the last dose. During these periods, use of other psychoactive

drugs (including alcohol) may be fatal. Unless adequately warned, individuals beginning LAAM treatment may become impatient with the slow onset of its effects and
self-administer other psychoactive medications with fatal results. Because of these
risks, take-home doses of LAAM are not permitted.

LAAM is used as an alternative to methadone in the maintenance treatment of
opioid-dependent individuals. It is important to note that LAAM is not a long-
acting form of methadone, but an entirely different medication. The recommended
initial dose is 20 to 40 mg. Subsequent doses should be administered at 48- or 72-hour
intervals and may be adjusted in increments of 5 to 10 mg until the desired steady
state is reached (usually within one to two weeks). Most patients can be stabilized on
doses in the range of 60 to 90 mg administered three times a week. The major advantage of LAAM over methadone is its less frequent administration schedule (i.e., every
two to three days, compared with methadone's daily administration). A three-times-
a-week dosing eliminates the need for take-home doses.

LAAM must never be administered on a daily basis. Daily dosing may result in excessive
drug accumulation and risk of fatal overdose. Patients may be started on LAAM
directly or they may transferred from methadone to LAAM. In this latter case, it is
recommended that the cross-over from methadone to LAAM be accomplished in a
single dose.

The side effects reported with LAAM are those generally seen with methadone and
include constipation, abdominal pain, excessive sweating, decreased sexual interest
and delayed ejaculation.

LAAM has been shown to be as effective as methadone in the maintenance treatment of opioid-dependent individuals with respect to reduction of illicit opioid use,
length of time patients stayed in treatment, employment, clinic attendance, involvement in illegal activities and interactions with the legal system. LAAM is thought to
be useful for clients who would benefit from fewer clinic visits.

LAAM is believed to have a low potential for abuse. The slow onset of action makes
it unattractive to opioid users who seek an immediate "high" and diminishes its street
value as well as its potential for diversion.

LAAM is currently not available in Canada. In the United States, it is used only for the management of opioid dependence and may be dispensed only by treatment programs approved by the Federal Drug Administration, the Drug Enforcement Agency and designated state authorities. It is available as an aqueous solution (ORLAAM), which is diluted for oral administration. LAAM is usually mixed with a fruit-flavored drink different in color from that used to dilute methadone.

Background Reading

LAAM — A long-acting methadone for the treatment of heroin addiction. (1994). *Medical Letter on Drugs and Therapeutics, 36 (924)*, 52.

National Institute on Drug Abuse, Medications Development Division. (1993). *Information on LAAM: Chemistry, Pharmacology and Clinical Trial Results*. Rockville, MD: National Institute on Drug Abuse.

Levallorphan

DRUG CLASS: Opioid Agonist/Antagonist

Levallorphan (Lorfan®) is a synthetic opioid antagonist that also possesses potent opioid agonist properties.[1] In the form of its tartrate salt, it is as a white odorless crystalline powder that is very bitter to the taste and is soluble in water and slightly soluble in alcohol. When opioids are not present in the body, a typical therapeutic dose of levallorphan (i.e., 1 mg administered by injection to a non-tolerant person) produces an analgesic effect equivalent to that of approximately 10 mg of morphine; levallorphan is thus a powerful analgesic in its own right. Most people receiving this drug also experience drowsiness and relaxation, while dysphoric reactions, such as anxiety and fearfulness, occur in many. Others compare the effects of a therapeutic dose to a state of alcohol intoxication and grogginess. Additional common side effects include dizziness, blurred vision, pupillary constriction, mild respiratory depression, nausea, upset stomach and sweating.

At doses higher than therapeutically indicated, psychotic-like effects may occur, including bizarre dreams, feelings of unreality, visual hallucinations and disorientation.[2] Serious overdose can cause coma, respiratory depression, lowered body temperature, abnormally low blood pressure and slowed heart rate, and toxic psychosis may precede coma.

The principal medical use of levallorphan has been to counteract (i.e., antagonize) the adverse effects of opioids. It can rapidly reverse most opioid effects, including such hazardous overdose effects as respiratory depression. Moreover, when used in appropriate doses, levallorphan can reverse or prevent opioid-induced respiratory depression without significant loss of analgesia.[3] Levallorphan has therefore been used

---

[1]   Opioid agonist and antagonist actions are discussed in the opioids chapter in Section 2.

[2]   These effects may also occur at therapeutic doses in some particularly sensitive individuals.

[3]   In some circumstances, levallorphan can also be used alone for relief of severe pain.

in pre- and post-operative situations, as well as during surgery and labor. However, levallorphan (and other opioid antagonists, such as naloxone) cannot reverse or prevent respiratory depression caused by overdose of other classes of drugs such as sedative/hypnotics. Caution must be exercised in administering levallorphan to patients who are physically dependent upon opioids, as it can produce a severe withdrawal reaction.

With the development of newer opioid antagonists such as naloxone that do not share levallorphan's agonist properties, levallorphan has been largely replaced in clinical practice.

Tolerance does not appear to develop to the opioid antagonist effects of this drug when it is taken chronically, although tolerance does develop to the agonist (e.g., analgesic) effects. Because of the unpleasant psychological consequences associated with its use at higher doses, levallorphan is rarely abused.

Background Reading

Reisine, T. & Pasternak, G. (1996). Opioid analgesics and antagonists. In J.G. Hardman, L.E. Limbird, P.B. Molinoff, R.W. Rudden & A.G. Gilman (Eds.), *Goodman and Gilman's The Pharmacological Basis of Therapeutics* (9th edition). (Chapter 23). New York/Toronto: McGraw-Hill Health Professions Division.

Lithium

DRUG CLASS: Mood Stabilizer

Lithium (e.g., Lithane®, Carbolith®, Duralith®) is used in psychiatry to stabilize mood in patients with bipolar disorder (manic-depressive illness). It is effective in calming acute manic episodes and in preventing the recurrence of mania and depression in these patients. Manic episodes are generally characterized by hyperactivity, flights of ideas, extreme and often compulsive talkativeness, highly accelerated rate of speech, excessive elation and irritability. Lithium can also be used to augment the effects of antidepressant agents in depressed patients. The dosage of lithium is individualized for each patient, usually based on lithium blood concentrations.

The most common early side effects of lithium include tremor, muscle weakness, upset stomach, diarrhea, thirst, increased urination and trouble concentrating. Long-term problems that may occur include weight gain, thyroid problems, kidney problems and acne.

Higher blood concentrations of lithium may produce a serious toxic reaction, early signs of which include sluggishness, drowsiness, confusion, coarse tremors, muscle twitching, loss of appetite, vomiting and diarrhea. Still higher blood levels can produce life-threatening effects such as seizures and coma. Many factors, including excessive dosage, dehydration, kidney problems and the presence of other medications, can cause increased lithium blood concentrations.

Lithium is not considered to be a drug of abuse.

Background Reading

Canadian Pharmaceutical Association. (1997). *Compendium of Pharmaceuticals and Specialties* (32nd edition). Ottawa: Canadian Pharmaceutical Association.

Meprobamate

DRUG CLASS: Anxiolytic

Meprobamate was the first drug to be labelled a "minor tranquillizer" (i.e., an anxiolytic). When it was introduced in the mid-1950s, it was marketed as a safe and non-addicting alternative to the barbiturates and other available sedative/hypnotic drugs. Although marketed as an anxiolytic, it also became popular for medical use as a sedative/hypnotic. It also achieved popularity among drug abusers because of its ability to produce barbiturate-like euphoria. Eventually it was realized that its properties are very similar to those of the barbiturates, and its use substantially declined with the introduction of the benzodiazepines.

Meprobamate is available alone (e.g., Equanil®, Miltown® [U.S.]) or in combination with ASA, caffeine citrate, and codeine phosphate (e.g., 282 Mep®).

At therapeutic low-dose levels (e.g., 400 mg/dose), meprobamate is effective in managing tension and non-psychotic anxiety. Its principal desired effects are feelings of calmness and relaxation, and it may also produce drowsiness sufficient to cause sleep. Other effects may include dizziness; weakness; mild impairment of co-ordination; visual disturbances; prickling, tingling or burning sensations on the skin; numbness; vertigo; sometimes overstimulation or paradoxical excitement; headache; palpitations; slight or sometimes significant drop in blood pressure; mildly irregular heartbeat; sometimes abnormally rapid heart rate; nausea; vomiting and diarrhea. At moderate dose levels (e.g., 800 mg/dose), its anti-anxiety effect is increased, and it can also induce sleep in many users. The side effects of moderate doses are generally similar to those produced by the barbiturates, although the degree of drowsiness and euphoria generated by meprobamate at equally effective doses tends to be less pronounced. At high doses, the intoxication produced by meprobamate and the barbiturates is almost identical. Unlike the barbiturates, meprobamate cannot produce anesthesia.

Extreme overdose of meprobamate results in respiratory depression, stupor, extremely low blood pressure, shock and coma. Death has resulted from doses as small as 12 grams (12,000 mg) but people have been known to survive doses as great as 40 grams. When the meprobamate overdose is taken with other CNS-depressant drugs, the risk of death is increased.

Regular users of meprobamate rapidly develop tolerance to its anxiety-relieving and sleep-inducing effects. Tolerance can also develop quite rapidly to the barbiturate-like euphoria it produces. There is a high degree of cross-tolerance between meprobamate and sedative/hypnotic drugs such as the barbiturates — once tolerant to a given effect produced by meprobamate, the user will also be tolerant to the same effect produced by an equivalent dose of these other drugs.

Chronic daily use of meprobamate can result in physical dependence. Generally, the greater the size of the daily dose and the longer the period of use or abuse, the more severe is the withdrawal syndrome resulting from abrupt abstinence. The onset of withdrawal usually occurs 12 to 48 hours after the last dose. The syndrome can range from relatively mild and temporary symptoms such as restlessness, anxiety and insomnia in mildly dependent users to potentially life-threatening complications in severely dependent users. The mild withdrawal syndrome also usually includes muscle twitching, impaired co-ordination, tremors, loss of appetite, nausea and vomiting. In severely dependent users (i.e., those who take several grams of meprobamate per day), withdrawal symptoms may be greatly intensified, and severe agitation, hallucinations and tonic-clonic (grand-mal) seizures may also occur. These severe symptoms also occasionally occur in physically dependent users of smaller daily doses. Death has been reported to occur during severe withdrawal.

Background Reading

American Hospital Formulary Service (AHFS) Drug Information 1991. (1991). Bethesda, MD: American Society of Health-Service Pharmacists.

Hardman, J.G., Limbird, L.E., Molinoff, P.B., Rudden, R.W. & Gilman, A.G. (Eds.) (1996). *Goodman and Gilman's The Pharmacological Basis of Therapeutics.* (9th edition). New York/Toronto: McGraw-Hill Health Professions Division.

Monoamine Oxidase Inhibitors
(MAOIs)

DRUG CLASS: Antidepressant

The group of drugs known as monoamine oxidase inhibitors (MAOIs) is used to treat depression. This group includes the irreversible inhibitors phenelzine (e.g., Nardil®), tranylcypromine (e.g., Parnate®), and isocarboxazid (e.g., Marplan® [not available in Canada]) and the newer, reversible inhibitor moclobemide (e.g., Manerix®). While the older agents are not used as first-line therapy for depression because of the related food restrictions, they are a valuable treatment option for some patients.

The irreversible MAOIs block the activity of the enzyme monoamine oxidase (MAO). This enzyme, which occurs naturally in the body, metabolizes certain amines that are present either in the body (particularly norepinephrine and related compounds) or in various common foods (e.g., aged cheeses, aged and cured meats, sauerkraut, soy sauce, wine, beer). Because MAOIs interfere with the activity of MAO, they indirectly prevent or slow the metabolism of such substances, with potentially serious consequences for the patient. Tyramine, for example, is a monoamine found in fermented foods and in particularly large amounts in aged cheese. Sufficient quantities of tyramine, if not adequately metabolized by MAO, can produce severely elevated blood pressure (hypertensive crisis) and other cardiovascular irregularities — effects that can be life-threatening. Furthermore, certain other drugs will, in the absence of MAO activity, produce more intense, long-lasting and sometimes dangerous effects. For these reasons, it is essential that patients be fully informed as to which foods and drugs they should avoid or use sparingly while undergoing irreversible MAOI therapy.

Moclobemide preferentially blocks the activity of one type of MAO (MAO-A). However, this inhibition is reversible within 24 hours. As a result, there is less potential for dangerous diet and drug interactions with moclobemide than with irreversible MAOIs.

Irreversible MAOIs can produce side effects even when patients carefully monitor their food and drug intake. Common side effects include insomnia, weakness, dizziness, dry mouth, upset stomach, constipation, postural hypotension (dizziness, as a result of suddenly reduced blood pressure, upon changing quickly from a lying to standing position) and sexual problems. The most common adverse effects of moclobemide are sleep disturbances, restlessness, dry mouth, dizziness, headache, sedation and nausea.

Symptoms of overdose with the irreversible MAOIs are similar to the drugs' adverse effects but are more intense, and may appear to be a combination of CNS and cardiovascular stimulation or depression. Symptoms include drowsiness, dizziness, agitation, severe headache, convulsions and coma. Deaths have been reported. Symptoms of overdose with moclobemide include nausea, drowsiness, disorientation and reduced reflexes.

Cases of withdrawal have been reported among patients who abruptly stop taking phenelzine. Withdrawal symptoms may include nausea, vomiting and malaise. More severe symptoms such as psychosis and convulsions have occurred rarely. A few cases of MAOI dependence and abuse have been reported for tranylcypromine and phenelzine. In general, however, the potential for abuse of these agents is very low.

Background Reading

Baumbacher, G. & Hansen, M.S. (1992). Abuse of monoamine oxidase inhibitors. *American Journal of Drug Alcohol Abuse, 18 (4)*, 399–406.

Canadian Pharmaceutical Association. (1997). *Compendium of Pharmaceuticals and Specialties* (32nd edition). Ottawa: Canadian Pharmaceutical Association.

Morning Glory Seeds

DRUG CLASS: Hallucinogen

Seeds of plants *Rivea corymbosa* and *Ipomoea violacea* of the *Convolvulaceae* (morning glory) family have long been used for their hallucinogenic effects in the sacred rituals of certain Mexican Indian tribes. The principal psychoactive components, which are structurally similar to LSD,[1] include *d*-lysergic acid amide (ergine) and *d*-isolysergic acid amide (isoergine). These alkaloids are substantially less potent psychoactively than LSD, ergines being approximately one-tenth as potent in doses of equal weight. However, when taken in sufficient quantities, these alkaloids produce effects quite similar to those produced by LSD (although nausea, vomiting and diarrhea are far more common with morning glory seeds). Approximately 100 seeds of *Rivea corymbosa*, for example, contain a hallucinogenic dose of these alkaloids comparable to 100 micrograms of LSD.

The traditional preparation involves pulverizing the seeds and then pouring the resultant powder into cold water. The solution is passed through a filter to remove impurities and is then drunk. Grinding the seeds is essential, because the seeds' hard, impervious coat would otherwise allow them to move unaltered through the gastrointestinal tract.

Morning glory seeds became a popular and easily available substitute for LSD during the 1960s and early 1970s. While nursery growers' exotic trade names, such as Heavenly Blue, Flying Saucer and Pearly Gates, inadvertently served to enhance the seeds' image as hallucinogens, many users were unaware that the concentrations of psychoactive constituents varied widely among the seeds of different botanical varieties of morning glory. Today, most seeds sold for horticultural purposes are coated with insecticides and/or fungicides that are extremely difficult to remove and cause

---

[1]   Certain other members of the *Convolvulaceae* family also contain the same alkaloids — e.g., *Argyreia nervosa* (Hawaiian baby woodrose).

considerable discomfort if ingested. These coatings therefore serve as a deterrent to the use of morning glory seeds as a drug.

Background Reading

Schultes, R.E. & Hoffman, A. (1980). *The Botany and Chemistry of Hallucinogens* (2nd edition). Springfield, IL: Charles C. Thomas.

MPPP and MPTP

DRUG CLASS: Opioid

"Designer" or "microchip" drugs such as MPPP are wholly synthetic substances that are intended to closely resemble controlled drugs in both chemical structure and effects. They are "designed" to take advantage of U.S. drug laws, under which their manufacture and use are not specifically prohibited. Despite the fact that it has become easier in recent years to prohibit manufacture and distribution of these substances in the United States, designer drugs have continued to appear on the street, especially in California.

MPPP (1-methyl-4-phenyl-4-propionoxypiperidine), called "synthetic heroin" or "new heroin," was among the vanguard of designer drugs in the opioid class. MPPP is similar to meperidine (e.g., Demerol®) both in structure and euphoric effect, but is reputed to produce effects that are more powerful. The ingredients and equipment needed to synthesize MPPP are relatively inexpensive, and the drug can be fairly easily manufactured by an experienced "basement" chemist. However, careless production of MPPP using excess heat or acid can produce a byproduct, known as MPTP (1-methyl-4-phenyl-1,2,5,6-tetrahydropyridine). MPTP is also produced legally in small quantities for research, and is commercially used to produce other industrial chemicals.

MPTP appears to lack the euphoric and analgesic effects of opiates, but has serious toxic effects on the central nervous system, causing irreversible brain damage. Some users of illicit MPPP that was contaminated with MPTP developed a syndrome resembling severe Parkinson's disease. These individuals showed difficulty in moving (in some cases, almost total immobility) and speaking, increased muscle tone, rigidity, pronounced tremor, constant drooling and flattened facial expression.

It has now been established that MPTP was the sole agent responsible for the onset of the symptoms of Parkinson's disease in street users, despite the fact that most had injected an MPPP/MPTP combination. It has been reported that an industrial chemist whose work routinely brought him into contact with MPTP also developed full-blown Parkinson's disease. This case suggests that absorption of MPTP, either through the skin or by passive vapor inhalation, may in the long run produce results similar to those of concentrated intravenous injection of the substance. MPTP-exposed patients who have sustained this type of permanent brain damage have responded favorably to anti-parkinsonism drugs, but the amount of medication taken regularly by these patients has been quite high.

One of the unanswered questions concerning MPTP is whether individuals who may have used relatively small quantities of the drug, but did not develop overt Parkinson-like signs and symptoms in the short term, will be at increased risk of developing Parkinson's disease in the long term.

Background Reading

Langston, J.W. & Ballard, P.A. (1983). Parkinson's disease in a chemist working with l-methyl-4-phenyl-1,2,5,6-tetrahydropyridine. *New England Journal of Medicine, 309, 310.*

Reisine, T. & Pasternak, G. (1996). Opioid analgesics and antagonists. In J.G. Hardman, L.E. Limbird, P.B. Molinoff, R.W. Rudden & A.G. Gilman (Eds.), *Goodman and Gilman's The Pharmacological Basis of Therapeutics* (9th edition). (Chapter 23). New York/Toronto: McGraw-Hill Health Professions Division.

Nitrous Oxide

DRUG CLASS: Inhalant Anesthetic

Nitrous oxide (N_2O; "laughing gas") is a colorless gas with low molecular weight that lacks the pungent odor typical of other inhalant anesthetic agents and has sometimes been described as "sweet" smelling. Nitrous oxide has a very rapid onset of action. Typical effects of this gas include euphoria, numbness of the body, giddiness and sometimes uncontrolled laughter. Perceptual distortion and a sense of floating have been described although true hallucinations are not typically reported. Some users experience anxiety or panic. All of these effects wear off within a few minutes after inhalation is discontinued.

Alone, at standard pressure, nitrous oxide is incapable of inducing general anesthesia. When mixed with oxygen in typical concentrations (50:50 ratio, e.g., Entonox®), it has excellent analgesic properties. Its primary medical use is as an adjunctive agent in anesthesia. It is widely used in dental surgery, and, to a lesser extent, in obstetrics for management of pain in early labor. It is also used in the food industry, as a gas in bottled whipped cream, and in the automotive industry, to enhance engine performance. When used for the latter purpose it is often tainted at its source with agents to make it unsuitable for human use — a measure clearly aimed at decreasing abuse as a result of diversion. The food grade nitrous oxide is sold over-the-counter in small cartridges that are designed for use in whipped cream dispensers. They also provide a cheap and ready supply of nitrous oxide gas for use on the street as a drug of abuse. Nitrous oxide is also readily available to many healthcare workers (dentists, anesthesia personnel etc.) and has been a primary drug of abuse in this population.

Street use of nitrous oxide, especially by unsophisticated users, often results in unconsciousness resulting from hypoxia due to the displacement of oxygen from the lungs of the user. The practice of releasing a whipping gas cartridge into a rubber balloon as a reservoir leads to the inhalation of 100 per cent nitrous oxide. Fatalities have been reported from the use of nitrous oxide primarily because of complications of low oxygen levels in the blood. These include cardiac dysrhythmias and aspiration, amongst others.

Little is known about the tolerance to or dependency on nitrous oxide as a drug of abuse. Chronic exposure to sub-toxic levels of nitrous oxide in the workplace has raised concerns about possible links to birth defects. Consequently, the use of nitrous oxide as a medical gas has been declining. It remains, however, a potential drug of abuse that is readily available to the public.

Background Reading

Stoelting, R.K. (Ed.). (1987). *Pharmacology and Physiology in Anesthetic Practice*. Philadelphia: J.B. Lippincott.

Nutmeg

DRUG CLASS:	Hallucinogen

Nutmeg is both a common household spice and a naturally occurring hallucinogenic material. Nutmeg is the seed of the East Indian tree *Myristica fragrans*, and has been used for its psychoactive and alleged aphrodisiac effects for centuries in some areas of Southeast Asia. The related spice, mace, is part of the fruit of the *Myristica fragrans* and has many of the same chemical constituents as nutmeg.[1] However, because the chemical constituents are present in different relative proportions in nutmeg and mace, the two spices have slightly different aromas and tastes, and are likely to have somewhat different pharmacological effects and/or potency.

Myristicin has long been believed to be the nutmeg's major psychoactive component, although elemicin and isoelemicin may also contribute to its activity. These substances are constituents of nutmeg's aromatic oil. A hallucinogenic dose of nutmeg ranges between 5 and 10 grams — approximately one teaspoonful or the equivalent of one to two nutmegs. Ground nutmeg, a coarse brown powder, may be taken alone or in a tea solution, or may be sniffed. Its psychoactive actions are usually experienced gradually, and two to five hours often pass before the full effects are perceived. Nutmeg intoxication can produce lethargy, marijuana-like euphoria, lightheadedness, uncontrolled giggling and laughter, feelings of detachment from one's surroundings, feelings of unreality and sensations of either heaviness or floating. Visual hallucinations at this dose level are less likely to occur than they are with LSD, although they do occur in some individuals. Other reported effects include auditory hallucinations, sensations of floating or flying and separation of limbs from the body, and distortions of time. Some users claim that nutmeg enhances sexual potency.

Hallucinogenic effects are typically preceded by severe nausea and vomiting, as well as diarrhea and transient headache. (As a result of the vomiting, the actual portion of the administered dose that is available to the body is unpredictable.) Other

---

[1]   Nutmeg and mace are also produced by other *Myristica* species, including *Myristica malabarica*.

physiological effects can include increased heart rate, dry mouth, impairment of motor co-ordination, and heaviness and tingling and/or numbness in the extremities, as well as facial flushing, urinary retention and constipation (which follows early diarrhea).

Several very unpleasant side effects are also, to a significant extent, dose-related. Doses of nutmeg greater than 15 to 20 grams can cause central nervous system excitation, agitation, frightening perceptual experiences, panicky feelings, delusions, pains in the chest and abdomen, abnormally rapid heartbeat, and parched mouth and throat. Very high doses can cause severe liver damage. Fatalities have resulted from overdose.

The duration of hallucinogenic effects is also dose-related. Effects may last from a few hours to 12 hours or more. In contrast to recovery from most other hallucinogens, recovery from nutmeg intoxication is slow, and the user may experience alcohol-like hangover and severe muscle and bone aches for several days. A chronic psychotic state associated with nutmeg use has been reported.

The abuse potential of nutmeg is lower than that of other common hallucinogens, despite its easy availability. In North America, it is rarely the first-choice drug for hallucinogen users because of its undesired side effects and the slow period of recovery following intoxication. It is used most commonly by prisoners and young teenagers because of its easy accessibility.

Background Reading

Brenner, N., Frank, O.S. & Knight, E. (1993). Chronic nutmeg psychosis. *Journal of the Royal Society of Medicine*, 86 (3), 179–80.

Schultes, R.E. & Hoffman, A. (1980). *The Botany and Chemistry of Hallucinogens* (2nd edition). Springfield, IL: Charles C. Thomas.

Opium

DRUG CLASS:	Opioid

Opium is a crude resinous preparation obtained from the thick white liquid found in the unripe seed pods (capsules) of the opium poppy, *Papaver somniferum*, which grows in some areas of Europe, the Middle East and southern Asia. Opium is prepared by collecting the liquid from scored poppy pods and allowing it to dry in a shady area for several days. The crude opium gradually darkens in color to chestnut or darker brown and hardens to a tar-like texture with an unpleasant odor and a bitter taste that typically produces nausea. The dried substance is then shaped into lumps or bricks for sale or shipment.

Opium contains a number of naturally occurring alkaloids, including morphine, codeine, papaverine, thebaine and narcotine. However, only morphine and codeine have psychoactive properties that attract abuse. Morphine comprises approximately 9.5 to 12 per cent (depending on source) of the bulk of crude opium, and codeine 0.5 to 1.5 per cent. Most of the total bulk, 75 to 80 per cent by weight, consists of a variety of substances that have little or no pharmacological activity.

Some opium smokers prepare a product enriched in active opioids by boiling the crude opium in water until it forms an aqueous solution. The mixture is then filtered, and the residue is boiled and filtered several more times to extract the maximum yield of opioids. The filtered solutions are combined and again boiled gently until only a black sticky paste (the purified opium) remains. The paste is then dried and smoked. Usually, the user lies down while smoking in order to lessen the impact of the nausea that smoking opium produces.

Smoking of opium for its euphoric and sedative properties was once widespread throughout the Middle East and Asia (particularly China). Today, the practice is much less frequently encountered and is largely confined to certain rural areas in these regions. During the latter half of the 19th century, opium smoking was also widely encountered in some areas of North America and Europe, where the habit had been imported by Chinese laborers.

Opium has a dependence liability similar to that of morphine. However, crude opium is rarely found on the North American and European street drug markets. Morphine and heroin, being far less bulky, are much easier to smuggle.

Opium as an analgesic in clinical medicine has largely been replaced by naturally occurring, semi-synthetic and wholly synthetic substitutes (such as morphine, hydro-morphone and meperidine respectively). Nonetheless, a few products containing opium or an extract of opium continue to be marketed for medicinal purposes. For example, a mixture of opium and belladonna is marketed in suppository form for relief of pain and spasm in the urinary tract. Further, a highly purified extract of opium, paregoric, is still occasionally used orally in place of morphine. Paregoric is a water and alcohol solution containing tincture of opium together with camphor, benzoic acid and anise oil, and is combined with various non-psychoactive substances in several products still widely used to treat diarrhea (e.g., Donnagel PG®). Opioid-dependent individuals may resort to paregoric products when other more potent drugs are not available.

Background Reading

Lewis, W.H. Elvin-Lewis, M.P.F. (1997). *Medical Botany. Plants Affecting Man's Health.* New York/Toronto: John Wiley and Sons.

Peyote

DRUG CLASS: Hallucinogen

The small brownish-grey peyote (peiotl) cactus *Lophophora williamsii* has been revered for centuries by a number of Indian tribes (including the Aztecs) in Mexico and the southwestern United States. The part of the cactus of interest for its psychoactive properties is often called the mescal button. This is tufted with whitish "hair" and is green-tipped. The button contains at least 15 pharmacologically active substances, the most important of which is the hallucinogen mescaline. Other alkaloids include a convulsant, a respiratory stimulant and a reflex stimulant. It is generally agreed that mescaline taken in combination with the many other alkaloids in the peyote button produces more intense effects than mescaline taken alone. The typical dose is three to six buttons.[1]

Traditionally, mescal buttons are dried until completely brown and then chewed and swallowed. Since the taste is extremely bitter, however, modern hallucinogen users often grind the material into a powder and ingest it either in capsule form or in a solution of tea or fruit juice. Irrespective of the method by which the substance is taken, it quickly produces severe nausea and vomiting. Other early effects include dizziness, anxiety and sometimes panic, rapid and deep respiration, elevated heart rate and blood pressure, dilated pupils, chills and profuse sweating.

Hallucinogenic effects usually begin within one or two hours after ingestion. Ordinarily trivial objects in the environment seem to take on vivid characteristics. The user also experiences intense visual "pseudohallucinations" (which the user knows to be unreal), often in geometric forms with strikingly brilliant colors.[2] Visual imagery predominates, although pseudohallucinations involving other senses (hearing, smell and taste) often accompany visual experiences and may also be intense. Synesthesias (i.e., the melding of one sense with another so that users "see" music or

---

[1]   Indians may use substantially more in religious ceremonies.

[2]   True hallucinations (i.e., hallucinations that the user believes to be real) are less common.

"hear" colors) frequently occur. Users also experience sensations of weightlessness, and distortions of time and space are common. There is a general feeling of detach-ment from worldly events, often accompanied by a prolonged exploration of the inner self. Some users report having experienced profound mystical revelations.

While these effects are generally desired by the user, a few people experience frightening hallucinations and are terrified by their loss of contact with reality.

Tolerance to the main psychoactive agent of peyote, mescaline, develops rapidly, within a few days of everyday use. Tolerant users must abstain for a period of several days in order to restore pre-tolerance sensitivity to the desired effects. This pattern of interrupted use reduces the likelihood of acquiring psychological dependence on peyote. Physical dependence does not occur.

Although peyote use is a traditional ritual of the Native American Church, the U.S. Supreme Court ruled in 1990 that states may prohibit its use for religious purposes. Its sacramental use has never been sanctioned in Canada.

Background Reading

Bullis, R.K. (1990). Swallowing the scroll: Legal implications of the recent Supreme Court peyote cases. *Journal of Psychoactive Drugs, 22 (3)*, 325–332.

Schultes, R.E. & Hoffman, A. (1980). *The Botany and Chemistry of Hallucinogens* (2nd edition). Springfield, IL: Charles C. Thomas.

Phentermine

DRUG CLASS: CNS Stimulant, Anorexiant

Phentermine (e.g., Ionamin®, Fastin®) is a synthetic central nervous system (CNS) stimulant produced through chemical synthesis. Phentermine is exclusively prescribed as a diet pill for the short-term management of obesity. The therapeutic dose range is 15 to 30 mg taken orally 10 to 14 hours before bedtime.[1] The effects produced are qualitatively similar to those produced by amphetamine, although the latter drug is significantly more potent. Common side effects of therapeutic doses of phentermine include increased heart rate and blood pressure, restlessness, insomnia, dry mouth and diarrhea. Higher doses may produce increased alertness, increased endurance and enhanced feelings of self-confidence. However, others may experience unpleasant overstimulation, anxiety, agitation, dizziness, tremors, abnormally rapid heart rate, abnormally high blood pressure and a toxic psychotic syndrome that may be manifested as hallucinations, confusion, delusional thinking and violent behavior. Extreme overdose can result in severe cardiovascular irregularities, seizures and coma.

Tolerance to the anorexiant (appetite-suppressant) effect of this drug can develop within a few weeks with regular use. Regular high-dose abuse can result in the rapid development of tolerance to the drug's desired euphoric and CNS-stimulant actions. Chronic use/abuse of phentermine can produce a state of psychological dependence. Physical dependence seems to occur in chronic high-dose abusers, who experience such withdrawal symptoms as extreme fatigue and emotional depression after abrupt abstinence.

Before fenfluramine was withdrawn from the market in 1997, the combination phentermine-fenfluramine ("phen-fen") had become widely prescribed for weight loss in the United States, although this combination had never officially been approved.

---

[1]   For example, a user who normally retires at 11 p.m. may take the drug at 9 a.m. The purpose of the timing is to ensure maximum daytime effects without interference with sleep.

The potential for abuse of phentermine is fairly high, although not as high as that of amphetamine. Phentermine is classified as a controlled drug in Canada, and these restrictions reduce its abuse potential.

Background Reading

Canadian Pharmaceutical Association. (1997). *Compendium of Pharmaceuticals and Specialties* (32nd edition). Ottawa: Canadian Pharmaceutical Association.

Gilman, A.G., Rall, T.W., Nies, A.S. & Taylor, P. (1990). (Eds.), *Goodman and Gilman's The Pharmacological Basis of Therapeutics*, (8th edition). New York: Pergamon Press.

Kalant, H. & Roschlau, W.H.E. (Eds.) (1989). *Principles of Medical Pharmacology*. (5th edition). Burlington: B.C. Decker Inc.

PMA
(Paramethoxyamphetamine)

DRUG CLASS: Hallucinogen with Stimulant Properties

PMA (paramethoxyamphetamine) is a synthetic amphetamine-type drug[1] with both stimulant and hallucinogenic properties. It has no medical use. Its effects are very similar to those of MDA (methylenedioxyamphetamine) and mescaline, although PMA is much more potent and far more toxic. PMA has an hallucinogenic potency approximately five times that of mescaline and three times that of MDA. PMA appeared as a recreational drug in the early 1970s and was often sold on the street as MDA. It appears that PMA itself was not generally sought after, but was used as a result of misrepresentation. It was associated with fatalities soon after it entered into street use. In Ontario, for example, the deaths of nine young people were confirmed to be attributable to PMA between March and August 1973.

The toxicity of PMA is related to excessive central nervous system (CNS) stimulation. Users may experience hallucinations, delirium, restlessness, agitation, muscle contractions, hyperactivity (thrashing around), rigidity, rapid heart rate, increased blood pressure, sweating, high fever, seizures, coma and death. It has been estimated that PMA's effects may be seen with approximately 50 mg.[2] PMA may be taken orally, "snorted" or injected.

Since PMA can be lethal even at moderate doses, its reputation discourages users and this limits the drug's potential for abuse.

---

[1]   This drug is a member of the family of hallucinogenic drugs sometimes referred to as ring-substituted amphetamines.

[2]   All doses refer to adults.

Background Reading

Buchanan, J.F. & Brown, C.R. (1988). "Designer drugs": A problem in clinical toxicology. *Medical Toxicology, 3,* 1–17.

Cimbura, G. (1974). PMA deaths in Ontario. *Canadian Medical Association Journal, 110,* 1263, 1265, 1267.

PPA
Phenylpropanolamine

DRUG CLASS: CNS Stimulant, Decongestant

Phenylpropanolamine (PPA) is a synthetic central nervous system (CNS) stimulant that is marketed in the form of its hydrochloride salt, phenylpropanolamine hydrochloride. In pure form, this salt is a white or almost white crystalline powder with a slight aromatic odor. Although phenylpropanolamine is closely related in structure to the amphetamines, it produces less CNS stimulation than many other stimulants.

Because of its ability to constrict blood vessels, phenylpropanolamine is an ingredient in many oral over-the-counter preparations marketed for the treatment of nasal or sinus congestion in Canada and the United States. These are generally combination products also containing antihistamines or pain relievers. Phenylpropanolamine has also been promoted in the United States as an appetite suppressant. In Canada it is not approved for this purpose, and is not sold as a single-ingredient product.

In the United States, pharmaceutical preparations contain up to 50 mg of phenylpropanolamine as a single ingredient, while sustained-release preparations contain up to 75 mg. The maximum therapeutic dose should not exceed 150 mg per day.[1]

Because of phenylpropanolamine's stimulant properties, its use by athletes during competition has been prohibited by the International Olympic Committee. Its presence in the body can be readily detected in urine.

Common side effects associated with therapeutic doses of phenylpropanolamine are qualitatively similar to those produced by the amphetamines, but are generally much less severe,[2] and their incidence is low in people receiving therapeutic doses. These

---

[1]   All doses refer to adults.

[2]   See the chapter on amphetamines in Section 3.

effects can include nervousness, insomnia, dizziness, headache, nausea and drowsiness. Some individuals may also experience severe reactions such as chest tightness, elevated blood pressure and irregular or rapid heartbeat at therapeutic doses. These effects may represent idiosyncratic reactions. At higher doses, abnormal heartbeat and heart rate, dilation of the pupils, seizures, anxiety, agitation and psychotic behavior can occur.

Hypertension (high blood pressure) and the consequences arising from hypertension are considered to be the most frequent and important adverse effects associated with phenylpropanolamine. Blood pressure increases are usually proportional to dose, but even a relatively low dose of 85 mg has been shown to cause very severe hypertension in some individuals. Cases of kidney failure, myocardial injury and stroke have been linked with use of phenylpropanolamine.

A review of cases involving single-ingredient phenylpropanolamine products reported to poison control centres in the United States concluded that phenylpropanolamine did not pose a serious public health hazard. However, individuals who are hypertensive, overweight and/or elderly may be at increased risk of adverse drug reactions caused by phenylpropanolamine.

Products that contain phenylpropanolamine in combination with other over-the-counter stimulants such as ephedrine and caffeine have been sold on the street as "look-alike" stimulants or "legal stimulants."[3] These combinations may increase the potential for phenylpropanolamine to produce serious reactions and account for most reports of toxicity due to over-the-counter stimulants. Animal studies in hypertensive rats suggest that phenylpropanolamine/caffeine combinations can lead to cerebral hemorrhage. Phenylpropanolamine has been shown to increase plasma concentrations of caffeine in humans.

Tolerance develops to phenylpropanolamine's nasal decongestant effects, and may develop to any appetite-suppressant effects.

The potential for abuse of phenylpropanolamine appears to be very low. At therapeutic dose levels, phenylpropanolamine appears to lack euphoric or amphetamine-like effects, and seems not to have adverse effects on cardiovascular or subjective

---

[3]   See the chapters on caffeine in Section 3 and ephedrine in Section 4 for a discussion of "look-alike" drugs.

functioning in most individuals. However, users taking phenylpropanolamine for its CNS stimulant effects are likely to take the drug in large amounts, increasing the risk of a toxic reaction. Other individuals who consider over-the-counter preparations to be innocuous may exceed the recommended dosage for phenylpropanolamine.

Background Reading

Lake, C.R., Gallant, S., Masson, E. & Miller, P. (1990). Adverse drug effects attributed to phenyl-propanolamine: A review of 142 case reports. *The American Journal of Medicine, 89,* 195–208.

Leo, P.J., Hollander, J.E., Shih, R.D. & Marcus, S.M. (1996). Phenylpropanolamine and associated myocardial injury. *Annals of Emergency Medicine, 28 (3),* 359–362.Mueller, S.M., Muller, J. & Asdell, S.M. (1984). Cerebral hemorrhage associated with phenylpropanolamine in combination with caffeine. *Stroke, 15 (1),* 119–123.

Pentel, P. (1984). Toxicity of over-the-counter stimulants. *Journal of the American Medical Association, 252 (1),* 1898–1903.

Veltri, J.C., Bradford, D.C., Dring, T., Kassner, S., McElwee, N.E. & Rollins, D.E. (1992). Acute exposure to phenylpropanolamine: An analysis of 5447 cases reported to poison control centers from 1984-1987. *Post Marketing Surveillance, 6,* 95–106.

Propylhexedrine

DRUG CLASS: CNS Stimulant, Decongestant

Propylhexedrine (e.g., Benzedrex®) is similar to amphetamine in its chemical structure, although at therapeutic dose levels it is a much weaker central nervous system (CNS) stimulant. The CNS-stimulating potency of propylhexedrine is estimated to be one-tenth that of amphetamine. However, propylhexedrine does possess potent local vasoconstricting properties, which can effectively relieve nasal congestion by shrinking congested mucous membranes.

Propylhexedrine was introduced in the United States as a nasal decongestant (in the form of a nasal inhaler) in 1949 and it is marketed under the trade name Benzedrex. Benzedrex replaced the amphetamine product Benzedrine®, which was intended for the same purpose but was widely abused. Benzedrex was removed from the Canadian market in 1988 due to insufficient sales.

Propylhexedrine is generally considered to be safe when used as indicated on the Benzedrex label. Adverse effects (if they occur) are ordinarily mild, although the following have been reported to occur occasionally: irritation of the lining of the nasal passages, sneezing, headache, increased blood pressure, nervousness and rapid heart rate. Continuous, long-term use of propylhexedrine can result in rebound nasal and sinus congestion (i.e., a recurrence of congestion).

Originally, it was assumed that the CNS-stimulating effects of propylhexedrine were so mild that the drug had no abuse potential. However, when taken in large amounts either orally (i.e., by ingesting the contents of an inhaler or by overdosing with oral tablets, which are available in Europe) or by injection (injection of a crude solution extracted from the inhaler, known as "stove-top speed" or "peanut-butter meth"), propylhexedrine produces effects similar to those of the more potent amphetamines. Therefore, it is attractive to some stimulant abusers, particularly as a substitute when amphetamines are unavailable.

High-dose abuse of propylhexedrine — either orally or, more frequently, by intra-venous injection — has proven to be dangerous. It has caused paranoid psychosis virtually identical to amphetamine psychosis, and a number of other serious toxic effects such as heart attacks or heart failure. At least 20 fatalities have been attributed to injected propylhexedrine, the majority of which were reported from the Dallas County area of Texas in the late 1970s and early 1980s. Further, when evaluating the toxicity of injecting the contents of an inhaler, one must consider not only the propylhexedrine but also the aromatics contained in the inhaler and the cotton fibres from the plug.

Although a limited number of drug users may abuse propylhexedrine, overall the potential for abuse of this drug is considered to be low. The Drug Abuse Warning Network in the United States did not detect a significant amount of propylhexedrine abuse over the seven-year period from 1983 to 1989. In 1991, the World Health Organization Expert Committee on Drug Dependence concluded that the incidence of propylhexedrine abuse and illicit trafficking was very low, and was unlikely to cause significant public health or social problems.

Background Reading

Smith, D.E., Wesson, D.R., Lea Sees, K. & Morgan, J.P. (1988). An epidemiological and clinical analysis of propylhexedrine abuse in the United States. *Journal of Psychoactive Drugs, 20 (4)*, 441–442.

Wesson, D.R., Smith, D.E. & Morgan, J.P. (1986). The international scheduling of OTC inhaler ingredients: An abuse perspective. *Journal of Psychoactive Drugs, 18 (2)*, 151–154.

World Health Organization. (1991). *WHO Expert Committee on Drug Dependence, 27th Report.* WHO Technical Report Series 808. Geneva: World Health Organization.

Selective Serotonin Reuptake Inhibitors (SSRIs)

DRUG CLASS: Antidepressant

The selective serotonin reuptake inhibitors (SSRIs) are a group of structurally diverse drugs that are used to treat depression. SSRIs include fluoxetine (e.g., Prozac®), fluvoxamine (e.g., Luvox®), sertraline (e.g., Zoloft®), paroxetine (e.g., Paxil®) and citalopram (e.g., Cipramil®). SSRIs are comparable to the older tricyclic anti-depressants in their antidepressant effect and speed of onset (several weeks after the beginning of treatment), but the newer drugs are generally better tolerated. As the name implies, these medications inhibit the reuptake of serotonin in the brain. Serotonin is believed to play an important role in modulating various functions including mood and sleep. The SSRIs have been found to be useful in treating bulimia, obsessive-compulsive disorder and panic disorder, as well as depression.

The primary adverse effects associated with the SSRIs involve the gastrointestinal system: nausea, diarrhea or constipation. Other side effects include insomnia or drowsiness, headache, nervousness, tremor, dizziness, dry mouth, sweating and weight loss. These effects tend to occur early in the course of treatment and are usually mild. Symptoms at higher doses include nausea, vomiting, tremor and irritability. The SSRIs are generally safer in overdose than are tricyclic antidepressants. When fluoxetine was first marketed, there were concerns that it induced violent and suicidal thoughts, but a causal link could not be established. Suicidal thoughts are a common symptom of depression itself and a significant concern in many depressed patients.

Users may develop tolerance to the therapeutic effect of SSRIs, although very few cases have been reported. Some patients may experience mild withdrawal reactions when they stop using one of these drugs. Reported withdrawal symptoms included anxiety, irritability, insomnia, headache, dizziness and gastrointestinal symptoms. These symptoms are less likely to occur with fluoxetine than with some of the other agents because of fluoxetine's longer duration of action.

There have been a few reports of abuse or dependence on fluoxetine in patients who have abused other substances, including one report of intravenous use. However, considering the extent of use of these agents (since their introduction in the late 1980s they have captured a significant proportion of the antidepressant market), their potential for abuse is low. Nevertheless, their widespread use has raised concerns over the potential for "misusing" SSRIs, for example, by medicating individuals to alter their personality, character or "self." These discussions have so far remained in the realm of anecdotal case reports and philosophical reflections. Research to date supports the role of SSRIs to treat psychiatric conditions such as depression, bulimia, obsessive-compulsive disorder and panic disorder.

Background Reading

Canadian Pharmaceutical Association. (1997). *Compendium of Pharmaceuticals and Specialties* (32nd edition). Ottawa: Canadian Pharmaceutical Association.

Pagliaro, L.A. & Pagliaro, A.M. (1993). Fluoxetine abuse by an intravenous drug user. *American Journal of Psychiatry, 150 (12)*, 1898.

Rapport, D.J. & Calabrese, J.R. (1993). Tolerance to fluoxetine. *Journal of Clinical Psychopharmacology , 13(5)*, 361.

Tinsley, J.A., Olsen, M.W., Laroche, R.R. & Palmen, M.A. (1994). Fluoxetine abuse. *Mayo Clinic Proceedings, 69*, 166–168.

STP; DOM

DRUG CLASS: Hallucinogen with Stimulant Properties

STP and DOM have come to be used as designations for the same potent halluci-nogenic compound — 2,5-dimethoxy-4-methylamphetamine. This compound is structurally related to the amphetamines. "DOM" is an abbreviation of the chemical name. The origin of the street designation "STP," however, is uncertain. Some writers believe it is an abbreviation of "serenity, tranquillity and peace." Others suggest that it is taken from the widely used motor oil additive of the same name — perhaps as a reference to the drug's stimulant properties.

STP was virtually unknown, except (as DOM) to a few researchers, prior to its dramatic entry into the street-drug subculture in the summer of 1967. During a period of a few days, several thousand STP tablets were distributed in the San Francisco area, apparently free of charge. The result was the admission of several users to local hospital emergency departments, all suffering a toxic psychosis. It was reported that the administration of the antipsychotic agent chlorpromazine in these patients "prolonged the disability of the patient under the influence of STP." However, this clinical observation was not supported by evidence from clinical trials.

Small doses of pure DOM (e.g., 1 to 2 mg)[1] can produce mild euphoria, talkativeness, and pleasant central nervous system stimulation. Higher doses (e.g., over 5 mg) tend to produce mescaline- or LSD-like effects, including vivid visual imagery, intense per-ceptual distortions, visual hallucinations and illusions. A number of unpleasant physical effects also occur and include nausea and vomiting, dry mouth, prickling or burning sensations on the skin, fatigue, tremors, muscle tension, increased reflex responses and abnormal sensitivity to light. Other side effects include increased heart rate and blood pressure, dilation of the pupils, increased body temperature, sweating and loss of appetite. Hallucinogenic effects last for approximately eight hours or

---

[1]   All doses refer to adults.

possibly longer (up to 24 hours) in higher doses. Acute adverse reactions to pure DOM — or "bad trips" — include intense anxiety, panic and occasionally psychotic reactions. "Bad trips" are more common with DOM than with most other hallucinogens.

Users rapidly develop tolerance to the subjective effects of pure DOM when taking the drug for as little as three days consecutively. However, users are not known to develop psychological and physical dependence on the drug. DOM has not become a popular hallucinogen, probably due to the duration and intensity of its effects and its reputation for producing "bad trips."

Background Reading

Meyers, F.H., Rose, A.J. & Smith, D.E. (1967-8). Incidents involving the Haight-Ashbury population and some uncommonly used drugs. *Journal of Psychedelic Drugs, 1 (2)*, 139–146.

Smith, D.E. (1969). The psychotomimetic amphetamines with special reference to STP (DOM) toxicity. *Journal of Psychedelic Drugs, 2 (2)*, 73–85.

Snyder, S.H., Faillace, L. & Hollister, L. (1967). 2,5-Dimethoxy-4-methyl-amphetamine (STP): A new hallucinogenic drug. *Science, 158*, 669–670.

Strychnine

DRUG CLASS: CNS Stimulant, Convulsant, Poison

Strychnine is a naturally occurring alkaloid that can be isolated from the dried ripe seed of *Strychnos nux-vomica*, a small tree native to Indonesia, Malaysia and other parts of the Asia. It can also be isolated from the seeds of the related plant *Strychnos ignatu* (St. Ignatius bean). In the past, it was widely used in "tonics" and laxatives, probably because of its reputation for stimulating the gastrointestinal tract and increasing voluntary muscle tone. However, these effects result only at unacceptably high doses. It continues to be used in rodent poisons.

Strychnine poisoning causes stiffening and twitching of the jaw, face and neck muscles followed by increased reflex excitability resulting in violent muscle responses to even very mild stimuli. There are powerful thrusts of the lower limbs and later severe seizures in which the whole body may arch so rigidly that only the heels and head touch the ground. Between seizures there may be several minutes of muscle relaxation.

Strychnine acts on certain areas of the brain and the spinal cord, where it appears to block normal inhibitory processes that control the voluntary muscles. Despite the extreme skeletal muscle disturbances, the higher brain centres of consciousness are not affected. Therefore the victim consciously experiences these very painful muscle contractions, and without immediate treatment can only apprehensively await the next severe spasm. Death is usually due to an oxygen deficit caused by severe contraction of the respiratory muscles (i.e., asphyxiation). The fatal overdose range for adults is 15 to 30 mg but any dose of strychnine should be considered life-threatening.

Treatment of strychnine poisoning usually includes the administration of diazepam intravenously. Artificial support of respiration is also essential if breathing is impaired, as is removing the patient from all avoidable sensory stimulation (e.g., light, sound and touch).

Strychnine has occasionally been included as an adulterant in street drug preparations.

TMA
(Trimethoxyamphetamine)

DRUG CLASS: Hallucinogen with Stimulant Properties

TMA (3,4,5-trimethoxyamphetamine) is a synthetic hallucinogen that is related to both MDA and mescaline in its chemical structure as well as to amphetamine.[1] TMA-2 (2,4,5-trimethoxyamphetamine), which also has been found to have hallucinogenic activity, is one of the six possible isomers of trimethoxyamphetamine. Hallucinogenic doses produce effects similar to those of mescaline, including intense visual imagery; perceptual distortions, including mainly visual pseudohallucinations (known to the user to be unreal); synesthesias (the perception that senses are melding with one another so that, for example, the user "sees" music); and dissociation from the environment. A number of amphetamine-like physiological effects occur prior to the onset of TMA's hallucinogenic actions. These can include behavioral arousal, slightly impaired motor co-ordination, increased reflex responses, slight tremor, dilation of the pupils, transient mild headache, nausea and vomiting, sweating, increased blood pressure and heart rate, loss of appetite and increased respiratory rate.

The amount of drug needed to produce hallucinogenic effects is similar to the amount of drug that will result in toxicity. This likely explains why TMA does not appear to be widely used by those seeking hallucinogenic experiences.

---

[1]   This drug is a member of the family of hallucinogenic drugs sometimes referred to as ring-substituted amphetamines.

Tricyclic Antidepressants

DRUG CLASS: Antidepressant

The tricyclic antidepressants are the some of the oldest and most widely used drugs for treating depression. While it is known how these drugs affect certain chemicals in the brain, such as norepinephrine and serotonin, it is not understood exactly how this eventually leads to an antidepressant effect. With everyday use of tricyclic antidepressants, mood improvement occurs gradually and may not be noticeable for several weeks. Although these drugs are ultimately effective for most depressed patients who take them, it is important for the physician and pharmacist to inform the patient that improvement does not occur immediately and that the drug therapy must be continued for the desired effect to be achieved.

Some of the more commonly used tricyclic antidepressants include amitriptyline (e.g., Elavil®), imipramine (e.g., Tofranil®), doxepin (e.g., Sinequan®), clomipramine (e.g., Anafranil®), desipramine (e.g., Norpramin®), nortriptyline (e.g., Aventyl®) and trimipramine (e.g., Surmontil®). Tricyclic antidepressants are used to treat moderate to severe depression, including that accompanied by anxiety or other mental illnesses. Clomipramine is also used for obsessive-compulsive disorder and imipramine is used for bedwetting in children and adolescents.

Even though it may take weeks for the full therapeutic effect of the drugs to be seen, a number of (usually mild) side effects may occur after the initial dose. These side effects vary somewhat among tricyclic antidepressants. Drowsiness is a common effect and may be desirable for those patients suffering from insomnia. Anticholinergic effects (e.g., blurred vision, dryness of the mouth, urinary retention, constipation) are also common. Other effects include cardiovascular symptoms (mildly irregular heartbeat and a drop in blood pressure, particularly when rising quickly to a standing position), sedative effects (confusion and disorientation, lack of motor co-ordination, concentration difficulties), sexual problems and, rarely, seizures. Some of these unwanted effects may persist in some patients. However, with regular daily use of tricyclic antidepressants, the patient usually acquires tolerance to most of the undesired effects.

At higher doses, any of the above symptoms may be intensified, and increasingly high doses may result in significant respiratory depression. However, the most important adverse effects are exerted on the brain and cardiovascular system. Very high doses (i.e., overdose) can cause restlessness, dilated pupils, reduced reflexes, seizures, coma, decreased blood pressure and serious abnormal heart rhythms. The margin of safety between daily therapeutic doses of tricyclic antidepressants and overdose sufficient to produce death can be relatively small.

Users do not appear to develop tolerance to the antidepressant effect of these drugs, even with extended use. When users abruptly stop taking tricyclic antidepressants, they may experience mild withdrawal symptoms including nausea, headache, muscle aches, runny nose and a general feeling of physical discomfort. Patients on long-term, high-dose therapy who abruptly discontinue the medication are at the greatest risk of experiencing this withdrawal syndrome.

Patients sometimes develop a psychological dependence on these drugs. Those with a history of drug abuse have been known to increase their daily dose of tricyclic antidepressants to excessive levels. Generally, however, antidepressants are rarely encountered on the street drug market. Considering the millions of patients who have regularly taken them as prescribed and the few who abuse them, these drugs appear to have a very low abuse potential.

Background Reading

Canadian Pharmaceutical Association. (1997). *Compendium of Pharmaceuticals and Specialties* (32nd edition). Ottawa: Canadian Pharmaceutical Association.

Cohen, M.J., Hanbury, R. & Stimmel, B. (1978). Abuse of amitriptyline. *Journal of the American Psychiatric Association, 240*, 1372–1373.

Wohlreich, M.M. & Welch, W. (1993). Amitriptyline abuse presenting as acute toxicity. *Psychosomatics, 34 (2)*, 191–193.

Valproic Acid and Carbamazepine

DRUG CLASS: Mood Stabilizer, Anticonvulsant

Valproic acid, or divalproex, (e.g., Epival® in Canada, Depakote® in the United States) and carbamazepine (e.g., Tegretol®) are anticonvulsant medications (first marketed for the treatment of epilepsy) that have been found to have mood-stabilizing properties. They are used in psychiatry to treat patients with bipolar disorder (manic-depressive illness), and represent alternatives to lithium, which was the mainstay of treatment for these patients for many years. Some patients do not respond to or cannot tolerate lithium. The dosages of valproic acid and carbamazepine are individualized for each patient, often based on blood concentrations.

The most common early side effects of valproic acid include drowsiness, upset stomach, diarrhea, dizziness and tremor. Over the long term, valproic acid may cause hair thinning and mild changes in liver function tests. It may also cause serious liver damage in rare cases.

Carbamazepine may cause drowsiness, dizziness, headache, blurry vision and upset stomach early in treatment. Long-term problems include lowered counts of white blood cells (which may be severe in rare cases) and mild changes in liver function tests. Carbamazepine can rarely cause a severe skin reaction.

Abuse of carbamazepine has been reported in a few alcohol-abusing individuals. In general, however, valproic acid and carbamazepine are not considered to be drugs of abuse.

Background Reading

Stuppaeck, C.H., Whitworth, A.B. & Fleischhacker, W.W. (1993). Abuse potential of carbamazepine. *Journal of Nervous & Mental Disease, 181* (8), 519–520.

Sullivan, G. & Davis, S. (1997). Is carbamazepine a potential drug of abuse? *Journal of Psychopharmacology (Oxford)* , *11* (1), 93–94.

Additional Drug Notes

Acamposate (calcium acetylhomotaurinate) —
A relatively new synthetic drug that appears
to reduce the probability of relapse in detoxified alcoholics by reducing the craving associated with withdrawal. Research evidence
suggests that acamposate acts by reducing the
hyperexcitability that develops in neurons in
the central nervous system during withdrawal
following long-term alcohol consumption.
Unlike CNS depressants that have been used
to treat withdrawal symptoms, acamposate
appears to have no hypnotic, antidepressant,
anxiolytic or muscle-relaxant effects. Adverse
effects include diarrhea and skin reactions,
but these have been observed to be mild
and of short duration. Acamposate has been
proposed as a complement to psychosocial
and behavioral therapies for people who are
physically dependent on alcohol.

*Alfentanil (Alfenta®, alpha-methylfentanyl,
AMF)* — Also called "China White" after a
particularly pure form of heroin from
Southeast Asia, AMF was among the first
"designer" opioids based on the chemical
structure of fentanyl. Its analgesic effect
occurs more rapidly than those of fentanyl
and sufentanil. Users have claimed that it
can produce a reasonably satisfactory "rush."
It is also said to relieve withdrawal symptoms
for a longer period than heroin. However,
dozens of deaths caused by AMF and other
structurally modified forms of fentanyl were

reported in the early 1980s. As a result, tight
controls were placed on AMF as a substance
with a high potential for abuse and without
recognized legitimate medical use. The risk of
fatal overdose appears to be greatest among
users who are intolerant of the toxic effects of
such potent opioid analgesics.

Although AMF and a few similar drugs are
now banned in the United States and
Canada, there are now more than 200 known
fentanyl congeners, some of which (e.g., PFF)
were unknown to professional chemists and
drug experts before they appeared on the
street. Some of the fentanyls appear to be
adequate substitutes for heroin. Furthermore,
unlike heroin, which must be imported (and
which is expensive), the fentanyls can be produced locally with relatively low-cost chemicals and equipment. For these reasons, and
despite the risks associated with the use of
such potent drugs, their abuse may continue.

Alphaprodine (Nisentil®) — A synthetic opioid
with an analgesic potency approximately
one-third that of morphine when equal doses
by weight are injected subcutaneously. Its
effects last only one to two hours, somewhat
briefer than those of other commonly used
opioids. The single therapeutic dose is 30 to
60 mg (administered by subcutaneous or
intravenous injection).

AMT (alpha-methyltryptamine) — A synthetic hallucinogen with psychic effects similar to, but milder than, those of psilocybin. Other effects are more intense than those of the latter drug, and AMT has a longer duration of action, up to 16 to 18 hours.

Amyl nitrite ("poppers") — A vasodilator (an agent that dilates blood vessels) that was used in the past to relieve severe constricting chest pain caused by angina pectoris. It is now used to treat cyanide poisoning. Amyl nitrite is prepared in vitrioles that are crushed, freeing the vapors to be inhaled. The effects are felt within 30 seconds of inhalation and last for two to three minutes. A typical therapeutic dose is 0.3 mL. The principal side effects are transient headache, increased heart rate, drop in blood pressure, dizziness and flushing of the face and upper torso. Large doses can cause nausea and vomiting, restlessness, abnormally low blood pressure, fainting, coldness of the skin, slowed heart rate and impaired respiration. The principal appeal of amyl nitrite to non-medical users lies in its reputation for enhancing sexual performance and orgasm — an effect believed to be caused by its vasodilator properties.

Angel's trumpet (Datura suaveolens, Brugmansia suaveolens) — Used for its hallucinogenic activity in the western Amazon and the Andes, this plant is also cultivated as an ornamental in Florida and other southeastern areas of the United States. Although occasional cases of accidental anticholinergic poisoning resulting from ingestion of the plant had occurred, a dramatic increase in the number of cases was noted in Florida in 1994. It appears that this problem resulted from an increase in the number of people experimenting with the plant for its hallucinogenic effects.

Betel nut — A preparation made from the seed of the *Areca catechu* or betel palm tree that is chewed (in a manner similar to tobacco chewing) for its mild euphoric and stimulating effects. Betel nut chewing is common throughout much of Southeast Asia and India, regions whose populations have a higher incidence of oral cancers and other mouth diseases than other areas. The principal psychoactive constituent in betel nut is the alkaloid arecoline which has anticholinergic properties.

Bromides (e.g., sodium bromide) — In the past, bromides were used as sedative/hypnotics as well as anticonvulsants. Because of their toxic effects at higher doses and/or with chronic administration, bromides have been replaced by safer and more effective drugs.

Bufotenin(e) (5-hydroxy-N,N-dimethyltryptamine) — This hallucinogenic alkaloid, closely related in chemical structure to psilocybin and DMT, is secreted by the skin glands of certain toad species. It is also found in the mimosa plant, *Piptadenia peregrina* or *Anadenanthera peregrina*, which grows in many areas of the West Indies and northern South America. Indians have used the plant for centuries in the form of a snuff that is widely known as "cohoba." Doses of 4 to 16 mg produce mescaline-like effects. In the late 1980s and early 1990s, toad venom was reported to have become a new illicit drug fad in the United States, Canada, Central America and Australia. "Toad licking" — the oral ingestion of toad venom, either directly from live toads or in solutions made by boiling the toads — was possibly inspired by media reports. It was viewed as a unique, and free, way of achieving the hallucinogenic effects produced by bufotenine (and possibly other hallucinogenic substances in toad venom). However, toad venom also contains other substances, including bufodienolides, that are highly toxic and produce symptoms similar to digoxin overdose, including vomiting and abnormal slowing of the heart rate. Deaths have been associated with use of toad-venom products represented as aphrodisiacs.

Bupropion (Zyban®) — An atypical antidepressant that primarily influences the neurotransmitters norepinephrine and dopamine, with little effect on serotonin. It has been associated with a higher incidence of seizures than other antidepressants. Bupropion is currently being investigated as a smoking cessation aid. In one study bupropion was shown to be an effective treatment for smoking cessation, although many participants in all groups were smoking after one year.

Calcium carbimide (Temposil®) — Now discontinued, this drug was formerly used to treat alcoholism. Consumption of alcohol when calcium carbimide is present in the body can cause a violent and unpleasant reaction, similar to that produced by disulfiram (Antabuse®).

Cantharides (Spanish fly) — Falsely identified as an aphrodisiac, this substance is prepared from the crushed wings of the insect *Lytta vesicatoria*. It is extremely toxic: even very small amounts can cause severe burning sensations and blistering in the upper gastrointestinal tract and the genitals, as well as irreversible damage to the genito-urinary tract and kidneys. Spanish fly has caused a number of deaths.

Catnip — An herb obtained from the plant *Nepeta cataria*, a member of the mint family. Catnip is known for producing playful behavior in cats. When smoked, catnip can produce mild euphoria and pseudohallucinations in humans, and for this reason has been passed off occasionally to unsophisticated street buyers as marijuana.

Clonidine (Catapres®) — Used primarily to treat high blood pressure. Clonidine has also been used experimentally to manage both opioid and alcoholic withdrawal. Methadone patients have occasionally abused this drug, either alone or with other drugs (to intensify their effects). Drowsiness and dry mouth are among its most common side effects.

Cyclazocine — A potent and long-acting opioid antagonist that can cause withdrawal symptoms in opioid-dependent people. It can also rapidly reverse the effects of opioid overdose. Cyclazocine is a powerful analgesic in its own right when opioids are not present in the body. Chronic administration can cause physical dependence. Cyclazocine is not legally available in Canada.

DET (N,N-diethyltryptamine) — A synthetic hallucinogen closely related chemically to DMT. A hallucinogenic dose is approximately 50 to 60 mg. DET produces effects similar to those of DMT, although DET's effects last longer (typically two to three hours).

DOB (4-bromo-2,5-dimethoxyamphetamine) — One of the most powerful of the phenylethylamine hallucinogens, a family that includes mescaline and MDA. It is at least 100 times more potent than mescaline. Doses of 2 to 3 mg produce peak intoxication after three to four hours. Overdose of DOB has been linked to deaths and a number of severe toxic reactions.

Dextromethorphan — Used widely as an antitussive (cough-suppressant) agent, dextromethorphan is included in many non-prescription cough and cold preparations, many of which include the suffix DM in their trade names. Dextromethorphan is chemically related to the opioid agonist levorphanol, but possesses little or no analgesic or respiratory depressant effects at usual therapeutic doses. The usual adult dose of dextromethorphan for temporary relief of cough is 10 to 20 mg every four hours or 30 mg every six to eight hours, to a recommended maximum of 120 mg per day. Dextromethorphan is generally very well tolerated with only occasional side effects such as nausea, slight drowsiness and dizziness.

There have been sporadic reports of teens and young adults using large quantities of preparations containing dextromethorphan (also referred to as "Robo", "X" and "rome" when used recreationally). Large doses of dextromethorphan (between 250 to 1,500 mg) have been reported to cause euphoria and visual, auditory and tactile hallucinations. Abruptly discontinuing chronic use of high doses of dextromethorphan may result in withdrawal symptoms including dysphoria and difficulty sleeping. Recent evidence has suggested that susceptibility to abuse is related to individual genetic differences in the liver's ability to convert dextromethorphan to its main metabolite dextrorphan. In the mid 1980s several deaths following ingestion of large doses of dextromethorphan prompted the Swedish government to restrict this compound to prescription-only status. Dextromethorphan is readily available in many non-prescription cough and cold remedies in Canada and the United States.

Dextromoramide — A synthetic opioid with an analgesic potency approximately twice that of morphine when equal doses by weight are injected subcutaneously. This drug is not legally available in Canada or the United States.

Dihydrocodeine — A semi-synthetic opioid derived from morphine with an analgesic potency approximately twice that of codeine when equal doses by weight are injected subcutaneously. This drug is not legally available in Canada. Elsewhere it has been used as both an analgesic and a cough suppressant.

Ethchlorvynol (e.g., Placidyl®) — Ethchlorvynol is no longer available in Canada. It was introduced in the mid-1950s and, like a number of other sedative/hypnotic drugs, was intended to be a safe, non-addicting alternative to the barbiturates. However, it possesses a dependence liability as great as that of the short-acting barbiturates and has caused a number of deaths

from overdose. With regular use, tolerance develops rapidly to its desired effects. Abrupt abstinence results in a serious withdrawal syndrome. This drug appears to have no therapeutic advantages over much safer and less addicting sedative/hypnotics such as the benzodiazepines.

Flumazenil (e.g., Anexate®) — Flumazenil is a benzodiazepine antagonist. It is used to completely or partially reverse the central nervous system (CNS) sedative effects of benzodiazepines. It may be used to reverse benzodiazepine-induced sedation after surgical or diagnostic procedures, or to diagnose or treat benzodiazepine overdose.

Flunitrazepam (e.g., Rohypnol®) — Flunitrazepam is not legally available in Canada. It is a benzodiazepine sedative/hypnotic that has been available in Europe for many years. Flunitrazepam is similar to other benzodiazepines in most respects. It is one of the most potent benzodiazepines, and is rapidly absorbed after oral administration, which may increase its risk of abuse. Some opioid abusers prefer flunitrazepam over other benzodiazepines. Street names include "roofies," "rope" and "the forget pill." It has been implicated in "date rape" because of its sedative, psychomotor impairment and amnesic effects. In these cases, the drug is typically added to the victim's beverage to reduce sexual inhibitions and facilitate sexual assault. If the beverage contains alcohol, the combined effects of flunitrazepam and alcohol result in CNS depression. The extent of use and uniqueness of flunitrazepam for these purposes is unclear.

GHB (gamma hydroxy butyrate) — A dopamine enhancer (i.e., it increases dopamine levels) that is structurally similar to gamma amino butyric acid (GABA). GHB is used clinically in certain European countries to treat narcolepsy and alcohol withdrawal. GHB possesses euphoric properties and is often used at "rave" parties where it is referred to as "Liquid Ecstasy" or "Liquid X." The following effects may be seen in an overdose situation: electrolyte imbalance, decreased respiration, bradycardia, vomiting, hypotension, seizure-like activity, confusion, delirium and death. This odorless and tasteless compound is often mixed with alcohol to potentiate the sedative effects of the latter.

Glutethimide (e.g., Doriden®) — Glutethimide is no longer available in Canada. It is a seda-tive/ hypnotic that was originally intended as a safe and non-addicting alternative to the bar-biturates. In fact, its dependence liability was later proven to be just as great as that of the latter drugs. At overdose levels, the respiratory depression caused by glutethimide is not nearly as great as that resulting from barbiturate over-dose. Nonetheless, a number of deaths have resulted from respiratory depression as well as from cardiovascular collapse. Chronic high-dose abuse results in severe physical depen-dence, and abrupt abstinence can produce a life-threatening withdrawal syndrome.

Ibogaine — A naturally occurring hallucinogenic alkaloid that is obtained from the roots of the West African plant *Tabernanthe iboga*. A hallucinogenic dose is approximately 300 mg, and its effects are similar to those produced by harmaline. Ibogaine is also a potent CNS stimulant. Overdose may result in seizures, paralysis and death from respiratory arrest. *Tabernanthe iboga* is used in some parts of Africa as an aphrodisiac and in religious rituals. Recently ibogaine has attracted interest as a possible treatment for opioid, stimulant and alcohol abuse, because of its reported ability to modify drug-seeking behavior. Biochemical studies have indicated that it may bind to N-methyl-D-aspartate (NDMA) receptors in a manner similar to a substance that is known to reduce development of tolerance to morphine and alcohol.

Isobutyl nitrite — A vasodilator (i.e., dilates blood vessels) that produces a spectrum of effects similar to those of amyl nitrite, although it is not specifically marketed to treat any medical disorder. It is sometimes sold as an odorizer. It has been abused for its intoxicating properties and its reputed ability to enhance sexual orgasm.

Kava-kava — A naturally occurring alkaloid obtained from the roots of the plant *Piper methysticum*, which grows on islands in the South Pacific. Small doses can produce mild euphoria. Larger doses produce a more intense euphoria, perceptual distortions and a pleasant state of lethargy, usually followed by sleep. Chronic use can produce depen-dence and adverse side effects.

Laudanum — A hydroalcoholic solution con-taining 10 per cent opium, widely used since the 16th century for various maladies. It is now rarely used.

Levorphanol (Levo-Dromoran®) — A powerful synthetic opioid with an analgesic potency approximately four times greater than mor-phine when equal doses by weight are injected subcutaneously. Levorphanol is reported to possess a very high dependence liability. The therapeutic dose range is 2 to 4 mg twice daily (taken by injection).

Lidocaine (Xylocaine®) — A synthetic local anesthetic used by injection in dental and other surgical procedures and topically (on the surface) to anesthetize mucous membranes for some medical procedures. Lidocaine is not abused for its own sake, since it has few sig-nificant psychoactive properties other than causing drowsiness. However, because sniff-ing lidocaine produces a freezing sensation in the nasal passages (mimicking the initial effect of cocaine), drug traffickers may use it to dilute cocaine.

Mazindol (Sanorex®) — An anorexiant (diet pill) used in the short-term management of obesity. Its effects are similar to, although milder than, those produced by amphetamines. The typical daily therapeutic dose is 1 to 3 mg taken orally. This drug has been subject to abuse. Tolerance develops to mazindol's main effects, and chronic abuse can result in dependence.

MDEA *(3,4-methylenedioxyethamphetamine, "Eve")* — One of a number of hallucinogens related to amphetamine. Its effects are similar to those of MDMA, and it appeared on the market following the restrictions placed on MDMA. Deaths associated with MDEA have been reported.

Methaqualone (e.g., Quaalude®) — Methaqualone is no longer available in Canada or the United States. Methaqualone was one of a number of sedative/hypnotic drugs synthesized during the past few decades. It was originally promoted as a safer and non-addicting alternative to the barbiturates. Methaqualone could rapidly produce intense euphoria even when taken orally, and therefore appeared to possess a dependence liability at least as great as that of the short-acting barbiturates such as secobarbital and pentobarbital. With regular use, tolerance developed rapidly to the sedative and euphoric properties of methaqualone. Chronic high-dose abuse caused profound barbiturate-like physical dependence, and abrupt abstinence produced psychotic symptoms and potentially life-threatening seizure activity.

Methcathinone ("cat") — A stimulant drug manufactured in clandestine laboratories. Methcathinone is reportedly highly potent, with long-lasting intoxicating effects. It is administered intranasally or intravenously. Methcathinone is similar to methamphetamine in both structure and stimulant effects. Cathinone, which is similar in structure to methcathinone, is the naturally occurring stimulant found in the fresh, young leaves of the khat *(Catha edulis)* bush.

Methyprylon (e.g., Noludar®) — Methyprylon is no longer available in Canada. It is one of a number of sedative/hypnotic drugs synthesized as alternatives to barbiturates. Methyprylon produces less euphoria than the barbiturates and is generally less toxic, although death from overdose has occurred. Physical dependence can result from chronic use. Withdrawal symptoms that occur after abrupt termination of regular use include insomnia and anxiety. Hallucinations and seizures may occur after regular use of very high doses is terminated abruptly. Methyprylon has generally been replaced in medicine by the benzodiazepines.

Methysergide maleate (Sansert®) — A semi-synthetic drug used on a maintenance basis to treat the pain and reduce the frequency of migraine and other forms of severe vascular headache in individuals who experience such headaches frequently (i.e., weekly). It is derived from an ergot alkaloid that is chemically related to LSD. The therapeutic dose is 2 mg taken orally, three times daily. Mild euphoria, dizziness, feelings of unreality and hallucinations are among the effects that sometimes occur at therapeutic dose levels. Higher doses may intensify these effects. Like LSD, methysergide tends to cause constriction of blood vessels, resulting in cold and numbness in the feet and hands.

Metopon (methyldihydromorphinone) — A powerful semi-synthetic opioid derived from morphine. When administered by subcutaneous injection in equal doses by weight, metopon's analgesic potency is approximately three times greater than that of morphine. It is not legally available in Canada or the United States.

Nabilone (Cesamet®) — A synthetic analogue of tetrahydrocannabinol that is used to manage severe nausea and vomiting associated with certain types of cancer chemotherapy. At therapeutic doses its effects may include drowsiness, dizziness, euphoria, dry mouth, impaired motor co-ordination, blurred vision and sensory disturbances. The usual dose of 1 to 2 mg twice daily produces significantly less euphoria than a comparable dose of THC.

Nalbuphine (Nubain®) — A semi-synthetic opioid agonist/antagonist, chemically related to the opioid oxymorphone and the opioid antagonist naloxone. Nalbuphine has analgesic potency equivalent to morphine by weight, and opioid antagonist potency approximately one-quarter that of nalorphine and 10 times that of pentazocine. It is used clinically to relieve moderate to severe pain. The recommended dose range is 10 to 20 mg by subcutaneous, intramuscular or intravenous injection every three to six hours. Nalbuphine is reported to have a low abuse potential, although physical dependence can develop with regular use.

Nalmephene (SumMon®) — A synthetic opioid antagonist used to treat respiratory depression induced by opioids and suspected opioid overdose. It is an orally active analog of naltrexone with a long duration of action. In one study, a single oral dose of 50 mg of nalmephene given to healthy volunteers could block the respiratory depression, analgesia and other agonist effects of intravenously administered fentanyl (2 mcg/kg) for 48 to 72 hours. Nalmephene is currently available only in the United States.

Nalorphine — A potent opioid antagonist that can precipitate withdrawal symptoms in opioid-dependent individuals and can also rapidly reverse the effects of narcotic analgesic overdose. Nalorphine can produce mild morphine-like effects when narcotic analgesics are not present in the body. It is not legally available in Canada.

Nefazodone (e.g., Serzone®) — A newer antidepressant classified as a serotonin-2 antagonist/reuptake inhibitor (SARI). Nefazadone is less sedating than the other current agent in this class, trazodone.

Noscapine (Noscatuss®) — A natural alkaloid obtained from opium that exerts no analgesic, sedating or euphoric effects. Since it suppresses the cough reflex, it is used for temporary relief of dry, irritating cough.

Oxymorphone (Numorphan®) — A powerful semi-synthetic opioid derived from morphine, with an analgesic potency approximately 10 times greater than that of morphine when administered by injection. The single therapeutic dose is 1.0 to 1.5 mg administered by intramuscular or subcutaneous injection, 0.5 mg by intravenous injection, or 5 mg by rectal suppository.

Paraldehyde — Paraldehyde is a sedative/hypnotic drug that has been used for sedation, induction of sleep and treatment of alcohol withdrawal symptoms since the 19th century. However, it has a very disagreeable taste and odor, is irritating to tissues and has various other toxic effects. It has been replaced — first by the barbiturates and more recently by the benzodiazepines.

PCE (cyclohexamine) — A synthetic dissociative anesthetic used in veterinary medicine. It is chemically related to phencyclidine (PCP) and produces effects that are similar but seemingly more potent, hence its street name: "rocket fuel." PCE has been sold as PCP, LSD and other drugs. A number of deaths have been attributed to PCE overdose.

Phenadoxone — A synthetic opioid with analgesic potency slightly less than that of morphine when injected subcutaneously. It cannot be regularly administered by needle because it produces marked irritation and pain at injection sites. Phenadoxone is not legally available in Canada or the United States.

Phenazocine — A powerful synthetic opioid with analgesic potency approximately three times as great as that of morphine when injected subcutaneously. Phenazocine is not legally available in Canada.

Phendimetrazine (e.g., Adipost®, Adphen®) — An anorexiant (diet pill) used in the short-term management of obesity. It produces effects similar to those of amphetamine, although it is not as potent. Chronic use can result in tolerance to its main effects and dependence. Since it was widely abused, and because it offers no special therapeutic advantages over other products used for the same purpose, phendimetrazine is no longer marketed in Canada.

Phenmetrazine (e.g., Preludin®) — A synthetic central nervous system (CNS) stimulant with effects similar to, although milder than, those produced by amphetamines. In the past, phenmetrazine was used clinically as a diet pill for the short-term management of obesity, but it has been withdrawn from the market in Canada. Regular use caused psychological and physical dependence in many users. The abuse potential of phenmetrazine is high, although not quite as high as that of amphetamine. Its actual abuse potential is now greatly reduced since its production and medical use have declined markedly.

Phenytoin (diphenylhydantoin; e.g., Dilantin®) — An anti-convulsant drug that is effective orally in controlling tonic-clonic (grand mal) and complex partial seizures in epileptic patients, and by intravenous injection to treat status epilepticus. It has been used extensively to minimize the risk of seizures associated with alcohol withdrawal. It has no abuse potential and, unlike the phenobarbital, which has also been used to control seizures, it does not produce dependence. Tolerance to its anti-seizure actions does not appear to develop. Most adult patients are maintained on 300 to 400 mg per day (taken orally in divided doses).

Pholcodine — A powerful semi-synthetic opioid that has traditionally been used as an antitussive (cough suppressant). It is not legally available in Canada or the United States.

PHP (phenylcyclohexylpyrrolidine) — Another one of many substances chemically related to PCP that also produces a similar spectrum of effects. Its attractiveness may be based on reports that its use is less readily detected in some routine urine screenings for PCP. Abuse of such substances has been reported in the western United States.

Remifentanil — Is similar to other fentanyl-type opioids in possessing potent analgesic and sedative effects resulting from its interaction with μ (mu) receptors. Its potency is somewhat less than that of fentanyl, and its rapid onset of action is similar to that of alfentanil. Like other members of this drug class, remifentanil has side effects that include respiratory suppression, nausea and vomiting, muscular rigidity, and slowing of heart rate. Because it is more rapidly metabolized in blood and tissues than other fentanyl-type opioids, it has been designated the first true ultra-short-acting opioid for use as a supplement to general anesthesia.

Reserpine (e.g., Serpasil®) — A naturally occurring alkaloid obtained from the plant *Rauwolfia serpentina*. It has been employed in the treatment of psychosis and hypertension (high blood pressure). Reserpine has been almost completely replaced in psychiatry by other available antipsychotic agents.

Sufentanil citrate (Sufenta®) — An extremely powerful opioid that is chemically related to, but five to seven times more potent than, fentanyl. This drug is used medically as an intravenous analgesic during surgery and as a primary anesthetic agent for induction and maintenance of anesthesia in certain major surgical procedures.

TMF (3-methylfentanyl) — A designer drug of the fentanyl family of opioids, it was implicated in the late 1980s in more than a dozen unintentional drug overdose deaths. It has been suggested that these deaths were the result of the combined respiratory depressant effects of TMF and other drugs.

Trazodone (e.g., Desyrel®) — An antidepressant with a different mechanism of action from the tricyclic antidepressants and the selective serotonin reuptake inhibitors. It is classified as a serotonin-2 antagonist/reuptake inhibitor (SARI) and is known for its sedation effects.

Venlafaxine (e.g., Effexor®) — A newer antidepressant classified as a serotonin-norepinephrine reuptake inhibitor (SNRI). This agent has a similar mechanism of action to the tricyclic antidepressants but is associated with fewer side effects.

Zolpidem (e.g., Ambien®) — A non-benzodiazepine sedative-hypnotic that is as effective as the benzodiazepines in shortening the time required for an individual to fall asleep and in lengthening total sleep time. The development of tolerance and physical dependence appears to occur infrequently. Zolpidem is not available in Canada.

6

Glossaries

Trade Names and Non-Proprietary Names of Selected Prescription and Over-the-Counter Drugs

The following table lists selected examples of products that contain at least one drug from a drug class discussed in *Drugs and Drug Abuse*. The table is not exhaustive. The proprietary trade names included in this table have been selected because they are widely known, while other trade names are not included for reasons of space. Trade names that include a manufacturer-specific prefix coupled with the common-use or non-proprietary name have also largely been excluded. While most of the products listed are available in Canada, many equivalent or similar products are marketed under similar names in the United States. The table also includes selected trade names of products that are available only in the United States, but are widely recognized in Canada, as well names of a few products that are discontinued from sale but are still widely recognized.

Trade names are capitalized and bear a registered trade mark symbol (®). To assist the reader, where there is no widely recognized trade name for a given drug preparation, the non-proprietary or common-use name has been included in the Trade Name column. Non-proprietary names are not capitalized. For combination products containing more than one drug, the Non-Proprietary Name/Chemical Form column includes names of the individual psychoactive drug constituents (and, in some cases, other therapeutically active constituents) separated by a + symbol. Equivalent names for individual substances are included in parentheses where appropriate. For products that contain psychoactive drugs from more than one class discussed in this book, the drug classes to which these psychoactive constituents belong are included in the Drug Class column, separated by a + symbol.

Throughout this table the term "hydrochloride" is abbreviated as HCl.

♦ indicates trade names that are available only in the United States.

Trade Name	Non-Proprietary Name / Chemical Form	Drug Class(es) of Psychoactive Drug Component(s)
A acamposate	acamposate (calcium acetylhomotaurinate)	Alcohol deterrent
Adipex-B® ♦	phentermine HCl	Stimulant (Appetite Suppressant)
Adipost® ♦	phendimetrazine tartrate	Stimulant (Appetite Suppressant)
Adphen® ♦	phendimetrazine tartrate	Stimulant (Appetite Suppressant)
Akineton®	biperiden HCl	Anticholinergic
Alert®	caffeine	Stimulant
Alfenta®	alfentanil HCl	Opioid
Ambien®	zolpidem	Sedative/Hypnotic
Amobarbital®	amobarbital (amylobarbitone)	Sedative/Hypnotic (Barbiturate)
Amytal®	amobarbital (amylobarbitone)	Sedative/Hypnotic (Barbiturate)
Anacin with Codeine®	ASA + caffeine + codeine phosphate	Stimulant + Opioid
Anacin®	ASA + caffeine	Stimulant
Anadrol® ♦	oxymetholone	Anabolic Steroid
Anafranil®	clomipramine HCl	Tricyclic Antidepressant
Anapolon 50®	oxymetholone	Anabolic Steroid
Anatest® ♦	testosterone propionate	Anabolic Steroid
Anavar® ♦	oxandrolone	Anabolic Steroid
Andriol®	testosterone undecanoate	Anabolic Steroid
Andronate® ♦	testosterone cypionate (testosterone cyclopentylpropionate)	Anabolic Steroid
Anexate®	flumazenil	Anxiolytic (Benzodiazepine)
Antabuse®	disulfiram	Alcohol deterrent
Aquachloral® ♦	chloral hydrate	Sedative/Hypnotic
Artane®	trihexyphenidyl HCl	Anticholinergic
Ativan®	lorazepam	Anxiolytic (Benzodiazepine)
Aventyl®	nortriptyline HCl	Tricyclic Antidepressant
Axid®	nizatidine	Histamine H2 Receptor Antagonist
B Barbilixir®	phenobarbital (phenobarbitone)	Sedative/Hypnotic (Barbiturate)
Barbita® ♦	phenobarbital (phenobarbitone)	Sedative/Hypnotic (Barbiturate)
Bellergal®	belladonna + ergotamine + phenobarbital	Anticholinergic + Sedative/ Hypnotic (Barbiturate)
Benadryl Decongestant®	diphenhydramine phosphate + pseudoephedrine HCl	Antihistamine + Stimulant (Decongestant)
Benadryl®	diphenhydramine HCl	Antihistamine
Brietal Sodium®	methohexital sodium	Sedative/Hypnotic (Barbiturate)
Buprenex® ♦	buprenorphine HCl	Opioid
Busodium® ♦	butabarbital sodium	Sedative/Hypnotic (Barbiturate)

continued ...

Trade Name	Non-Proprietary Name / Chemical Form	Drug Class(es) of Psychoactive Drug Component(s)
Buspar®	buspirone HCl	Anxiolytic
Butalan® ♦	butabarbital sodium	Sedative/Hypnotic (Barbiturate)
butalbital	butalbital (allylbarbituric acid)	Sedative/Hypnotic (Barbiturate)
Butisol Sodium®	butabarbital sodium	Sedative/Hypnotic (Barbiturate)
Cafergot PB®	belladonna + caffeine + ergotamine + pentobarbital	Anticholinergic + Stimulant + Sedative/Hypnotic (Barbiturate)
Cafergot®	caffeine + ergotamine tartrate	Stimulant
Carbolith®	lithium carbonate	Mood Stabilizer
Cesamet®	nabilone	Antiemetic, Hallucinogen
Chlor-Tripolon Decongestant®	chlorpheniramine maleate + pseudoephedrine sulphate tablet or phenylpropanolamine (syrup)	Antihistamine + Stimulant (Decongestant)
Chlor-Tripolon®	chlorpheniramine maleate	Antihistamine
Chlorprom®	chlorpromazine HCl	Typical Antipsychotic
Cipramil®	citalopram	Antidepressant (SSRI)
Claritin®	loratidine	Antihistamine
Clopixol Acuphase®	zuclopenthixol acetate	Typical Antipsychotic
Clopixol®	zuclopenthixol dihydrochloride	Typical Antipsychotic
Clopizol Depot®	zuclopenthixol decanoate	Typical Antipsychotic
Clozaril®	clozapine	Atypical Antipsychotic
cocaine HCl	cocaine HCl	Stimulant
codeine	codeine phosphate	Opioid
Codeine Contin®	codeine sulphate	Opioid
Cogentin®	benztropine mesylate	Anticholinergic
Contac C®	chlorpheniramine maleate + phenylpropanolamine HCl	Antihistamine + Stimulant (Decongestant)
cyclazocine	cyclazocine	Opioid Antagonist
Cyclomen®	danazol	Steroid
Dalmane®	flurazepam HCl	Anxiolytic (Benzodiazepine)
Danocrine® ♦	danazol	Steroid
Dapex® ♦	phentermine HCl	Stimulant (Appetite Suppressant)
Darvon Pulvules® ♦	propoxyphene HCl	Opioid
Darvon-N®	propoxyphene napsylate	Opioid
Deca-Durabolin®	nandrolone decanoate	Anabolic Steroid
Delatestryl®	testosterone enanthate	Anabolic Steroid
Demerol®	meperidine HCl (pethidine HCl; isonipecaine HCl)	Opioid
Depakene®	valproic acid	Anticonvulsant
Depakote® ♦	divalproex sodium	Mood Stabilizer
Depotest® ♦	testosterone cypionate	Anabolic Steroid
Deprenyl®	selegiline HCl (l-deprenyl HCl)	Antidepressant (MAOI)
Desoxyn® ♦	methamphetamine HCl (desoxyephedrine HCl)	Stimulant
Desyrel®	trazodone HCl	Antidepressant (Serotonin Antagonist/Reuptake Inhibitor)

continued ...

Trade Name	Non-Proprietary Name / Chemical Form	Drug Class(es) of Psychoactive Drug Component(s)
Dexedrine®	dextroamphetamine sulphate	Stimulant
dextromoramide	dextromoramide tartrate	Opioid
dihydrocodeinone	dihydrocodeinone phosphate (hydrocodone phosphate) or dihydrocodeinone bitartrate (hydrocodeine bitartrate)	Opioid
Dilantin®	phenytoin (diphenylhydantoin)	Anticonvulsant
Dilaudid®, Dilaudid-HP®, Dilaudid-HP Plus®, Dilaudid-XP®	hydromorphone HCl (dihydromorphinone HCl)	Opioid
Dimetane®	brompheniramine maleate	Antihistamine
Dimetane Expectorant-DC®	hydrocodone bitartrate + brompheniramine maleate + phenylephrine HCl + phenylpropanolamine HCl + guaifenesin	Opioid + Antihistamine + Stimulants (Decongestants)
Dolophine HCl® ♦	methadone HCl	Opioid
Doloral®	morphine HCl	Opioid
Donnagel-PG®	opium	Opioid
Donnatal®	belladonna alkaloids (hyoscyamine sulphate + atropine sulphate + scopolamine hydrobromide) + phenobarbital	Anticholinergics + Sedative/Hypnotic (Barbiturate)
Doryx®	doxylamine hyclate	Antihistamine
Duragesic®	fentanyl	Opioid
Duralith®	lithium carbonate	Mood Stabilizer
Duramorph® ♦	morphine sulphate	Opioid
E Effexor®	venlafaxine HCl	Antidepressant (Serotonin-Norepinephrine Reuptake Inhibitor)
Elavil®	amitriptyline HCl	Tricyclic Antidepressant
Elavil Plus®	amitriptyline HCl + perphenazine	Tricyclic Antidepressant, Typical Antipsychotic
Eldepryl®	selegiline HCl (l-deprenyl HCl)	Antiparkinsonism Agent (MAOI)
Endep® ♦	amitriptyline HCl	Tricyclic Antidepressant
Enovil® ♦	amitriptyline HCl	Tricyclic Antidepressant
ephedrine	ephedrine	Stimulant
Epitol® ♦	carbamazepine	Mood Stabilizer, Anticonvulsant
Epival®	divalproex sodium	Anticonvulsant
Equanil®	meprobamate	Anxiolytic
Equipoise®	boldenone undecylenate	Anabolic Steroid (veterinary)
Ergodryl®	ergotamine tartrate + caffeine citrate + diphenhydramine HCl	Stimulant + Antihistamine
Etrafon®	amitriptyline HCl + perphenazine	Tricyclic Antidepressant + Typical Antipsychotic
Excedrin®	acetaminophen + caffeine	Stimulant
F Fastin®	phentermine HCl	Stimulant (Appetite Suppressant)
Fentanyl Citrate Injectable® ♦	fentanyl citrate	Opioid
Fentanyl Oralet® ♦	fentanyl citrate	Opioid
Fiorinal®	ASA + caffeine + butalbital	Stimulant + Sedative/Hypnotic (Barbiturate)

continued ...

Trade Name	Non-Proprietary Name / Chemical Form	Drug Class(es) of Psychoactive Drug Component(s)
Fiorinal® C1/4, C1/2	ASA + caffeine + codeine phosphate + butalbital	Stimulant + Opioid + Sedative/Hypnotic (Barbiturate)
Fluanxol Depot Injection®	flupenthixol decanoate	Typical Antipsychotic
Fluanxol Tablets®	flupenthixol dihydrochloride	Typical Antipsychotic
Frisium®	clobazam	Anxiolytic (Benzodiazepine)
G Gen-XENE® ♦	clorazepate dipotassium	Anxiolytic (Benzodiazepine)
Gravol®	dimenhydrinate	Antihistamine
H Habitrol®	(S)- nicotine	Stimulant
Halcion®	triazolam	Anxiolytic (Benzodiazepine)
Haldol®	haloperidol	Typical Antipsychotic
heroin (diamorphine)	heroin HCl	Opioid
Hismanal®	astemizole	Antihistamine
Hycodan®	hydrocodone bitartrate	Opioid
Hycomine®	pyrilamine maleate + hydrocodone bitartrate + phenylephrine HCl	Opioid + Antihistamine + Stimulant (Decongestant)
Hydromorph Contin®	hydromorphone HCl (dihydromorphinone HCl)	Opioid
HydroStat® ♦	hydromorphone HCl (dihydromorphinone HCl)	Opioid
hyoscine hydrobromide	hyoscine hydrobromide	Anticholinergic
I Impril®	imipramine HCl	Tricyclic Antidepressant
Infumorph® ♦	morphine sulphate	Opioid
Ionamin®	phentermine resin complex	Stimulant (Appetite Suppressant)
K Kadian®	morphine sulphate	Opioid
Kemadin®	procyclidine HCl	Antiparkinsonism Agent (Anticholinergic)
Ketalar®	ketamine HCl	Hallucinogen, Dissociative Anesthetic
Klonopin® ♦	clonazepam	Anxiolytic (Benzodiazepine)
L LAAM	levomethadyl acetate (l-alpha-acetylmethadol)	Opioid
Lanorinal® ♦	butalbital + ASA + caffeine	Stimulant + Sedative/Hypnotic (Barbiturate)
Largactil®	chlorpromazine HCl	Typical Antipsychotic
Lectopam®	bromazepam	Anxiolytic (Benzodiazepine)
Leritine Injection®	anileridine phosphate	Opioid
Leritine Tablets®	anileridine HCl	Opioid
Levate®	amitriptyline HCl	Tricyclic Antidepressant
Levo-Dromoran® ♦	levorphanol tartrate (levorphan tartrate)	Opioid
Levoprome® ♦	methotrimeprazine (levomepromazine)	Typical Antipsychotic
Librax®	chlordiazepoxide HCl + clidinium bromide	Anxiolytic (Benzodiazepine) + Anticholinergic
Librium®	chlordiazepoxide HCl	Anxiolytic (Benzodiazepine)
Lithane®	lithium carbonate	Mood Stabilizer
Lithizine®	lithium carbonate	Mood Stabilizer
Lomotil® Tablets	diphenoxylate HCl + atropine sulphate	Opioid + Anticholinergic
Lomotil® Liquid	diphenoxylate HCl	Opioid
Lorfan®	levallorphan	Opioid Agonist/Antagonist
Loxapac®	loxapine (oxilapine)	Typical Antipsychotic

continued ...

Trade Name	Non-Proprietary Name / Chemical Form	Drug Class(es) of Psychoactive Drug Component(s)
Loxitane® ♦	loxapine (oxilapine)	Typical Antipsychotic
Ludiomil®	maprotiline HCl	Tricyclic Antidepressant
Luminal® ♦	phenobarbital	Sedative/Hypnotic (Barbiturate)
Luvox®	fluvoxamine maleate	Antidepressant (SSRI)
M-Eslon®	morphine sulphate	Opioid
M-Orexic® ♦	diethylproprion HCl (amfepramone)	Stimulant (Appetite Suppressant)
M.O.S.-SR®	morphine HCl	Opioid
M.O.S.-Sulfate®	morphine sulphate	Opioid
M.O.S.®	morphine HCl	Opioid
Malogen Aqueous®	testosterone	Anabolic Steroid
Malogen® (oil)	testosterone propionate	Anabolic Steroid
Manerix®	moclobemide	Antidepressant (MAOI)
Marplan® ♦	isocaboxazid	Antidepressant (MAOI)
Maxibolin® ♦	ethylestrenol	Anabolic Steroid
Mazanor® ♦	mazindol	Stimulant (Appetite Suppressant)
Mazepine®	carbamazepine	Anticonvulsant + Mood Stabilizer
Meditran®	meprobamate	Anxiolytic
Mellaril®	thioridazine HCl	Typical Antipsychotic
Metandren®	methyltestosterone	Anabolic Steroid
methadone HCl	methadone HCl	Opioid
Methadose® ♦	methadone HCl	Opioid
methandrostenolone	methandrostenolone	Anabolic Steroid
Midol Multi-Symptom® Extra Strength	acetaminophen + caffeine + pyrilamine maleate	Stimulant + Antihistamine
Miltown® ♦	meprobamate	Anxiolytic
Modecate®	fluphenazine decanoate	Typical Antipsychotic
Moditen Enanthate®	fluphenazine enanthate	Typical Antipsychotic
Moditen HCl®	fluphenazine HCl	Typical Antipsychotic
Mogadon®	nitrazepam	Anxiolytic (Benzodiazepine)
Morphine-HP®	morphine sulphate	Opioid
Morphitec®	morphine HCl	Opioid
MPPP	l-methyl-4-phenyl-4-propionoxypiperidine	Opioid
MS Contin®	morphine sulphate	Opioid
MS-IR®	morphine sulphate	Opioid
Myproic Acid® ♦	valproic acid	Mood Stabilizer
nalorphine	nalorphine HCl	Opioid Antagonist
Nandrobolin®	nandrolone laurate	Anabolic Steroid (veterinary)
Narcan®	naloxone HCl	Opioid Antagonist
Nardil®	phenelzine sulphate	Antidepressant (MAOI)
Navane®	thiothixene	Typical Antipsychotic
Nembutal Sodium®	pentobarbital sodium	Sedative/Hypnotic (Barbiturate)

continued ...

Trade Name	Non-Proprietary Name / Chemical Form	Drug Class(es) of Psychoactive Drug Component(s)
Nicoderm®	nicotine	Stimulant
Nicorette®, Nicorette (Plus)®	nicotine	Stimulant
Nicotrol®	nicotine	Stimulant
Nisentil® ♦	alphaprodine HCl	Opioid
Nobesine®	diethylproprion HCl (amfepramone)	Stimulant (Appetite Suppressant)
Noctec® ♦	chloral hydrate	Sedative/Hypnotic
Norfranil® ♦	imipramine HCl	Tricyclic Antidepressant
Norpramin®	desipramine HCl	Tricyclic Antidepressant
Novahistex DM with Decongestant®	dextromethorphan hydrobromide + pseudoephedrine HCl	Cough Suppressant + Stimulant (Decongestant)
Novahistex DH Expectorant®	hydrocodone bitartrate + guaifenesin + phenylephrine HCl	Opioid + Stimulant (Decongestant)
Novahistex DH®	hydrocodone bitartrate + phenylephrine HCl	Opioid + Stimulant (Decongestant)
Novahistine DH®	hydrocodone bitartrate + phenylephrine HCl	Opioid + Stimulant (Decongestant)
Nozinan®	methotrimeprazine (levomepromazine)	Typical Antipsychotic
Nubain®	nalbuphine HCl	Opioid Agonist/Antagonist
Numorphan®	oxymorphone HCl	Opioid
Nytol®	diphenhydramine HCl	Antihistamine
Obephen® ♦	phentermine HCl	Stimulant (Appetite Suppressant)
Obermine® ♦	phentermine HCl	Stimulant (Appetite Suppressant)
Obestin-30® ♦	phentermine HCl	Stimulant (Appetite Suppressant)
Oby-Trim® ♦	phentermine HCl	Stimulant (Appetite Suppressant)
opium tincture (laudanum)	opium tincture	Opioids
Oramorph SR®	morphine sulphate	Opioid
Oranabol®	oxymesterone	Anabolic Steroid
Ormazine® ♦	chlorpromazine HCl	Typical Antipsychotic
Ornade®	chlorphenaramine + phenylpropanolamine (PPA)	Antihistamine + Stimulant (Decongestant)
OxyContin®	oxycodone HCl (dihydrohydroxycodeinone HCl)	Opioid
Oxydess II® ♦	dextroamphetamine sulphate	Stimulant
Pamelor® ♦	nortriptyline HCl	Tricyclic Antidepressant
Panshape® ♦	phentermine HCl	Stimulant (Appetite Suppressant)
Paral® ♦	paraldehyde	Sedative/Hypnotic
Paregoric®	camphorated opium tincture	Opioids
Parnate®	trancyclpromine sulphate	Antidepressant (MAOI)
Paxil®	paroxetine HCl	Antidepressant (SSRI)
Paxipam® ♦	halazepam	Anxiolytic (Benzodiazepine)
Pentothal®	thiopental sodium	Sedative/Hypnotic (Barbiturate)
Pepcid®	famotidine	Histamine H2 Receptor Antagonist
Peptol®	cimetidine	Histamine H2 Receptor Antagonist
Percodan®	oxycodone HCl (dihydrohydroxycodeinone HCl)	Opioid
Periactin®	cyproheptadine HCl	Antihistamine

continued ...

Trade Name	Non-Proprietary Name / Chemical Form	Drug Class(es) of Psychoactive Drug Component(s)
Permitil Concentrate® ♦	fluphenazine HCl	Typical Antipsychotic
Pertofrane®	desipramine HCl	Tricyclic Antidepressant
Phenaphen with Codeine® No.2, No.3, No.4	ASA + codeine phosphate + phenobarbital	Opioid + Sedative/Hypnotic (Barbiturate)
Phenazine®	perphenazine	Typical Antipsychotic
Phentride® ♦	phentermine HCl	Stimulant (Appetite Suppressant)
Phentrol® ♦	phentermine HCl	Stimulant (Appetite Suppressant)
Phetercot® ♦	phentermine HCl	Stimulant (Appetite Suppressant)
Placidyl®	ethchlorvynol	Sedative/Hypnotic
Ponderal Pacaps®	fenfluramine HCl	Stimulant (Appetite Suppressant)
Ponderal®	fenfluramine HCl	Stimulant (Appetite Suppressant)
Pondimin®	fenfluramine HCl	Stimulant (Appetite Suppressant)
Prelu-2® ♦	phendimetrazine tartrate	Stimulant (Appetite Suppressant)
Primazine® ♦	promazine HCl	Typical Antipsychotic
Proavil®	amitriptyline HCl + perphenazine	Tricyclic Antidepressant + Typical Antipsychotic
Prolixin® ♦	fluphenazine HCl	Typical Antipsychotic
Prosom®	estazolam	Anxiolytic (Benzodiazepine)
Prostep®	nicotine	Stimulant
Prozac®	fluoxetine HCl	Antidepressant (SSRI)
Prozine® ♦	promazine HCl	Typical Antipsychotic
Pyribenzamine®	tripelennamine HCl	Antihistamine
Q Quaalude®	methaqualone HCl	Sedative/Hypnotic
R Razepam® ♦	temazepam	Anxiolytic (Benzodiazepine)
Redux® ♦	dexfenfluramine	Stimulant (Appetite Suppressant)
Restoril®	temazepam	Anxiolytic (Benzodiazepine)
ReVia®	naltrexone HCl	Opioid Antagonist
Rhotrimine®	trimipramine maleate	Tricyclic Antidepressant
Risperdal®	risperidone	Atypical Antipsychotic
Ritalin (SR) ®	methylphenidate HCl (methylphenidylacetate HCl)	Stimulant
Rivotril®	clonazepam	Anxiolytic (Benzodiazepine)
RMS-Uniserts® ♦	morphine sulphate	Opioid
Robidone®	hydrocodone bitartrate (dihydrocodeinone bitartrate)	Opioid
Rohypnol® ♦	flunitrazepam	Anxiolytic (Benzodiazepine)
Roxanol® ♦	morphine sulphate	Opioid
Roxicodone® ♦	oxycodone HCl (dihydrohydroxycodeinone HCl)	Opioid
S Sanorex®	mazindol	Stimulant (Appetite Suppressant)
Sarisol No.2® ♦	butabarbital sodium	Sedative/Hypnotic (Barbiturate)
Seconal Sodium®	secobarbital sodium (quinalbarbitone sodium)	Sedative/Hypnotic (Barbiturate)
Seldane®	terfenadine	Antihistamine
Serax®	oxazepam	Anxiolytic (Benzodiazepine)

continued ...

Trade Name	Non-Proprietary Name / Chemical Form	Drug Class(es) of Psychoactive Drug Component(s)
Serpalan® ◆	reserpine	Mood Stabilizer
Serpasil®	reserpine	Mood Stabilizer
Serzone®	nefazodone HCl	Antidepressant (Serotonin-2 Antagonist/Reuptake Inhibitor)
Sinequan®	doxepin HCl	Tricyclic Antidepressant
642®	ASA + caffeine + propoxyphene HCl	Stimulant + Opioid
Sleep-Eze®	diphenhydramine HCl	Antihistamine
Solfoton® ◆	phenobarbitone	Sedative/Hypnotic (Barbiturate)
Sominex®	diphenhydramine HCl	Antihistamine
Somnol®	flurazepam HCl	Anxiolytic (Benzodiazepine)
Sopor® ◆	methaqualone HCl	Sedative/Hypnotic
Spancap No. 1® ◆	dextroamphetamine sulphate	Stimulant
Stadol NS®	butorphanol tartrate	Opioid Antagonist/Agonist
Statex®	morphine sulphate	Opioid
Stay Alert®	caffeine	Stimulant
Stay Awake®	caffeine	Stimulant
Stelazine®	trifluoperazine HCl	Typical Antipsychotic
Sublimaze®	fentanyl citrate	Opioid
Sudafed®	pseudoephedrine HCl	Stimulant (Decongestant)
Sufenta®	sufentanil citrate	Opioid
Supeudol®	oxycodone HCl (dihydrohydroxycodeinone HCl)	Opioid
Surmontil®	trimipramine maleate	Tricyclic Antidepressant
T-Diet® ◆	phentermine HCl	Stimulant (Appetite Suppressant)
Tagamet®	cimetidine	Histamine H2 Receptor Antagonist
Talwin Injection®	pentazocine lactate	Opioid Agonist/Antagonist
Talwin Tablets®	pentazocine HCl	Opioid Agonist/Antagonist
Tecnal®	butalbital + ASA + caffeine	Sedative/Hypnotic (Barbiturate), Stimulant
Tecnal® C1/4, C1/2	ASA + caffeine + codeine phosphate + butalbital	Stimulant + Opioid + Sedative/Hypnotic (Barbiturate)
Tegretol®	carbamazepine	Anticonvulsant, Mood Stabilizer
Temposil®	calcium carbimide (calcium cyanamide)	Alcohol Deterrent
Tenuate®	diethylproprion HCl (amfepramone)	Stimulant (Appetite Suppressant)
Tepanil® ◆	diethylproprion HCl (amfepramone)	Stimulant (Appetite Suppressant)
Teramin® ◆	phentermine HCl	Stimulant (Appetite Suppressant)
Testex® ◆	testosterone propionate	Anabolic Steroid
Testos 100® ◆	testosterone	Anabolic Steroid
Thor-Prom® ◆	chlorpromazine HCl	Typical Antipsychotic
Thorazine® ◆	chlorpromazine HCl	Typical Antipsychotic
Tipramine® ◆	imipramine HCl	Tricyclic Antidepressant
Tofranil®	imipramine HCl	Tricyclic Antidepressant
Tranxene®	clorazepate dipotassium	Anxiolytic (Benzodiazepine)

continued ...

Trade Name	Non-Proprietary Name / Chemical Form	Drug Class(es) of Psychoactive Drug Component(s)
Trexan® ♦	naltrexone HCl	Opioid Antagonist
Triadapin®	doxepin HCl	Tricyclic Antidepressant
Triaprin® ♦	butalbital + acetaminophen	Sedative/Hypnotic (Barbiturate)
Triavil®	amitriptyline HCl + perphenazine	Tricyclic Antidepressant + Typical Antipsychotic
Trilafon®	perphenazine	Typical Antipsychotic
Triptil®	protriptyline HCl	Tricyclic Antidepressant
Tualone®	methaqualone HCl	Sedative/Hypnotic
Tuinal®	amobarbital sodium + secobarbital sodium	Sedative/Hypnotics (Barbiturates)
222®, 282®, 292®	ASA + caffeine citrate + codeine phosphate	Stimulant + Opioid
282 Mep®	ASA + caffeine citrate + codeine phosphate + meprobamate	Stimulant + Opioid + Anxiolytic
Tylenol® No.1,2,3	acetaminophen + caffeine + codeine phosphate	Stimulant + Opioid
U Unisom®	doxylamine HCl	Antihistamine
Unitest® ♦	testosterone	Anabolic Steroid (veterinary)
V Valium®	diazepam	Anxiolytic (Benzodiazepine)
Versed®	midazolam HCl	Anxiolytic (Benzodiazepine)
Vesprin® ♦	triflupromazine HCl	Typical Antipsychotic
Vibutal® ♦	butalbital + ASA + caffeine	Sedative/Hypnotic (Barbiturate), Stimulant
Vivactil® ♦	protriptyline HCl	Tricyclic Antidepressant
Vivol®	diazepam	Anxiolytic (Benzodiazepine)
W Wake-Ups®	caffeine	Stimulant
Wellbutrin® ♦	bupropion HCl	Atypical Antipsychotic
Wilpowr® ♦	phentermine HCl	Stimulant (Appetite Suppressant)
Winstrol V®	stanozolol	Anabolic Steroid (veterinary)
X Xanax®	alprazolam	Anxiolytic (Benzodiazepine)
Xylocaine®	lidocaine HCl (lignocaine HCl)	Local Anesthetic
Xylocard®	lidocaine HCl (lignocaine HCl)	Local Anesthetic
Z Zantac®, Zantac-C®	ranitidine HCl	Histamine H2 Receptor Antagonist
Zantryl® ♦	phentermine HCl	Stimulant (Appetite Suppressant)
Zoloft®	sertraline HCl	Antidepressant (SSRI)
Zonalon®	doxepin HCl	Tricyclic Antidepressant
Zyban® ♦	bupropion HCl	Atypical Antipsychotic
Zyprexa® ♦	olanzapine	Atypical Antipsychotic

Glossary of Medical and Scientific Terms

 A

abstinence	cessation of intake of a given drug following a period of prolonged use.
acidosis	abnormal metabolic state caused by the accumulation of acidic components in, or the loss of basic components from, the body. Body function, and especially brain function, may be severely disrupted.
acquired immune deficiency syndrome (AIDS)	immune disorder caused by infection with the human immunodeficiency virus (HIV) leading to decline in immune function, increased susceptibility to opportunistic infections and, eventually, death. (*See* human immunodeficiency virus.)
acute	rapid; sudden; short term (contrast with chronic).
addiction, drug	(obsolete); state of dependence on a drug substance that shapes a pattern of self-administration that is harmful to physical and/or mental health, social well-being and economic functioning.
adjunctive	supportive; complementary; e.g., adjunctive treatment: the use of a medication or other therapeutic measure to enhance the effects of another.
affect	outward expression of emotion or feeling, may differ from an individual's described emotion.
AIDS	*See* acquired immune deficiency syndrome.
akathesia	compulsive need to move about constantly.
alkaloid	substance, chemically an organic base, found in various parts of some plant materials; many are pharmacologically active, accounting for the drug effects of some plant materials, such as morphine and codeine in the opium poppy, caffeine in coffee beans, nicotine in tobacco leaves.
allergy	hypersensitivity reaction to a specific substance, or allergen.
alveolar-capillary membrane	membrane consisting of the cells lining the alveoli and the pulmonary capillaries in the lungs, across which gas exchange and drug absorption occur.

alveoli   small air sacs of the lung.

amnesia   partial or total loss of memory.

analgesic   drug that can lessen pain without causing unconsciousness; e.g., ASA (as in Aspirin®), acetaminophen (as in Tylenol®).

analogue   with respect to drug structure, a drug that differs from another in some aspects of structure, but is similar in others; both drugs may have similar functions; e.g., codeine is an analogue of morphine.

anesthesia   loss of feeling or sensation in part or all of the body; especially in relation to drug-induced insensitivity to pain; may be accompanied by unconsciousness (general anesthetic vs. local anesthetic).

anorexia   marked loss of appetite; may be induced by drugs, psychological disorders or physical illness.

antagonist   substance that specifically blocks or opposes the effects of another substance; e.g., naloxone is an opioid antagonist.

anticholinergic   drug that blocks the passage of impulses through certain nerves in which acetylcholine is the neurotransmitter.

anticholinergic effects   effects resulting from the antagonism of the neurotransmitter acetylcholine. Low-dose effects typically include reduced stomach motility and gastric secretion, dry mouth, dilation of the pupils, blurring of near vision, relaxation of smooth-muscle spasms and increased heart rate; much higher-dose effects may include intensification of low-dose effects and CNS effects such as hallucinations, mild euphoria, disorientation, confusion, delirium, memory loss, paranoid thinking, agitation, speech disturbances, impaired motor co-ordination and sometimes seizures. The latter effects may be accompanied by abnormally high blood pressure, headache, high fever, flushing of the skin, nausea and vomiting.

anticonvulsant (anti-epileptic, anti-seizure)   drug that prevents or relieves seizures (convulsions), e.g., phenytoin (as in Dilantin®).

antiemetic   drug that prevents or relieves nausea and vomiting; e.g., dimenhydrinate (Gravol®).

anti-inflammatory   drug that reduces tissue inflammation; e.g., ASA (as in Aspirin®), ibuprofen (as in Advil® and Motrin®).

antipyretic   drug that reduces abnormally high body temperature or fever; e.g., acetaminophen (as in Tylenol®), ASA (as in Aspirin®) and ibuprofen (as in Advil® and Motrin®).

antitussive	drug that suppresses the cough reflex, e.g., codeine, dextromethorphan (the latter often indicated by the letters DM, as in Benylin DM®).
apnea	cessation of breathing.
asthma	condition of the lungs characterized by wheezing, coughing and labored breathing; associated with inflammation of the airways and tightening or constriction of the muscles in the breathing passages. May be induced by allergen exposure, exercise, irritant particles or psychological stress.
ataxia	impaired ability to co-ordinate the voluntary muscles such as those involved in walking or driving.
atrophy	wasting away of a previously normal organ or tissue; may be caused by a number of factors including aging, disease or toxic drug reactions.
attention-deficit hyperactivity disorder (ADHD)	behavioral disorder characterized by age-inappropriate attention span and/or hyperactivity and impulsivity that cause impairment in social or academic functioning. Onset of symptoms occurs before age seven. This disorder was formerly known as attention deficit disorder with hyperactivity (ADDH) and has also been termed "hyperkinetic syndrome" or "minimal brain dysfunction."
autism	condition characterized by impaired social interaction and communication and restricted, stereotypical behavioral patterns. Ability to respond to or communicate with the outside world is impaired and use of language is often minimal or absent. Onset of symptoms occurs before age three. Mental retardation is present in over two-thirds of patients but some may exhibit normal intelligence. Above-average abilities, especially in calculation or rote memory, may be present in some patients, even with overall mental retardation (so-called "idiot savants").
autonomic nervous system	the part of the nervous system that is not under voluntary or conscious control.

B

bipolar affective disorder (bipolar I disorder)	psychiatric diagnosis; a mood disorder characterized by cyclical patterns of depression and mania. Formerly called "manic-depression" or "manic-depressive disorder."

blood doping	procedure in which an athlete's blood is removed, stored and transfused back into the body prior to competition or during training to enhance oxygen delivery and improve athletic performance.
bradycardia (brachycardia)	abnormally slow heart rate (contrast with tachycardia).
bradykinesia	describes slowness of voluntary movements (e.g., walking), difficulty in getting movements started (e.g., getting up from a chair), and sometimes completing movements that have been started.

© C

cardiac arrest	complete cessation of heart activity.
cardiac arrhythmia	irregular beating of the heart.
cardiovascular system	the heart and blood vessels.
central nervous system (CNS)	the brain and spinal cord.
cerebellum	the part of the brain that controls voluntary muscle co-ordination.
cerebral cortex	the thin grey matter covering the upper surface of the brain; its three major functions are sensory perception (sensation), association (thought) and motor control (movement).
chronic	of long duration (contrast with acute).
cirrhosis	replacement of normal liver tissue with dysfunctional fibrous tissue; a progressive degenerative disease frequently associated with chronic alcoholism, hepatitis.
CNS	*See* central nervous system.
coma	state of profound unconsciousness from which the individual cannot be roused.
congener	chemical compound that is closely related to another in chemical composition and pharmacological effect.
convulsion	violent uncontrolled muscle spasm(s); involuntary generalized contraction or series of contractions of the voluntary muscles.
cross-dependence	condition in which one drug suppresses withdrawal symptoms in an individual who is physically dependent on another drug of

similar pharmacological effects; e.g., various opioids (e.g., heroin and methadone) share cross-dependence, as do many CNS depressants (e.g., alcohol and benzodiazepines).

cross-tachyphylaxis   loss of sensitivity to the effects of other drugs with similar pharmacological effects following short-term, repeated administration of a drug.

cross-tolerance   reduced sensitivity to the effects of a drug due to acquired tolerance to another drug that produces similar pharmacological effects; e.g., opioids share cross-tolerance, as do CNS depressants such as barbiturates.

cyanosis   bluish discoloration of the skin or mucous membranes caused by insufficient oxygen in the blood and/or markedly insufficient blood in the capillaries.

delirium tremens (DTs)   late and prolonged phase of alcoholic withdrawal characterized by acute mental disturbances including frightening hallucinations, delusional thinking, extreme mental confusion, disorientation, severe agitation and abnormally high body temperature; most severe form of alcohol withdrawal symptoms, occurring after cessation of heavy alcohol consumption.

delusion   false belief, set of beliefs or impression that an individual adamantly insists is true irrespective of evidence to the contrary.

dependence, drug/substance   state of dependence on a drug substance in which the individual continues substance use despite significant substance-related problems that may include harm to physical and/or mental health, social well-being and/or economic functioning.

dependence liability   tendency of a drug to produce dependence in the user.

depersonalization   change in self-perception so that the usual sense of one's own reality is lost, manifested in a sense of unreality or self-estrangement, in a change in body image, or in a feeling of loss of control over one's actions or speech.

depressant   drug that causes the functions of an organ system to slow down; with reference to psychoactive substances, a drug that causes central nervous system functions to slow down; e.g., benzodiazepines, barbiturates.

depression	1. drug's effect in slowing down the functions of an organ system;
	2. emotional state (or mood) characterized by feelings of despair and unhappiness; may be normal or abnormal depending on its cause, severity and chronicity.

derivative	substance derived from another substance by chemical manipulation, e.g., heroin is derived from morphine by reaction of morphine with acetic anhydride.

detoxification (or detoxication)	1. process of removal or neutralization of toxic (harmful) drug effects;
	2. care and supportive services provided to persons recovering from psychoactive drug intoxication (as in detoxication centres).

diffuse	pass through or spread widely through a tissue or medium.

disinhibition	reduction or loss of inhibition; e.g., emotional disinhibition results in greater freedom of emotional expression after alcohol consumption; some individuals' usual inhibitions are so reduced that they exhibit emotion or aggression that is otherwise suppressed.

disinhibitor	drug that facilitates the loss of inhibitions; e.g., alcohol is an emotional disinhibitor causing greater than normal freedom in emotional expression.

dissociative agent	drug that produces feelings of isolation or remoteness from the environment; e.g., PCP.

diuretic	drug that is capable of increasing urine flow; e.g., caffeine.

dopamine	a chemical that is produced naturally by certain brain cells, and that, in appropriate concentrations at particular brain sites, allows nerve cells to transmit messages as part of normal CNS functioning. Some drugs block specific effects of dopamine, while others act like dopamine at specific receptors or increase the availability of dopamine at receptors in particular areas of the brain, thereby altering brain functioning and producing various effects, e.g., producing feelings of euphoria, and reducing tremor, rigidity, and slowness of movement in patients with Parkinson's disease.

drug	any chemical agent that affects living processes.

dysfunction	abnormal or impaired function.

dysphoria	unpleasant emotional state; e.g., anxiety, depression; (contrast with euphoria).

dystonia	acute, involuntary, painful muscle contractions, usually of the neck or eyes.

E

electroencephalogram (EEG)	electrophysiological recording of brain activity, obtained through the process of encephalography using electrodes attached to various areas of the scalp; often used in sleep research and in detecting and diagnosing brain disorders such as epilepsy.
endogenous	originating within the body (contrast with exogenous).
ergogenic	performance-enhancing.
ergogenic drug use	defined by the International Olympic Committee (IOC) as "the administration of or use by a competing athlete of any substance foreign to the body, or of any physiological substance taken in an abnormal quantity or by an abnormal route of entry into the body with the sole intention of increasing in an artificial manner his/her performance in the competition."
erythema multiforme	a symptom complex representing a reaction pattern of the skin and mucous membranes to various factors, including substances ingested; the rash is characteristically sudden in onset, with reddening and raised lesions that have concentric rings.
euphoria	a highly exaggerated feeling of well-being (contrast with dysphoria).
euphoriant	drug that produces euphoria; e.g., cocaine.
exacerbation	intensification; making worse.
exogenous	originating outside of the body; i.e., related to external events (contrast with endogenous).
extrapyramidal symptoms (EPS)	a group of effects including dystonias, akathesia and parkinsonism; may be precipitated by typical antipsychotic agents. *See* dystonia, akathesia, parkinsonism.

G

grand mal seizure	*See* tonic-clonic seizure.

half-life	(usually with respect to a drug's half-life in plasma) time required for the concentration of a substance to be reduced by one-half through elimination and/or conversion to another substance.
hallucination	mental impression having no real stimulus, i.e., no basis in reality; may involve any of the senses, so that hallucinations may be visual, auditory or tactile; a belief that one sees, hears or feels something that is not really present.
harmful use	pattern of psychoactive substance use that causes damage to physical or mental health.
hemorrhage	escape of blood from blood vessel(s); bleeding.
hepatitis	inflammation of the liver, usually, but not always, caused by viral infection; a form of hepatitis can be caused by chronic exposure to toxic substances such as alcohol.
human immunodeficiency virus (HIV)	the virus that causes AIDS; may be acquired through sexual contact, sharing of unclean intravenous (IV) needles or syringes, contaminated blood products and maternal-fetal transfer (mother-to-child prenatally).
hyperreflexia	exaggerated reflex response to one or more stimuli.
hypersensitivity	abnormally increased sensitivity; hypersensitivity reaction is an extreme reaction to a stimulus, such as to a drug.
hypertension	abnormally high blood pressure (contrast with hypotension).
hypertensive crisis	extremely elevated blood pressure.
hyperthermia (hyperpyrexia)	abnormally high body temperature (contrast with hypothermia).
hypnotic	drug that induces sleep; e.g., benzodiazepines such as lorazepam (e.g., Ativan®), barbiturates.
hypotension	abnormally low blood pressure (contrast with hypertension).
hypomania	an abnormality of mood resembling mania but of a lesser intensity.
hypothermia	abnormally low body temperature (contrast with hyperthermia).

iatrogenic	resulting from an action or attitude of a physician or other health care provider; caused by medical examination or treatment.
idiopathic	of unknown causation.
illusion	altered interpretation of a real external sensory stimulus, believed by the individual to be an accurate interpretation; faulty perception of an external object.
inhibitor	substance that blocks certain physiological processes, usually in relation to enzymatic processes; e.g., a monoamine oxidase inhibitor (MAOI) blocks the metabolism of monoamines by the enzyme monoamine oxidase (MAO).
intoxication (acute)	1. transient condition following the administration of a psychoactive substance, resulting in disturbance in level of consciousness, cognition, perception, affect or behavior; inebriation; 2. state of poisoning.
intramuscular (im)	within a muscle.
intravenous (iv)	within a vein.

L

lethality	capacity to kill.
libido	life force; usually in reference to sexual drive.

M

mania	mood disorder characterized by expansiveness, elation, agitation, hyperexcitability, hyperactivity and increased speed of thought and speech (flight of ideas).
manic-depressive psychosis	*See* bipolar affective disorder.
metabolism	process by which drug substances are converted in the body into different substances (metabolites), biotransformation.

narcotic	1. literally, that which benumbs or deadens, relating to the term "narcosis";
	2. drugs that have actions similar to morphine and heroin, and are classified in this book as opioids;
	3. (when spelled with capital "N") drugs formerly regulated under the *Narcotic Control Act* in Canada, including cannabis and cocaine in addition to the opioids. (In 1995 the *Narcotic Control Act* was replaced by the *Controlled Drugs and Substances Act*.)

opioid	drug with morphine-like activity, whether naturally occurring, or produced semi-synthetically or synthetically.
osteomalacia	condition marked by softening of the bones, with pain, tenderness, muscular weakness, anorexia and loss of weight.
overdose	any dose in excess of that therapeutically indicated; often used to describe a life-threatening dose.

palpitation	subjective sensation of rapid, irregular or strong pulsation of the heart.
paranoia	condition of abnormal suspiciousness, not warranted by the real situation.
paradoxical reaction	reaction to a drug that is the opposite of the anticipated effect.
parenteral	by injection.
parkinsonian	related to parkinsonism. *See* parkinsonism.
parkinsonism	a group of disorders in which patients experience tremor, slow movements (bradykinesia), stiffness of the limbs and difficulty walking. The four main types of parkinsonism are classical (or idiopathic) Parkinson's (Parkinson's disease), essential tremor, drug-induced parkinsonism and pseudo- (or atypical) parkinsonism. Drug-induced parkinsonism often occurs in psychiatric patients

because the drugs used in the treatment of some mental illnesses may block the action of dopamine in the brain, and disability may develop quite quickly compared with the slow progression of classical Parkinson's.

Parkinson's disease	an idiopathic form of parkinsonism that progresses relatively slowly. The five main signs and symptoms of Parkinson's disease are resting tremor, rigidity, bradykinesia, gait disorder and loss of balance. *See* parkinsonism.
pathology	1. the study of diseases; 2. the symptoms of a disease; e.g., renal pathology would describe the effects or symptoms of a disease process on the kidney.
peripheral neuropathy	disease or damage to nervous tissue other than the brain and spinal cord; characterized by loss of sensation (numbness) or tingling.
polyneuropathy	disease condition involving several nerves.
premorbid	preceding a disease state or psychological disorder.
pseudohallucination	hallucination known to the individual to be unreal.
pseudoillusion	illusion known to the individual to be unreal.
psychoactive drug	any drug that affects perception, thoughts, emotions and/or behavior.
psychomotor	concerning voluntary muscular movement.
psychopathology	1. the study of mental and emotional disorders; 2. symptoms associated with a psychological disorder.
psychopharmacology	the study of the actions and effects of drugs on perception, thoughts, emotions and behavior.
psychotic disorder	(with respect to psychoactive drug effects) — a cluster of major mental phenomena that occur during or immediately after psychoactive substance use and may be characterized by vivid hallucinations, misidentifications, delusions, psychomotor disturbances (excitement or stupor) and an abnormal affect (ranging from fear to ecstasy).
psychotomimetic (psychotogenic)	causing psychological reactions that mimic natural forms of psychosis.
psychotropic drug	drug exerting an effect on the mind; psychotherapeutic drug.

pulmonary	relating to the lungs.
pulmonary artery	the artery that carries blood from the heart to the lungs.
pulmonary hypotension	abnormally low blood pressure in the pulmonary artery.

receptors, receptor sites (target sites)	specific sites in the body with which a drug interacts to produce its effects.
recidivism	tendency to repeat past socially unacceptable behavior; sometimes used as the equivalent of relapse to drug use following treatment.
REM (rapid eye movement) sleep	recurring phase of normal sleep associated with dreaming, characterized by constant, irregular movement of the eye under the eyelid; necessary to the body which, if deprived through poor sleep, drugs or disease, will attempt to "catch up" on REM sleep, leading to vivid dreams and overall less restful sleep.
respiratory arrest	cessation of breathing.

schizophrenia	psychiatric disorder characterized by severe disturbances of thought, mood and behavior; behavior may be regressive and bizarre, and delusions and hallucinations are often (but not always) present.
sedation	state of quiescence and relaxation that may progress to sleepiness; reduction of irritability or excitement, especially in response to drug administration.
seizure	pattern of abnormal rhythmic electrical activity in the brain and its sequelae. The manifestations can be motor (i.e., as in convulsions), sensory, autonomic or psychic.
sequela (plural: sequelae)	condition following or occurring as a result of another condition or event; e.g., individuals experiencing a tonic-clonic seizure commonly experience sequelae such as loss of consciousness, generalized movements of the limbs, tongue-biting and incontinence.

side effect	drug-induced effect that accompanies the intended effect(s) of a drug; side effects are often undesired, but sometimes beneficial.
skeletal muscle	elongated muscle fibres attached to skeletal structures and under voluntary control.
smooth muscle	muscle tissue different in structure to skeletal muscle and not under voluntary control, found in visceral structures; e.g., heart and stomach.
solvent	1. substance that can dissolve other substances; 2. often used as shorthand terminology to describe organic solvents (e.g., toluene) that are sniffed to achieve intoxication.
soporific	sleep-inducing.
status epilepticus	persistent and severe seizure activity with little or no interruption.
stupor	extreme lethargy; partial or nearly complete unconsciousness.
subcutaneous (s.c., subq, subc)	beneath the skin.
syncope	fainting; temporary loss of consciousness resulting from a sudden drop in blood pressure.
synesthesia	the paradoxical melding of one sensory modality with another such that the individual feels able to "see" music or "hear" colors. Many hallucinogenic substances produce synesthesia.

tachycardia	abnormally rapid heart rate (contrast with bradycardia).
tachyphylaxis	state of tolerance to certain psychoactive drugs, such as some hallucinogens, which develops either during the course of acute intoxication or when the drug is used repeatedly; additional doses of the drug will produce no additional effect until the body's sensitivity is restored by a period of abstinence.
tolerance	reduced sensitivity to a drug resulting from the adaptation of the body to repeated exposure to that drug; thus, higher doses become necessary to maintain the body's original response to the drug.

tonic-clonic seizure	generalized seizure resulting in loss of consciousness and intense muscular spasm (tonus) followed by a series of convulsive twitches (clonus). Formerly called "grand mal."
topical	(pertaining to drugs) applied locally to the area being treated; e.g., to the skin, eye, etc.
toxic psychosis	psychotic state caused by drugs or other foreign agents, e.g., lead; normally disappears when the psychosis-inducing substance is eliminated from the body.
toxicity	1. state of being poisoned; 2. adverse effects created by a drug.

ulcer	lesion on the skin or on any mucosal surface in the body.

vasoconstriction	constriction of the blood vessels.
vasodilation	dilation of the blood vessels.
voluntary muscle	muscle over which a person can exert control, such as those involved in conscious activities such as movement, walking (contrast with involuntary muscles such as those involved in breathing or heart contraction).

W

withdrawal	physical and psychological symptoms created by abstinence from, or much reduced exposure to, a drug upon which an individual is physically dependent.

Glossary of Street Drug Language

The colorful terminology that comprises street drug language is derived from the attributes or characteristics of the drugs, drug-related activities and users. In addition, drug terms often have several meanings depending on the geographical location and the given drug-using population. In most cases, knowing the attributes of a drug (e.g., its actions, common appearance) or the characteristics of a user (e.g., type of drug used, pattern of use) provides enough information to understand a given street term. Methamphetamine, for example, is commonly called "speed," an obvious reference to the intensity of its stimulating effects. Users are often called "speeders." And the derogatory term "speed freak" is applied to the heavily dependent user whose behavior is often unpredictable and erratic, and sometimes bizarre. "Ripped" and "wrecked" graphically describe the exhausted condition of a methamphetamine user after several consecutive days of heavy use.

Many street terms move into general use through frequent public exposure in the media and through use by popular personalities such as entertainers. The term "pusher," for example, brings to mind one who sells drugs illicitly, and is the most widely accepted term, as is "junkie" for a user who is heroin dependent and "cold turkey" for abrupt discontinuation of drug use, especially opioid use.

Street drug language is constantly changing. New terms come rapidly into vogue. Others become obsolete just as rapidly, and still others that have fallen into disuse can return to popularity. This list does not attempt to provide a complete glossary of all terms currently in use. Instead, it aims to provide an overview of some of the more commonly used terms. More complete lists are available from such sources as the World Wide Web.

Glossary

A-Bomb	marijuana and heroin smoked in a cigarette.
Acapulco gold	marijuana.
ace	marijuana.
acid	LSD (*d*-lysergic acid diethylamide).
acid freak	*See* head. Synonym for acid head.
ack-ack; **firing the ack-ack gun**	method of smoking heroin by dipping the tip of a tobacco cigarette in heroin (Asian slang).
Adam	MDMA.
amoeba	PCP.
amped	stimulated by drugs, especially cocaine or amphetamine.
amped out	fatigued after using amphetamines.
angel dust	1. phencyclidine (PCP) 2. PCP sprinkled on marijuana in powdered form and smoked. Synonym for supergrass.
animal tranquillizer	PCP.
avenging angel	*Amanita phalloides*, a mushroom in the *Amanita* family.

babysit, babysitter	guide someone through a first drug experience, particularly with the use of hallucinogens such as LSD; provide reassurance and reality contact for the inexperienced user.
back to back	smoking crack after injecting heroin or using heroin after smoking crack.

back-up; backtrack	procedure permitting blood to flow back into a syringe to ensure that the needle is in a vein (a precaution often taken by veteran heroin addicts).
bad trip	unpleasant, frightening or even terrifying experience occurring after taking a drug with hallucinogenic effects properties (e.g., PCP). Synonym for bummer, bum trip.
bag	quantity of drug purchased in an envelope or folded paper; "nickel" bags ($5.00) and "dime" bags ($10.00) describe prices of some years ago, which have substantially increased; when applied to heroin usually refers to highly diluted street heroin, possibly as low as one to three per cent pure.
bagging	inhaling a drug, usually from a bag.
bananas	Talwin Nx®, a pentazocine and naloxone combination that is not marketed in Canada.
barbs	barbiturates. Synonym for goofballs, downers, sleepers.
barrels	LSD.
baseball	freebase cocaine.
basement chemist	illicit, usually small-scale, drug manufacturer. Synonym for kitchen chemist, underground chemist.
bazooka	cocaine; crack.
beautiful	description of a drug of an unusually good quality, producing exceptionally intense euphoria ("The stuff is beautiful.")
bebe	crack.
bennies	amphetamine sulphate tablets, in reference to a specific pharmaceutical product, Benzedrine® tablets.
bhang	marijuana.
big C	cocaine.
big T	pentazocine.
bindle	small packet of drug powder; heroin.
binge	usually refers to a sustained period (i.e., several days) of uninterrupted heavy alcohol consumption; occasionally refers to sustained use of other drugs.

biscuits	Dolophine® tablets (methadone).
black acid	may refer to LSD or a combination of LSD and PCP.
black beauties	capsules containing a combination of *d-* and *dl-*amphetamine; in reference to the color of a specific pharmaceutical product that is not legally available in Canada.
black gold	high potency marijuana.
black hash	opium and hashish.
black tar heroin	potent heroin from Mexico.
blackjack	paregoric cooked to a concentrated form and injected; used mainly when other opioids are unavailable.
blackout	amnesia for events occurring while heavily intoxicated with alcohol or other sedative/hypnotic drugs.
blast	*See* rush.
blotter; blotter cube	paper on which LSD has been absorbed to aid distribution without detection.
blow	sniff or snort; nasal inhalation; also inhalation of smoke ("blowing grass").
blow a fill	smoke opium.
blow a stick	smoke marijuana.
blow smoke	inhale cocaine.
blue cheer	combination of LSD, methamphetamine and strychnine.
blue heaven	LSD.
blue heavens	amobarbital, a barbiturate.
blue velvet	1. combination of paregoric with tripelennamine (an antihistamine) crushed and combined in solution for needle administration, to produce an intensely euphoric high; used as a weak heroin substitute; 2. combination of elixir of terpin hydrate with codeine and tripelennamine (an antihistamine) used as a weak heroin substitute.

blues	amobarbital capsules, blue in color. Synonym for blue heavens, blue birds. See the chapter on barbiturates in Section 3. (Not to be confused with Heavenly Blues, a variety of morning glory.)
blunt	marijuana or marijuana with cocaine inside a cigar.
body packer	person who transports a drug in a package taped or otherwise attached to the body, to avoid detection of the drug. *See* body stuffer.
body stuffer	person who ingests crack or cocaine in a moisture-proof or moisture-resistant packaging to avoid detection of the drug, e.g., when passing through customs or facing law enforcement investigation.
bombed	high or intoxicated on alcohol or other drugs.
bombita	heroin and cocaine combined. Synonym for dynamite, speedball.
bong	water-cooled pipe used to smoke marijuana, often made of glass or bamboo.
booze	ethyl alcohol.
brick	(from shape) compressed block of opium, morphine or hashish, usually a kilogram.
bring down	1. precipitate a "crash" from the excessive agitation produced by stimulants, by ingesting CNS depressants (usually barbiturates or similar drugs); 2. help reduce highly adverse effects produced in some hallucinogen users by talk, reassurance and (sometimes) minor tranquillizers. Synonym for talk down.
bubble gum	cocaine; crack.
buda; buda stick	1. high-grade marijuana cigarette (Thai stick); 2. marijuana cigarette filled with crack.
buddha	potent marijuana spiked with opium.
bump	1. crack; fake crack; 2. boost a high; 3. hit of ketamine.
burned	cheated by a pusher through misrepresentation of the true identity, quantity and/or purity of the purchased drug; having purchased fake drugs.

burned out	1. in a state of brain or chronic behavioral impairment resulting from chronic heavy drug use; 2. collapse of veins from repeated injections.
businessman's lunch; **businessman's LSD;** **businessman's trip;** **businessman's special**	DMT (dimethyltryptamine), a hallucinogen with potent effects lasting 30 to 60 minutes.
butterballs	Talwin Nx®, a pentazocine and naloxone combination not marketed in Canada.
button	peyote cactus button containing mescaline.
butts	tobacco cigarettes.

Cs	cocaine.
cactus	mescaline, from peyote cactus.
cadillac	PCP.
California sunshine	LSD.
cancer sticks	tobacco cigarettes.
candy	cocaine; crack; depressants; amphetamines.
candy cane	cocaine.
candy flip	one "hit" of ecstasy (MDMA) for every three hits of LSD.
candy flipping	mixing ecstasy (MDMA) with other drugs.
cap; caps	1. capsule containing drugs in granule, crystal, liquid or powdered form; 2. crack; LSD; heroin; psilocybin/psilocin.
cap up	transfer bulk-form drugs into capsules.
channel	vein used for injecting drugs.
charge	*See* rush.

charged up	*See* amped.
chasing the dragon	inhaling the vapors of heroin or cocaine heated on tin foil.
chemicals	synthetic drugs (e.g., amphetamines, LSD, crack).
chiba chiba	high potency marijuana from Colombia.
chicken scratch; henpicking	searching on hands and knees for crack.
China white	1. very pure form of heroin, term originally referred to particularly pure heroin from Southeast Asia 2. fentanyl analogue used as heroin substitute.
chipping	use drugs occasionally.
cigs	tobacco cigarettes.
CJ	PCP.
clean	drug free ("I've been clean for over three years"). Synonym for straight.
clean up; clear up	quit using drugs.
coast	tranquil state occurring shortly after heroin injection, characterized by mild dozing and lolling of the head.
coasting	under the influence of drugs.
cocaine blues	emotional depression after extended cocaine use or following abstinence from cocaine.
cocktail	1. cigarette laced with cocaine or crack; 2. partially smoked marijuana cigarette inserted in a regular tobacco cigarette.
coffin nails	tobacco cigarettes.
coke	cocaine.
coke bugs	hallucination after using cocaine, which creates the sensation of bugs, burrowing under the skin.
cold turkey	stop or withdraw abruptly from drug use through total abstinence. The term is believed to be related to the highly prominent goose-flesh during heroin (or other opioid) withdrawal, giving the appearance of a plucked turkey. Synonym for kicking the habit.

Colombian red	potent strain of marijuana, its name designating its origin (Colombia) and its hue.
Colombian	marijuana.
Columbus black	marijuana.
come down	experience the gradual wearing-off of the effects of a drug after achieving a "high."
come home	end a "trip" from LSD.
connect	make an illicit drug purchase.
connection	1. pusher; 2. intermediary between street pusher and higher-level drug source; 3. in the plural, refers to the complex network from local producer (or grower) to street user.
contact high	mild euphoria occurring in non-smokers and believed by them to be the result of inhalation of the marijuana fumes produced by smokers. Actually, the individual's mental set and positive response to the elevated mood of the smokers are probably the most significant contributors.
cook	prepare powdered opioids or other drugs for injection by dissolving them with water and heating the solution in a spoon or similar container over a flame.
cook down	the process of placing heroin into a liquid preparation by heating to allow it to be injected.
coolie	tobacco cigarette laced with cocaine.
cop	purchase or otherwise obtain drugs. Synonym for buy.
copilot; co-pilot	1. guide for first drug experience; *see* babysit, babysitter; 2. amphetamine.
cotton	1. small amount of cotton batting used to filter impurities from dissolved heroin as it is drawn into the syringe; 2. currency.
cotton shooter; cotton picker	desperate or impoverished heroin addict who is unable to afford a "buy" who injects a weak heroin solution made from the residue on cotton used by other addicts to filter a heroin preparation.

crack	freebase cocaine that is sold in lump form and ready for smoking.
crack house	place where crack cocaine is sold and smoked.
crackers	a mixture of pentazocine and methylphenidate.
crank	methamphetamine; amphetamine; methcathinone.
crash	1. sleep off the effects of drugs; 2. pronounced and often rapid transition, produced by abrupt abstinence from amphetamines, cocaine or other stimulants, from a state of CNS overstimulation to a state of CNS depression, initially characterized by prolonged sleep and followed by emotional depression and often extreme hunger. Sometimes it is deliberately precipitated by administration of barbiturates or similar drugs.
crystal	methamphetamine (crystal meth); PCP; amphetamine; cocaine.
crystal joint	PCP.
cube	1. sugar cube containing LSD, a convenient form in which to distribute and ingest the minute quantity of the substance required to produce hallucinogenic effects; 2. one ounce.
cut	adulterate or dilute drugs. Synonym for shave.
cycling	use of anabolic steroids in cycles, with several weeks of use followed by a steroid-free period.
cyclone	PCP.

Ds	hydromorphone.
daily fix	methadone dispensed once daily in maintenance programs.
dead on arrival (DOA)	PCP; crack; heroin.
deadly amanita	*Amanita phalloides*, a mushroom from the *Amanita* family.
dealer	one who sells drugs. Synonym for pusher.
destroying angel	*Amanita phalloides*, a mushroom from the *Amanita* family.

dexies	dextroamphetamine.
dillies	hydromorphone.
dime-store high	glue sniffing.
dime	1. ten dollars worth of drugs (dime bag); 2. crack; 3. ounce of marijuana.
do a line	inhale cocaine, especially when the drug is laid out in a narrow line.
dollies	methadone.
domes	LSD.
doobie; doubie	marijuana cigarette.
dope	initially in reference to heroin or marijuana; now a general term for drugs of abuse.
dope fiend	crack addict.
dot; dots	dose of LSD so small that it is difficult to see with the naked eye, typically distributed as an almost invisible spot on absorbent paper produced by dropping a small quantity of drug solution on to the paper (typically 50 to 75 micrograms).
doub	twenty-dollar rock of crack.
dove	thirty-five-dollar piece of crack.
down and dirtys	methaqualone.
downer	broadly used to refer to depressants, barbiturates, tranquillizers and other drugs that produce sedation and/or sleep.
dreamers	morphine; opioid drugs.
drop	1. ingest a pill, tablet or capsule orally; most closely identified with LSD ("to drop acid"); 2. dry out; 3. abstain from drugs or alcohol after prolonged use to the point of substantial or complete loss of tolerance.

drug-store dope	morphine.
dry up	refers to the situation when illicit drugs, usually heroin or other opioids, are not available at any cost; for example, when the authorities intercept usual supplies. When the street "dries up," panic often ensues among physically dependent users. Pharmacy thefts tend to peak at such times.
dust	1. drug in powder form; 2. heroin; cocaine; PCP; 3. marijuana mixed with various chemicals.
dusting	adding PCP, heroin or another drug to marijuana, which is then rolled into a smokable form.
dusty roads	cocaine and PCP mixture for smoking,
dynamite	a mixture of heroin and cocaine.

echoes	LSD flashbacks that persist for an extended period after using the drug.
ecstasy	1. MDMA; 2. formerly MDA.
eightball	crack and heroin.
eighth	1. measure of drug by weight, equal to one-eighth of an ounce; analogously, a "sixteenth" is a weight of drug equal to one-sixteenth of an ounce, and so on; 2. heroin; marijuana.
electric kool aid	LSD.
elephant; **elephant tranquillizer**	phencyclidine (PCP).
embroidery	scars left over veins from frequent injections of drugs.
euphoria	MDMA.

eye opener; eyeopener	1. the first heroin (or other opioid) injection of the day, without which withdrawal may rapidly ensue. Synonym for morning shot;
	2. the first alcoholic beverage of the day;
	3. crack; amphetamine.

factory (underground factory; basement laboratory)	location where illicit drugs are synthesized or otherwise processed for street sale.
fantasia	dimethyltryptamine.
fiend	1. term for compulsive drug user. *See* "dope fiend";
	2. person who smokes marijuana alone.
fix	1. quantity of drugs, usually heroin, necessary to satisfy the immediate needs of a physically dependent user
	2. drug injection.
flake	cocaine. Synonym for Big C, snow, coke.
flaky	addicted to cocaine.
flashing	inhaling glue or other products containing solvents.
flats	LSD.
floating (high; stoned; flying)	under the influence of drugs; intoxicated, usually in reference to drugs other than alcohol.
flow	"give in" to the psychic effects of a drug rather than fight them.
flying	*See* floating.
footballs	Talwin Nx®, a pentazocine and naloxone combination that is not marketed in Canada.
freebase	smoking cocaine; crack.
freeze	1. cocaine;
	2. renege on a drug deal;
	3. situation of unavailability of drugs.
frogs	LSD.

G

G	1. $1,000; 2. gram of drugs; 3. term used for an unfamiliar male; 4. GHB (gamma hydroxy butyric acid).
g-rock	one gram of rock cocaine.
gaggers	methcathinone.
ganja; ganga; ghanja; ghana	marijuana.
gank	fake crack.
garbage head	1. users who buy crack from street dealers instead of cooking it themselves; 2. (outdated) indiscriminate polydrug user.
garbage	inferior quality drugs. *See* junk.
gas	1. nitrous oxide; 2. commercial or aerosol volatile solvents.
gee	opium.
gee gee	opium pipe.
get off	1. inject a drug; 2. get "high"; 3. quit using drugs.
glass; glass gun	hypodermic needle.
glue	commercial volatile solvents.
God's drug (God's own medicine)	morphine (a reference to its natural rather than synthetic origin).
gold	1. particularly potent marijuana; 2. marijuana from southwestern Mexico (Acapulco) or Colombia, which is yellowish in color.
gold dust	cocaine.
gong	marijuana; opium.

goofball	cocaine and heroin; barbiturate or other depressant; a combination of amphetamines and barbiturates.
goon	PCP.
grass	marijuana. Synonym for pot, weed, etc.
guide	*See* babysitter, copilot.

Ⓗ

H	heroin.
habit	state of physical dependence, usually on opioid analgesics.
hard candy	heroin.
hard drugs	opioids; also used in reference to any drug that is restricted under federal statutes (including, in Canada, cocaine and cannabis, even though cannabis is often referred to as a "soft" drug because of the nature of its effects and its low dependence liability).
hash	hashish.
hash oil	highly purified oil of hashish, which has the highest concentration of THC among cannabis-derived products.
Hawaiian salt	smokable methamphetamine.
head	a heavy regular user of a drug. Refernce is often made to a specific drug, e.g., "acid head."
hearts	amphetamine (in reference to the triangular shape of a specific product, Dexedrine® tablets).
Heavenly Blue	1. trade name for a specific type of morning glory seed that has hallucinogenic properties, and produces blue flowers when cultivated; 2. LSD.
hemp	marijuana.
high	drug-induced euphoria.
highbeams	the wide eyes of a person on crack.

hit	single puff on a marijuana cigarette; single puff on a pipe; (any drug) injection of drugs.
hog	phencyclidine (PCP). Synonym for angel dust, animal tranquillizer, elephant.
honey oil	hash oil; ketamine; inhalant.
hookah	Middle-Eastern water pipe used for smoking tobacco or marijuana.
hooked	physically dependent on a drug; "addicted."
hop	opium for smoking.
horse	heroin.
horse tranquillizer	PCP.
hot dope	heroin.
hot ice	smokable methamphetamine.
hot shot	dose of an unusually pure form of heroin (which can produce dangerous effects in users who are tolerant only to weak street heroin).
huffer; huffing	glue sniffer; use of an inhalant.
hug drug	MDA or MDMA.
hunting	desperate drug-seeking just prior to and at onset of withdrawal.
hustling	1. the heroin addict's daily routine of illegal activities to obtain sufficient money to buy more heroin; 2. attempting to obtain drug customers.

I

ice	cocaine; methamphetamine; smokable amphetamine; MDMA; PCP.
Indian	marijuana.

J	marijuana cigarette. Synonym for joint.
jag	1. keep a high going, maintain a high; 2. (outdated) the state of being under the influence of solvents; 3. (outdated) the state of being under the influence of amphetamines.
Jamaican	marijuana.
jive; jive sticks	marijuana; marijuana cigarettes.
joint	marijuana cigarette.
juice	1. a cough syrup containing an opioid or opioids; 2. anabolic steroids.
junk	diluted heroin.
junkie	heroin addict.

kicking the habit	abruptly abstaining from a physically addicting drug, used most commonly in reference to heroin. Term is believed to be related to the uncontrollable spasmodic jerking and kicking occurring during the peak period of heroin withdrawal. Synonym for going cold turkey. Term may also refer more generally to overcoming any drug habit.
kiddie dope	1. prescription drugs; 2. general name for look-alikes.
killer weed	a mixture of marijuana and PCP.
kit	paraphernalia for injecting drugs.
kitchen chemist (basement chemist; underground chemist)	illicit drug manufacturer.
KJ	PCP.

lace	1. deliberately add one drug to another to produce a different or more potent effect (e.g., marijuana laced with powdered PCP or cocaine); 2. cut; dilute a drug with non-psychoactive adulterants often without the buyer's knowledge (e.g., heroin laced with quinine).
laughing gas	nitrous oxide.
leaf	marijuana. Synonym for grass, pot, weed, smoke and so on.
leapers	amphetamines.
legal high	high produced by legally available substances (other than alcohol) not requiring a prescription, such as certain solvents, herbs (e.g., dill), spices (e.g., nutmeg), and over-the-counter preparations containing codeine.
lemons	methaqualone.
lid	quantity of marijuana for street sale, approximately one ounce.
lid poppers	amphetamines.
lids	LSD.
line	unit dose of cocaine, typically $\frac{1}{30}$ gram, arranged in a thin strip for snorting.
lines	1. plural of line; *see* above 2. *see* tracks.
liquid ecstasy	GHB (gamma hydroxy butyric acid).
loco weed	marijuana.
love drug	MDA; MDMA; methaqualone.
lovely; lovely high	PCP.
ludes	methaqualone, in reference to a specific pharmaceutical product, Quaalude®, which is no longer marketed.

M	morphine.
M & M	MDMA.
magic dust	PCP.
magic mushroom, sacred mushroom	usually refers to psilocybin /psilocin, but has also been used to refer to other hallucinogenic mushrooms, or ordinary mushrooms to which PCP or an other psychoactive drug has been added.
mainline	inject intravenously; common term with heroin and amphetamine users. Synonym for shoot up.
Mary Jane; maryjane	(outdated) marijuana.
Maui wowie, Maui wauie	potent form of marijuana from the Hawaiian island of Maui.
MDM	MDMA.
mesc, mescal, mescap	mescaline.
meth	1. methamphetamine; synonym for speed; 2. methadone.
Mexican	marijuana grown in Mexico. Mexican red, Mexican brown and Mexican green are specific grades, the first being the most potent.
Mexican valium	rohypnol (flunitrazepam).
Mickey Finn	chloral hydrate.
Miss Emma	morphine. Synonym for M, morph, soldier's drug.
mist	PCP.
monkey	1. drug dependency; (outdated) the state of being in withdrawal from heroin ("to have the monkey on my back"); 2. cigarette made from cocaine paste and tobacco.
moonrock	heroin and freebase cocaine.
morph	morphine.
mule	drug carrier or drug smuggler.

munchies	intense hunger and constant snacking, often characteristic of marijuana intoxication.
mushroom	psilocybin.

Ⓝ

needle freak	refers to individuals who achieve such gratification from the act of injection that they will sometimes inject non-psychoactive substances for the pleasure of the injection experience.
Needle Park	formerly infamous traffic island in New York City where heroin addicts and pushers were known to congregate.
nod	tranquil state occurring shortly after heroin injection, characterized by mild dozing and lolling of the head ("He's on a nod," "He's nodding.")
nuggets	crack.

Ⓞ

OD	take an overdose, usually of a very serious nature.
OJ	a mixture of cannabis and opium, from "opium joint."
on a trip	under the influence of drugs.
One and Ones	a mixture of pentazocine and methylphenidate.
opium joint	a mixture of cannabis and opium.
outfit	paraphernalia for injecting drugs. Synonym for fit, kit, works.
overamped	experiencing agitation and other negative symptoms (possibly as severe as toxic psychosis) resulting from an excessive dose of amphetamines. Synonym for overcharged.
overcharged	*See* overamped.

Panama, Panama gold, Panama red	marijuana grown in Panama. Panama gold and Panama and Panama red are considerably more potent than marijuana grown in the United States or Canada.
panic	1. acute state of fear precipitated by the onset of withdrawal and frantic action to acquire drugs; 2. abrupt drying-up of heroin sources, affecting all local addicts.
peace, peace pill	PCP.
peace weed	a mixture of marijuana and PCP.
peaches	amphetamine tablets, in reference to the color of a specific pharmaceutical product containing amphetamine in tablet form.
peaking	at the period of the most intense effects during an LSD trip.
peanut butter	1. type of methamphetamine that is brown in color; 2. by-product of the reaction between propylhexedrine and hydrochloric acid; has been injected intravenously.
peanut butter meth	a crude solution of propylhexedrine extracted from an inhaler.
pearls	amyl nitrite. Synonym for poppers.
pep pills	amphetamines. Synonym for peppers, uppers.
percs	oxycodone-containing tablets, derived from the name of a specific pharmaceutical products.
peter pan	PCP.
pink panthers, pink robots, pink wedges	LSD.
pipe	1. crack pipe; pipe used for smoking crack or freebase cocaine; 2. marijuana pipe; pipe used for smoking marijuana; 3. vein into which a drug is injected; 4. mix drugs with other substances.
pocket rocket	marijuana.
pop	1. take a tablet or capsule orally; 2. inject subcutaneously; synonym for skin pop; 3. inhale cocaine.

poppers	amyl nitrite, which is administered by crushing (popping) the small vial in which it is contained and immediately inhaling the vapors.
poppy	opium.
pot	marijuana.
purple hearts	in reference to the color and shape of specific products: phenobarbital; LSD; amphetamine.

Q

qat	khat.

R

ragweed	inferior quality marijuana; heroin.
rainbows	capsules containing a combination of amobarbital and secobarbital, in reference to the red and blue capsules of a specific pharmaceutical product containing these drugs. Synonym for reds and blues.
rave	1. large party, designed for young people to enhance a hallucinogenic experience through music and behavior; 2. sometimes used in reference to a large party in which drug use is not encouraged, but that otherwise mimics (1) above; 3. MDMA.
red devil	depressant; PCP.
reds	secobarbital capsules, in reference to the red capsules of a specific pharmaceutical product containing this drug. Synonym for pinks, secos, red birds, red devils.
reds and blues	capsules containing a combination of amobarbital and secobarbital, in reference to the red and blue capsules of a specific pharmaceutical product containing these drugs. Synonym for rainbows.
reefer	marijuana cigarette.

ripped	1. under the influence of drugs; 2. exhausted after an amphetamine run of several days; 3. adversely affected by a drug.
rippers	amphetamines.
rits	methylphenidate, from the trade name Ritalin®.
roach clip	used to hold partially smoked marijuana cigarette.
roach(es)	1. butt of marijuana cigarette; 2. rohypnol (flunitrazepam).
road dope	amphetamine.
rock	freebase cocaine.
rocket fuel	PCE (cyclohexamine).
roid (roids)	anabolic steroids.
roid rage	aggressive behavior caused by steroid use.
roofie (rophy; roopies; ropies; ruffies)	rohypnol (flunitrazepam).
rope	1. low-grade marijuana (from the Indian hemp plant, which contains THC); 2. rohypnol (flunitrazepam).
run	period of several consecutive days during which an individual injects methamphetamine ("speed") several times a day, usually with little or no food or sleep for the duration.
rush	intense orgasm-like sensation that rapidly follows intravenous administration of such drugs as heroin, amphetamines or cocaine.

sativa	marijuana.
scag	heroin.
schoolboy	codeine.
score	succeed in making a drug purchase.

scuffle	PCP.
seams	PCP.
shave	1. adulterate, dilute or short-weight a drug; 2. literally shave off minute quantities (e.g., of a block of hashish) and thereby short-weight the buyer.
sheet	PCP.
shoot, shoot up	inject a drug intravenously.
shooting gallery	place where drugs are injected, particularly for heroin.
shotgun	inhaling marijuana smoke forced into one's mouth by another's exhaling through the marijuana cigarette.
shrooms	psilocybin/psilocin. Synonym for magic mushrooms.
sinse	marijuana.
sketching	coming down from a speed-induced high.
skin popping	injecting subcutaneously.
sleepers	sedative/hypnotic drugs, such as barbiturates.
smack; schmeck; schmeek	heroin.
smokes	tobacco cigarettes.
sniff	commercial volatile solvents.
snort	inhale cocaine or another powdered drug; use inhalant.
snorts	PCP.
snow	cocaine; heroin; amphetamine.
snow light	visual hallucinations after cocaine use, image of flashing bright lights.
snow bird; snowflake(s)	cocaine; a person dependent on cocaine.
snowball	cocaine and heroin.

soft drugs	term used in some circles to describe drugs of abuse perceived to have low toxicity and/or dependence liability; sometimes used to differentiate such drugs from "hard drugs" including opioids and potent stimulants such as cocaine and methamphetamine.
space blasting	smoking cocaine and PCP together.
space cadet	PCP and freebase cocaine.
space dust	crack dipped in PCP.
special "k"	ketamine.
speckled eggs	amphetamines.
speed	methamphetamine; amphetamine; crack.
speed freak	habitual or heavy regular user of methamphetamine; usually, a user who exhibits paranoid thinking and is often aggressive and/or unpredictable.
speedball	injection of heroin mixed with cocaine or methamphetamine.
stacking	1. taking several different anabolic steroids in cycles to enhance muscle-building and performance effects while minimizing adverse effects; 2. taking steroids by prescription.
stacking the pyramid	progressively increasing the dose and numbers of anabolic steroids used before decreasing the doses for a drug-free period.
stardust	cocaine; PCP.
step on	dilute a drug.
steroids	anabolic steroids.
stove top speed	a crude solution of propylhexedrine extracted from an inhaler.
sugar	cocaine; LSD; heroin.
super acid	ketamine.
super rods	PCP.
super weed	a mixture of marijuana and PCP.
supergrass	marijuana on which PCP has been sprinkled.

Superman	LSD-impregnated paper bearing a "Superman" imprint.
surfer	PCP.
synthetic heroin	MPPP. Synonym for new heroin.
synthetic marijuana	PCP.
synthetic morphine	pentazocine.
synthetic THC	PCP.

Ts	pentazocine.
Ts and blues (**Ts and Bs; tease and bees; tease and blues; teddies and bettys; tops and bottoms; tricycles and bicycles**)	pentazocine mixed with tripelennamine, prepared in solution and injected intravenously as a heroin substitute.
Ts and Rs; Ts and Rits; Ts and Ritz	a mixture of pentazocine (Talwin®; "Ts") and methylphenidate (Ritalin®; "Rs").
tapping the bags	removing small amounts of heroin from a bag before selling it, thus "short-weighing" the buyer.
tea	1. pentazocine 2. marijuana.
tee	pentazocine.
Thai sticks	marijuana cigarettes.
THC	Δ 9-tetrahydrocannabinol (delta-9-tetrahydrocannabinol), also known as Δ 1-tetrahydrocannabinol, the most active chemical component in marijuana and hashish.
three hundreds	methaqualone.

toad licking	orally ingesting the venom of certain toad species, either in solutions made from boiling these toads or occasionally directly from live toads, to achieve hallucinogenic effects caused by bufotenin in the venom.
toke	1. puff of a marijuana cigarette; 2. take a puff of a marijuana cigarette; 3. inhale cocaine.
tootsie roll	heroin.
totalled	exhausted after an acute drug experience. Synonym for wasted.
tracks; track marks	1. collapsed veins resulting from chronic injection (lines); 2. discoloration and scars, resembling a tattoo in appearance, resulting from chronic injection.
tragic magic	PCP and freebase cocaine.
tranks	benzodiazepines.
traveller	user of hallucinogenic drugs.
trip	1. the experience produced by a hallucinogenic drug; 2. take a hallucinogenic drug.
tripping	intoxicated on psychedelic drugs, especially LSD.
trippers	LSD.
tschat	khat.
tumor candy	tobacco cigarettes.
turnarounds	amphetamines, especially d-amphetamine in combination with dl-amphetamine.
tweaking	drug-induced paranoia; peaking on speed.
tweek	methamphetamine-like substance.

up against the stem   addicted to smoking marijuana.

uppers   general term for most stimulant drugs of abuse, such as amphetamines and related drugs; despite cocaine's stimulant effects, it is not usually included under this group name.

V

Vs   benzodiazepines; from the brand name Valium®.

W

wacky dust   cocaine.

wake-ups   amphetamines. ("Wake-Ups®" is a trade name for a caffeine preparation that does not include amphetamines.)

wedges   LSD.

weed   marijuana.

weed oil   oil derived from marijuana leaf material.

white cross   methamphetamine; amphetamine.

white lady   cocaine; heroin.

white sugar   crack.

whizbang   a mixture of cocaine and heroin.

windowpane   LSD.

wired   1.   chronically dependent on amphetamines
              2.   physically dependent on heroin.

woollies   marijuana and crack or PCP.

works   paraphernalia for injecting drugs. Synonym for fit, kit, outfit.

X	ecstasy (MDMA).
X&L	a combination of MDMA and LSD.
XTC	MDMA.

yellow footballs   propoxyphene napsylate.

yellows; yellow jackets; yellow jacks   capsules containing pentobarbital sodium, in reference to the yellow capsules of a specific pharmaceutical product containing this drug.

Common "street names" of drugs appear within quotation marks in the index. For less common street names, see also the glossary of street drug language on pages 603 to 630 or the chapters on individual drugs.

TRADE NAMES appear in small capitals in the index. See also the glossary on pages 579 to 588.

Medical and scientific terms are explained briefly in the glossary on pages 589 to 602.

Boldface type is used to indicate main references within an index entry.

Footnotes are indicated by "n" following a page reference (e.g., 34n).

Users of the book will soon notice that each of the drugs in Section 3 is described under the following headings: Synopsis; Drug source; Trade names; Street names; Combination products; Medical uses; Physical appearance; Dosage; Routes of administration; Effects of short-term use: low doses; Effects of short-term use: moderate doses; Effects of short-term use: higher doses; Effects of long-term use; Lethality; Tolerance and dependence; Patterns of use; and Abuse potential. This order is followed for the description of each drug in Section 3, but these subheadings have not generally been repeated in the index entries.

B

N